Lethal Spots, Vital Secrets

LETHAL SPOTS, VITAL SECRETS

Medicine and Martial Arts in South India

ROMAN SIELER

OXFORD
UNIVERSITY PRESS

OXFORD
UNIVERSITY PRESS

Oxford University Press is a department of the University of Oxford. It furthers the University's objective of excellence in research, scholarship, and education by publishing worldwide.

Oxford New York
Auckland Cape Town Dar es Salaam Hong Kong Karachi
Kuala Lumpur Madrid Melbourne Mexico City Nairobi
New Delhi Shanghai Taipei Toronto

With offices in
Argentina Austria Brazil Chile Czech Republic France Greece
Guatemala Hungary Italy Japan Poland Portugal Singapore
South Korea Switzerland Thailand Turkey Ukraine Vietnam

Oxford is a registered trademark of Oxford University Press in the UK and certain other countries.

Published in the United States of America by
Oxford University Press
198 Madison Avenue, New York, NY 10016

Cataloging-in-Publication data is on file at the Library of Congress
ISBN 978–0–19–024385–2 (hbk.); 978–0–19–024386–9 (pbk.)

1 3 5 7 9 8 6 4 2
Printed in the United States of America
on acid-free paper

For Harini and Nilan

Contents

Acknowledgments

NUMEROUS PEOPLE HAVE contributed to this book in manifold ways and therefore deserve my deepest gratitude. To begin with, I want to thank Bo Sax for his continued support and interest in my research. Moreover, his enthusiasm for anthropology has doubtlessly had a strong impact on me. I also wish to express my gratitude to Gabi Alex, who was crucial in enhancing my interest in the region and culture of Tamil Nadu, and to whom I am also indebted for her support and guidance. I am obliged to numerous people at the French Institute (IFP), Pondicherry—for countless discussions, invaluable suggestions, and the friendships I made while being there. Most notably, I wish to thank Laurent Pordié, who provided his guidance for the field and beyond. I am also thankful to Guy Attewell and Harilal Madhavan for engaging discussions over tea or *cāppāṭu*. Thanks are moreover due to IFP researchers and staff M. Kannan, Brigitte Sébastia, Audrey Richard-Ferroudji, N. Murugesan, G. Muthusankar, B. Murugan, and librarians Anurupa Naik, K. Ramanujam, R. Narenthiran, and G. Saravanan, as well as to Harish Naraindas, Jawaharlal Nehru University, who all contributed by providing help, valuable information and insights, or by commenting on early versions of this book. I am indebted to many people at the South Asia Institute, Heidelberg, as well, such as my fellow doctoral candidates.

I owe my gratitude to those who have sparked my interest in learning the Tamil language. Thomas Lehmann started this process, and I am also grateful to several teachers of the Pondicherry Institute of Linguistics and Culture—T. Parasuraman, L. Ramamoorthy, and G. Ravishankar—and to S. Arokianathan of Pondicherry University. I have found and keep finding other teachers as well: Tamils, old and young, encountered in day-to-day situations and places, who are happy to learn that a *veḷḷaikkāraṉ* appreciates their beloved Tamil.

I am grateful to Cynthia Read at Oxford University Press, New York, to her whole team, to everyone involved in the copy-editing and review process, and to two anonymous reviewers who provided excellent critiques of an earlier version of this book. Financial support was provided by a DAAD research scholarship and a writing scholarship of the Graduate Academy of Heidelberg.

This book would not have taken shape without the loving support of my family. I am thankful to my parents for their constant support, despite my being far away most of the time. And I am most grateful to my wife for her love and perpetual encouragement and for enduring all the shortcomings and grievances that working on this project entailed. Finally, I want to thank all *ācāṉs* whom I met in Kanyakumari. Though all faults of this book are entirely my own, they have decisively contributed to shaping this project and to stimulating me to write about this intriguing and important subject.

Earlier versions of parts of this book were published in 2014 as "Patient Agency Revisited: 'Healing the Hidden' in South India," in *Medical Anthropology Quarterly* 28 (3): 323–341 (DOI: 10.1111/maq.12067), © Koninklijke Brill NV, and in 2012 as "Kaḷari and Vaittiyacālai: Medicine and Martial Arts Intertwined," in *Asian Medicine* 7 (1): 164–195. I would like to thank the publishers for permission to reprint revised parts of these essays.

Note on Transliteration

I HAVE TRANSLITERATED all Tamil words following the scheme used by the Madras *Tamil Lexicon* (1924–1936) and the Romanization system of Tamil of the Library of Congress. Words common to Tamil and other Indian languages are generally rendered in their respective Tamil forms (such as, for example, *tōcam* instead of *doṣa*), except where noted otherwise, or where the Sanskrit equivalent is given in parenthesis (Skt.). For reasons of comprehensibility, I have reproduced some terms according to their more common scholarly usage in their Sanskrit spelling (such as *guru, guru-śiṣya-paramparā*, Śiva, and so on). All such transliterations of Sanskrit terms follow standard lexicographical usage. Plural forms of Indian terms are rendered by the suffix -s (*ācāṉ*s as plural of *ācāṉ*, instead of *ācāṉkaḷ*). For ease of reading, I have decided to render certain words in their usual English spellings without the use of diacritics, such as in the case of toponyms (such as Kanyakumari instead of *kaṉṉiyākumari* and Nagercoil instead of *nākarkōvil*), terms commonly deployed in standard or official usage (including siddha medicine instead of *citta maruttuvam* and Siddhar instead of *cittar*), and personal names. When quoting direct speech, I provide the transcription of only selected passages of the Tamil original in order not to overburden nonspecialist readers. All translations from Tamil sources, both oral and textual, are mine.

Lethal Spots, Vital Secrets

Introduction

THE VITAL SPOTS

A SEEMINGLY FRAGILE old man strikes out with his bare hand at his opponent with lightning speed. During this action, the index and middle finger of his charging hand are kept intertwined in an intriguing *mudrā*, a hand gesture, in which his fingers point toward the opponent like the tip of a needle. In fact, the old man only just touches his adversary's forearm lightly, but the man thus touched stares in disbelief at his now paralyzed arm. Before the victim can even think about using his other arm to retaliate, he receives a similar attack on his other wrist; he is now completely debilitated. A similar, well-aimed blow to the larynx takes away his voice, and, utterly helpless, he numbly watches the old man drive a knife deep into his stomach.

We have just seen the opening sequence of the 1996 Tamil movie *Indian* (*Intiyaṉ*), which has several scenes depicting fictional combat techniques of *varmakkalai*, the "art of the vital spots," a South Indian tradition which popularly is depicted as mysterious and secretive. The old man, the main character of the movie, played by Tamil actor Kamal Haasan, is a Gandhian freedom fighter who feels driven to punish corrupt government officials by deploying this secret and dangerous art, in which he had been instructed as a young man. The police are unable to catch this vigilante killer in the absence of clues which may help trace his identity, since he skillfully makes use of the vulnerable points of the body in order to kill his victims. The plot of *Indian* is typical of how vital spot practices are commonly perceived in present-day South India.

However, *varmakkalai*, literally "the art [*kalai*] of the vital spots [*varmam*]," found mainly in southern parts of Tamil Nadu, South India, includes martial and healing practices as well. I translate *varmam* as "vital spots," hoping to capture the fact that such loci are particularly vulnerable spots of the body, injury to which can lead to serious life-threatening effects, but which are also utilized for therapeutic interventions. "Hitting the vital spots," *varma aṭi*, is the name given to the bare-handed form of combat, which targets these loci. The movie, in which the scene above is found, reflects the stereotypical perception of vital spots and its practitioners: with lengthy training, enemies can be stunned and even killed empty-handed through "hitting the vital spots." But at the same time, the art of the vital spots provides the therapeutic means in handling cases of trauma suffered in combat but also of injuries and other ailments. "Vital spot medicine," *varma maruttuvam*, is the name given to the healing component of *varmakkalai*. Skilled practitioners of both vital spot combat and therapeutic techniques, called *ācāṉs*,[1] are generally reluctant to provide explanations or definitions of their practices, except for one: "the vital spots are secret" or "*varmam* means secret" (Maṇiyaṉ 2012, 9). *Ācāṉs* have therefore been described as shrewd and mysterious persons and as keenly concealing their knowledge, since they practice in secrecy and pass on their knowledge only to a chosen few, if at all. Several authors have reported *ācāṉs* as using blankets for covering patients and the specific manipulations, which they administer away from the eyes of others (Zarrilli 1992b), or as notorious drunkards and unreliable, wayward persons (Langford 2002, 214).

Released in 1996 and having been dubbed in several other Indian languages,[2] the movie *Indian* gained a considerable degree of attention, won three national film awards, and was chosen as the Indian submission for the Academy Award for Best Foreign Language Film of the year 1996. Aside from *Indian*, the vital spots are increasingly present in public popular culture, as several movies, novels, and since recently even comic strips

1. And, less frequently, *varmāṇi* (Maṇiyaṉ 2012, 9).

2. The movie was dubbed into Hindi and called *Hindustani*. It may seem ironic that the picturization of a practice that is found regionally concentrated in the extreme South of India is titled "Indian/Hindustani." Maybe an underlying intention here was to de-regionalize, de-provincialize and thus to promote the vital spots by making a principally South Indian practice stand for the whole of India. It must be noted, however, that the title *Indian* also refers to the Gandhian (albeit very un-nonaggressive!) nationalist protagonist of the movie.

document.[3] It must therefore strike one as extraordinary that *varmam* spots have provoked little academic attention, barring a few studies, which bear only marginal references to the subject. The general perception of the discipline is clearly flawed; scholarly accounts, alongside the popular reception, have emphasized a secretive, almost mystical character of the vital spots and their practitioners, and thus have rendered the related practices as mysterious and lopsided as depicted above. It is this situation that the present study attempts to address. In doing so, it draws on participant observation and experience as gathered from intensive engagement with *ācāṉ*s, and their practices in the southernmost regions of mainland India: Kanyakumari district. The main questions, which I try to pursue in the following chapters, include: What are the specific practices related to the vital spots, and why are they shrouded in secrecy? And, coming to terms with the simultaneously martial and medical characteristic of practices concerned: What does healing and harming mean for the persons involved? In other words: How are both medicine and combat compatible, and what does this have to say with regard to healing and martial arts as categories and practices? Lastly, if *varmakkalai* indeed is a secret tradition, what are the reasons for it being so and what does secrecy mean for its practitioners? What challenges do they face, and how is the knowledge transmitted within the peculiar environment of secrecy, which by definition restricts flow and exchange of information? In other words: How does one learn a secret practice?

Some Vital Spots of This Study

Varmam are the "vital spots," or rather, as one might argue as well, the "mortal" or "lethal spots." That is to say that such spots are perceived as locally demarcated, extremely vulnerable points of the body (human as well as animal) which, when injured by an impact—mostly in physical form, such as a hit or through falling from heights—cause medical conditions of severe, possibly even lethal, nature. These points therefore have

3. The novel *Pēcum kaṅkaḷ* (Telling eyes), which was serialized in the popular magazine *Āṉanta vikaṭaṉ*, takes the vital spots as a red thread of its plot. Prolific author Rajesh Kumar is said to have consulted with *ācāṉ*s (Rājēntiraṉ 2009, 17) for his novel *Tiṉam Tiṉam Tikil Tikil* (Terror everyday), which describes gruesome scenes of mysterious killings. The Internet comic *Kinnari*, by Meenakshi Krishnamoorti, prominently features *varmakkalai* (see http://www.kinnaricomic.com/?id=1).

been described as the body's "Achilles heel, . . . located in different spots" (Balakrishnan 1995, 143). Any trauma caused to such loci has to be met with immediate therapeutic techniques, which also deploy vital spots. These points and the underlying theory therefore encompass therapeutic and combat importance at the same time. Not only can physical traumata be healed, but they can be caused deliberately by someone who knows locations and related stimulation techniques; *varmakkalai* embraces the skills of both *healing and harming* (see Zarrilli 1992b). Therapeutic practices (*varma maruttuvam*, "vital spot medicine") include manipulations, massages, setting of fractures, and emergency revival methods for unconscious persons. These are regarded as part of siddha medicine, one of the codified, indigenous medicines practiced largely in Tamil Nadu and recognized by the Indian government today.

At the same time, vital spots are the focus of attention of combat exercises, called *varma aṭi*, literally "hitting the vital spots," a martial art in which adepts learn to protect their own spots, while targeting an opponent's *varmam*. In this regard, *varma aṭi* practice can be seen as closely related to the popular martial arts form of Kerala, *kaḷarippayaṭṭu*, which makes use of sets of vulnerable spots as well (Zarrilli 1992a; 1992b). Both medical and martial aspects of vital spots are not regarded to conflict, but, on the contrary, as mutually supportive and are performed side by side by hereditary practitioners. While to a casual observer the martial aspect of vital spot practices alongside its healing component may appear a strange juxtaposition, if not a downright contradiction in terms, the knowledgeable take a different, holistic view of the two aspects. It is in fact usual to find exponents simultaneously maintaining a dispensary for offering medical services to patients suffering from different ailments and a training ground, on which they practice and impart martial techniques.

The majority of vital spot practitioners are male. The term *ācāṭṭi* is the female variant of *ācāṉ* (Immanuel 2002, 146),[4] and, albeit rarely encountered, there are a number of female practitioners. Nevertheless, I have been largely involved with male *ācāṉ*s in Kanyakumari and was able to meet only one female practitioner. She assisted in the dispensary of a male practitioner and was deployed for massaging female patients. I have not

4. The Madras *Tamil Lexicon* ([1924–1936] 1982, 211) notes *ācāḷ* as female variant of *ācāṉ*. Besides this dictionary entry, I have however not come across this term in writing or in spoken discourse.

encountered a female practitioner who has set up her own vital spot dispensary or training ground. While it is likely that there are fewer female practitioners, this only gives reason to suspect that *ācāṭṭis* are less visible than their male counterparts, since they may be "merely" assistants to male practitioners. This would evidence a male-dominated field, and should not imply gender-based differences in knowledge and practice, but only in terms of social position. Also, this should not deceive into mistaking vital spot practice, though apparently a male-dominated field, for an all-male one.[5]

Most *ācāṉs* have never visited an officially recognized education institution for learning their particular skills, but have instead received instruction from accomplished practitioners, often their own kin. It is difficult to precisely estimate the number of practitioners, who may be registered as siddha medical practitioners (or as other alternative Indian medical practitioners). More often, however, *ācāṉs* are not registered or licensed with any medical practitioners' boards at all, and hence governmental records provide no numerical data on *varmakkalai* exponents as such. In the case of a practice being located between healing (*varma maruttuvam*) and harming (*varma aṭi*), between a codified, recognized indigenous medical system (siddha medicine) and hereditary, noncodified forms of practice, this state of affairs should surprise no one. *Varmakkalai* is moreover characterized by a high degree of concealment of knowledge and practice. Thus the practices under scrutiny, the bodily loci alongside their practitioners, suffer from a number of ambiguities. Some of these include the challenge that instructing or learning restricted information poses to practitioners and students, and the seemingly paradoxical situation of therapeutically applying a practice which is supposed at the same time to be kept concealed and of communicating and justifying it to patients and to inquisitive authorities. It is these ambiguities which I am concerned with in this study.

Themes of the Study, State of Research, and Data Used

The *varmam* vital spots have hitherto been covered only marginally by scholarly research. Phillip Zarrilli's (1998) seminal work on *kaḷarippayaṭṭu* martial arts in Kerala, *When the Body Becomes All Eyes*,

5. Balasubramaniam and Dharmalingam (1991, 41) mention that some *dais* or traditional midwives utilize vital spots for inducing delivery or for regulating blood flow.

alone has ventured for one chapter across the border to Tamil Nadu and has briefly described Tamil *ācāṉs*' practices (see also Zarrilli 1992b). But even with regard to nonscholarly textual sources, vital spot practices remain poorly understood. This is for several reasons. Manuscripts on *varmam*, mostly in Tamil with some in Malayalam, and typically inscribed on palm-leaf bundles, are often in the possession of hereditary practitioners. These manuscripts are difficult to date reliably, judging from the language used—most such texts range from the fourteenth to the eighteenth centuries (Krishnamurthy and Chandra Mouli 1984). These texts moreover embrace a kind of jargonistic code, called *paripāṣai* (Skt. *paribhāṣā*), a feature common to most siddha manuscripts, and, in fact, common to most tantric traditions in South Asia (Urban 2001b). It has been speculated that such codes have been deliberately deployed by authors of manuscripts so as to conceal their contents, which in this way remain incomprehensible to uninitiated persons (Zvelebil 1973, 21; Trawick 1983, 939). Due to this reduced textual accessibility, which is exacerbated by the fact that most manuscripts remain in the private possession of practitioners while only few have been edited and published, information on the vital spots is sparse, especially in English-language publications. In Tamil and Malayalam, there are a number of cheap booklets, mainly sold at railway stalls or small, often mobile bookshops at fairs and festivals, which focus on the more esoteric aspects of vital spots and on mysterious, occult powers of practitioners. These tend to be stereotypical or fictitious stories. Other accounts in the Tamil vernacular exist, which have to be acknowledged as attempts to convey precise enumerations and as efforts to name and locate the spots. Some of these have been compiled in order to help institutionalize and standardize vital spot therapies for a curricular framework of contemporary instruction of siddha medicine, yet do not include the cultural or social circumstances or records of practitioners. While the different forms of published material are proof of the increasing popularity which *varmakkalai* enjoys within Tamil Nadu as part of siddha medicine, information on the subject proper remains scarce.

Unfortunately, a similar dearth of literature and understanding holds true for siddha medicine itself. Of the few studies on the social and cultural relevance of siddha medicine, most have tended to either focus on theoretical aspects and/or practice (Sujatha 2003; 2007; 2009), or on its discourse (Hausman 1996; Weiss 2003; 2009), but seldom have both been analyzed in a combined way. This is not the only compartmentalization prevalent in cultural studies. Medicine is largely treated as a discrete and self-contained concept. The same is true for aspects of astrology or physical exercises such as yoga or martial arts. However, such practices may not always be the detached, discrete wholes, as depictions lead us to believe, but may overlap considerably in discourse, theory, and practice. Prevalent academic compartmentalization, I believe, has created diverse problems, such as the scarcity of historical sources regarding vital spot practices.[6] A historiographical tendency has been to consider medical and martial practices separately. To combine the two, the antecedents of both would have to be painstakingly reconstructed: a monumental piece of work which exceeds the limits of this study. But an eclectic approach is nonetheless required to describe the broader tradition of not only the vital spots, but also of healing practices in India in general, which are known for their incorporation of astrological factors or physico-philosophical theories such as yoga. Moreover, vital spots and the related manual, martial or medical aspects do not appear to be an exclusively South Indian phenomenon. A review of primary sources and secondary literature on classical ayurveda, Indian healing practices, yoga, esoteric traditions, and fighting arts reveals an intriguing, recurrent theme of bodily loci throughout various times in India and wider South Asia. As is the case with the *varmam* loci, these topics, often characterized by the interplay of martial and medical concepts, open up a rich field for research, which scholars have so far neglected.[7] The in-depth research such a project would demand falls beyond the scope of this study, but I provide a preliminary outline of the vital spot traditions in India in chapter 1.

It is necessary to address the relationship between siddha medicine and other Indian healthcare practices, especially ayurveda, and the connection of the vital spots with these. Siddha medicine is today recognized as one of the indigenous, codified medicines of India. It is close to ayurveda in its theoretical content and therapeutic application, but deviates both in being regionally confined to the South of India and the state of Tamil Nadu in particular, and in the language of most of its textual sources, namely Tamil. Like other Indian medicines, including ayurveda, yoga and naturopathy,

---

6. Practitioners often offer another possible explanation for the scarcity of historical records of vital spot practices. For fear of the military skills of *ācāṉs*, British colonial authorities allegedly prosecuted vital spot experts and prohibited their trade.

7. A short article in French on vital spot traditions in South Asia by Arion Roşu (1981) is an exception.

yunani, and homoeopathy, siddha receives focused attention with regard to development, regulation, and education. The Department of AYUSH (Ayurveda, Yoga & Naturopathy, Unani, Siddha and Homeopathy), which is part of the Ministry of Health and Family Welfare of the government of India, is responsible for quality control, standardization, centralization, and all matters of instruction in all these medical systems. However, siddha medicine lags behind the better-known ayurveda with regard to standardization, institutionalization, and promotion. This is reflected in a comparatively lower number of professionalized practitioners as against hereditary, noninstitutionally trained ones, as well as of medicine-manufacturing units for both the domestic and the global market. Especially in terms of standardization of medical knowledge, the design of a curriculum and formal education, siddha falls considerably behind other Indian medicines. One need only note that there are merely two government and five private siddha colleges, as opposed to 200 such institutions for ayurveda (Department of AYUSH 2010). Moreover, these specialized colleges for siddha were started only in 1964, alongside the introduction of a distinct degree course, Bachelor of Siddha Medicine and Surgery, BSMS (Sébastia 2010, 1). Prior to this, siddha medicine had been taught jointly with ayurveda. One reason for this might be seen in the fact that heightened interest in siddha is a recent phenomenon, and clear demarcations vis-à-vis ayurveda were drawn increasingly only from the beginning of the twentieth century onwards (Hausman 1996, 250). Earlier, the two medicines appear not to have been strictly delineated by their physicians or textual sources (Krishnamurthy and Chandra Mouli 1984). Therefore, the promotion and institutionalization of siddha medicine during the twentieth century have been described as resembling and as influenced by the Tamil language revivalist rhetoric, since practitioners and policy makers have argued that siddha is a medical science in its own right, distinct from both ayurveda and biomedicine (Weiss 2003; 2009). As will be seen, siddha medicine is not merely a medical system, but indeed a rhetoric and a strategy for promotion as well. The category of siddha as a medical system has been utilized to mark certain sets of practices and practitioners—those in Tamil South India—as distinct from other Indian medical practitioners, mainly ayurvedic ones, but also as distinct from biomedical doctors. In fact, *ācāṉ*s may define their practice as part of siddha medicine, as ayurvedic, or as not related to either but distinct from other Indian forms of therapy altogether. It is therefore more helpful to recognize the vital spots as a manifestation of an Indian concept of health and the body.

One ambiguity surrounding the vital spots, and simultaneously one more gap in scholarly description and analysis, has to do with the particular physical nature of related practices. *Ācāṉs* diagnose and treat ailments by using their bodies: their hands and senses. Manual therapies however have not received much scholarly attention. Moreover, despite the obviously important role musculoskeletal or massage therapists and "bonesetters" play the world over,[8] physical, therapeutic attention to the individual body has been devalued in many societies, and physicians involved in it receive less respect than their counterparts in bodily detached forms of medicine (Van Dongen and Elema 2001; Hinojosa 2004b). Similarly, *ācāṉs* face not only the scrutiny of other practitioners but they often have to cope with strict administrative regulations. And while there is a small but increasing number of studies on manual therapies or "bonesetting" in Central and South America (Huber and Anderson 1996; Hinojosa 2002; 2004a; 2004b; Oths and Hinojosa 2004), Africa (Onuminya 2004; Nyamongo 2004), Southeast Asia (Anderson and Klein 2004), Europe (Anderson 2004), and North America (Walkley 2004), it is not the case for South Asia, in which manual modes of healing are sadly both underrated and underrepresented.[9] Both medicine-based and ritual forms of healing have in the past attracted comparably more attention, especially from anthropologists, than manual medicine has. This is all the more surprising as the body and the sense of touch have become increasingly noticed fields of study of the social sciences in general and of anthropology in particular (Classen 2005; Alex 2008; Hsu 2008). The present study attempts to fill this apparent gap.

Academic writing, moreover, though largely neglectful of manual healthcare modalities, has further tended to reduce such practices structurally. This is best illustrated by the appellation "bonesetting," often used for vital spot healing practices (Zimmermann 1978). I try to avoid such reductionist denominations when directly referring to therapeutic concepts, preferring "vital spot practices" over "bonesetting," to include the martial-cum-medical character of *varmakkalai*, or manual medicine. Indeed, many manual practitioners attend to much more than bones and hence the description "bonesetter" is inadequate (Hinojosa 2002; Oths

8. See especially Majno (1975, 73) and Hinojosa (2002, 23). Though statistical numbers are scarce, it has been estimated that in rural India, every cluster of twenty to twenty-five villages has a bonesetter, roughly totaling about 60,000 hereditary, manual physicians (Shankar and Unnikrishnan 2004, 24, 84).

9. Helen Lambert's work (1995; 2012) must be mentioned as an exception in this regard.

and Hinojosa 2004). In eschewing the word "bonesetter," I also reflect the feelings of *ācāṉ*s toward this term and its Tamil equivalent, *elumpu-vaittiyar*, "bone-doctor," which they despise, precisely for its limited and pejorative nature. By describing their therapies as manual medicine, I try to acknowledge the way in which *ācāṉ*s perform their occupation, namely manually, and physically, a crucial aspect of their practices, as will be seen.

Another vital theme to be explored is secrecy. Asked what *varmam* is or how it works, *ācāṉ*s may answer with: "It is secret." Vital spot practices are constantly subjected to concealment: practitioners may use covers while treating patients, they teach their martial art only in private, and emphasize their occupation's secret nature. The most common explanation for this is that vital spot practice is potentially dangerous, as it may simultaneously comprise healing and harming. But secrecy, although the object of a long tradition of theorizing since at least Georg Simmel (1906; 1907; 1950), has been mostly investigated partially, thus conveying an incomplete picture. By analyzing the particular expressions of secrecy present in vital spot practices, this book provides one explanation for the inaccessibility of texts mentioned above and also demonstrates why siddha medicine and *varmakkalai* are understudied or misunderstood by scholars. Both are to a considerable extent corporeal forms of practice; for both, textual components are ancillary and secondary, as compared to experiential and tacit knowledge, I argue. Since scholarly research has tended to focus on written sources, the understanding and analysis of practices such as siddha medicine and the vital spots have been fragmentary as a matter of course. It is important to recognize that both texts and physical practice exist in parallel and, importantly, their forms and interpretations inform one another. Much of this study therefore argues for a combined analysis of text and practice, explicit and tacit information, and of conscious and corporeal knowledge, in order to arrive at a, hopefully, more inclusive understanding of such esoteric, secretive practices.

Geographical Setting: Kanyakumari

The term *ācāṉ* as a designation for medical and martial practitioners of the vital spots is most commonly used in the southernmost portions of Tamil Nadu. Another designation for such practitioners is *varmāṇi* (Maṇiyaṉ 2012, 9), the meaning of which, though not found in dictionaries, can be deduced as "one who takes care of vital spots." Both the terms *ācāṉ* and *varmāṇi* are rarely found in most of North and Central Tamil Nadu, however, where people are not normally aware of its meaning. It is rather the regions of mainland India's extreme south—the Kanyakumari and Tirunelveli districts in Tamil Nadu state—but also some southern parts of Kerala, where vital spot practices are found (figure 0.1).

Almost every publication and every author appear to agree that the southernmost part of India is the most prominent place of practice and place of origin of vital spot practices (Irācāmaṇi 1996, 2), and that all distinguished *ācāṉ*s belong to this region (Balasubramaniam and Dharmalingam 1991, 27). Accordingly, many Tamil practitioners living and practicing elsewhere claim ancestry and origin from Kanyakumari district (Citamparatāṇupiḷḷai 1991, 76). Whether this is done on the basis of an actual relation to Kanyakumari or not, it further substantiates this region's strong connection with vital spot practices. Many manuscripts on vital spots reproduce myths explaining the origin or discovery of vital spots, which further connect these with the extreme South of India. Some of these myths ascribe the descent of *varmam* loci to the people of Kanyakumari as a gift from god Śiva, in order to bestow upon the righteous of this area both martial prowess and medical skills.[10] Other myths connect the vital spots closely to the Siddhars, the alleged founding fathers of siddha medicine, who are here accredited with having discovered these vulnerable spots and having developed related therapies. In Kanyakumari district today, these Siddhars are understood to have been active almost exclusively in this region; several hill caves and temples bear the inscription "abiding place of Siddhars."[11] The whole Kanyakumari district is generally portrayed as the abiding place of Siddhars and as the cradle of *varmakkalai* (Balasubramaniam and Dharmalingam 1991, 26; Immanuel 2007, 110). It is from here, most *ācāṉ*s imagine and state, that teachings on the vital spots were diffused to other parts of South India, most notably to present-day Kerala, but also to China and Japan, where the techniques are today more popularly known as acupuncture and acupressure, respectively. Kanyakumari is hence home to numerous *ācāṉ*s and the setting of much of this book.

---

10. See, for instance, the myth of the celestial twins Ayyaṉ and Kaiyaṉ, who were sent to instruct the Cēra kings in vital spot combat in order to balance the supremacy of the Northern Tamil dynasties (Irājēntiraṉ 2006; Chidambarathanu Pillai 1991; 1994a; 2008, 3–4).

11. Such as the famous "medicine hill," Maruthuvāḻmalai, not far from the tip of the subcontinent.

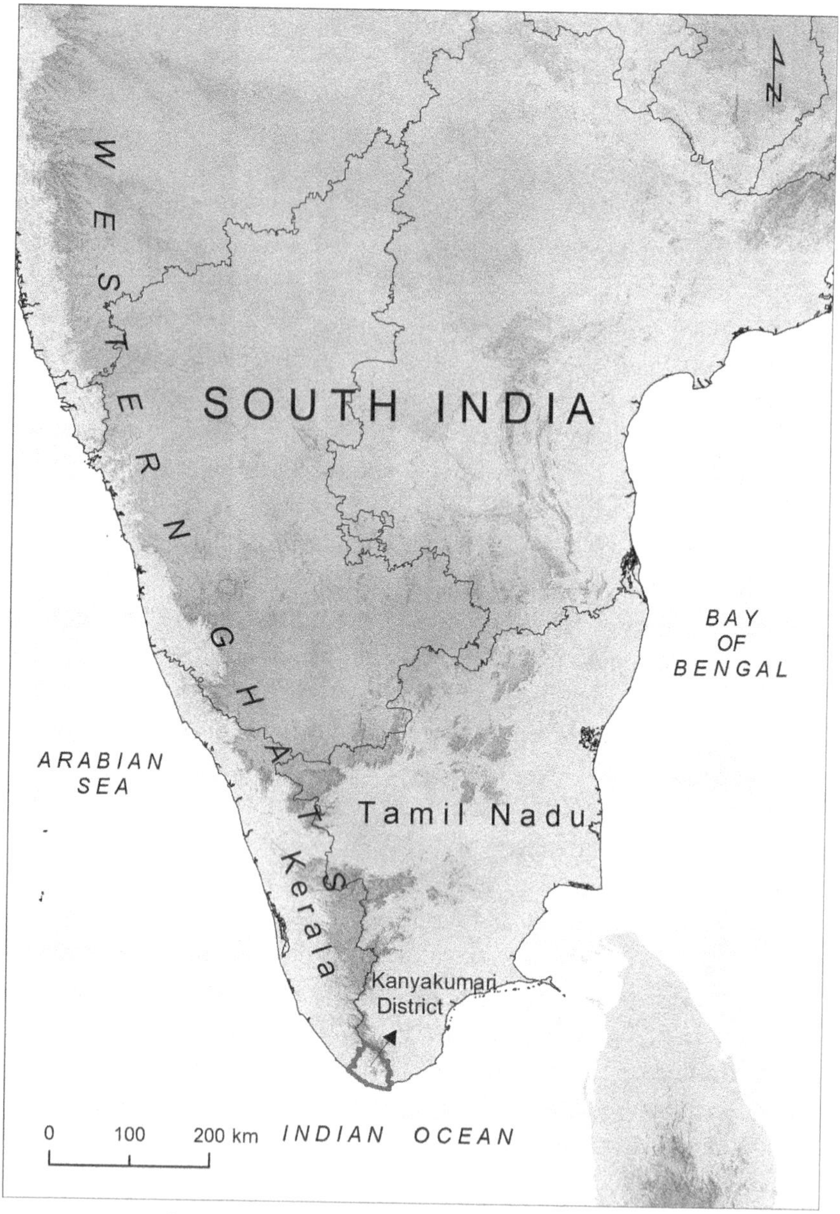

FIGURE 0.1 A The region: Kanyakumari. Maps created by G. Muthusankar, Department of Geomatics, Institut Français de Pondichéry

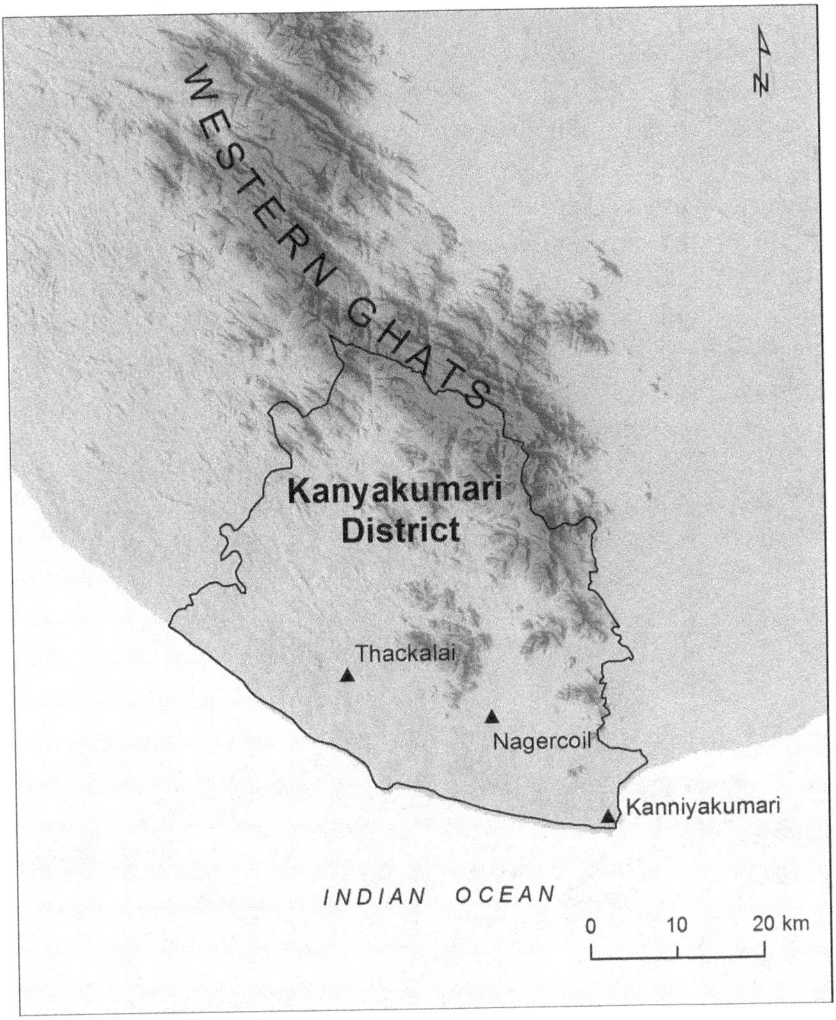

FIGURE 0.1 B *(see 0.1 A)*

Kanyakumari is the smallest district of Tamil Nadu after Chennai. With an area of 1,684 km^2 and a population amounting to 1,870,374, it is one of the most densely populated regions of India, according to the 2011 census. Kanyakumari has been termed "Lands End," as it is the southernmost district of the landmass of India. Nagercoil town, its administrative capital, is situated only about 20 km from the tip of the subcontinent, where Kanyakumari town is located. The district is well developed in many regards, and features as one of the most advanced districts, which is attested to by a literacy rate of 91.75 percent and a high female sex ratio.[12] It borders on Tirunelveli district of Tamil Nadu in the north and east and to Thiruvananthapuram district of Kerala state in the west, and with the latter Kanyakumari has a lot in common. In the first place, Kanyakumari shares Kerala's climatic conditions and tropical vegetation, which allow for two to three rice harvests a year, abundant coconut groves and banana fields, and a lush green appearance, as water is not the rare commodity it is in other parts of Tamil Nadu (figure 0.2). Kanyakumari receives good rains from both the northeast and the southwest monsoons and temperatures are mild during the whole year, allowing for a rich and intensive agricultural utilization. Therefore, lush green paddy fields and coconut topes feature as major marks in the landscape, as do the hilly slopes of the Western Ghats, one of the botanically richest areas of the Indian peninsula, which provide for a diverse medicinal flora (Kingston et al. 2007, 32) (figure 0.3).

Kanyakumari district is one of the oldest geocultural regions of South India (Ram 2008, 137), and a geographically isolated one, moreover,

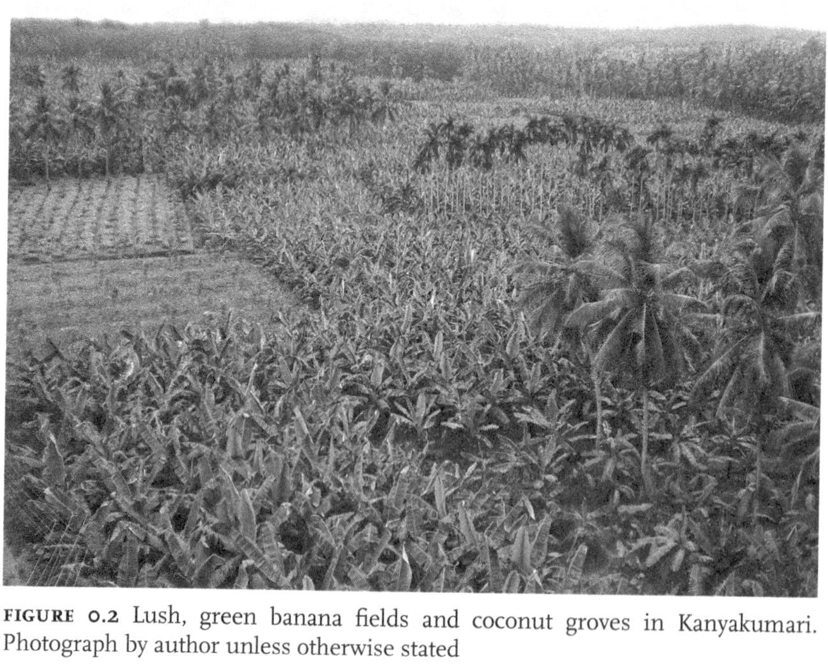

FIGURE 0.2 Lush, green banana fields and coconut groves in Kanyakumari. Photograph by author unless otherwise stated

12. http://www.census2011.co.in/census/district/51-kanniyakumari.html.

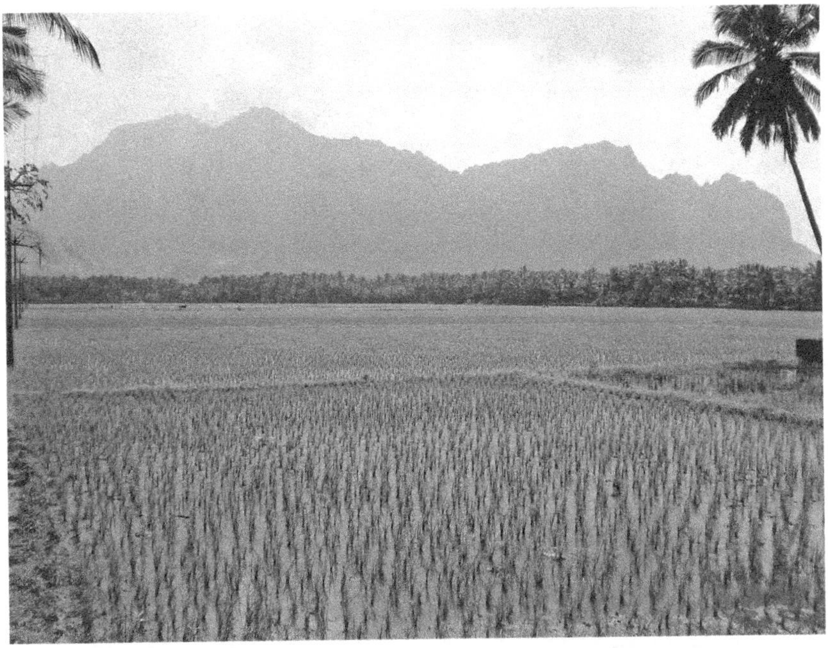

FIGURE 0.3 Rice fields and steep mountain ranges of the Western Ghats

a fact which according to Stuart Blackburn (1988, xxiii) has contributed to maintaining a strong sense of regional identity. The district is circumscribed by natural borders: surrounded by ocean on three sides—the Arabian Sea on the southwest, the Bay of Bengal on the east, and the Indian Ocean on the south. Partly steep mountain ranges of the Western Ghats to its western and its northern sides further provide for a natural border. Fights for supremacy characterize the history of this fertile and bounded region, with different regional dynasties holding sway over it at different periods: Vēnād, Cōḻa, Pāṇṭiyaṉ, and lastly Tiruvitāṅkūr or Travancore claiming supremacy. These dynasties were both Tamil and Malayali, and the alternating rule within this area and its situation of Tamil and Malayali rulers contributed to a mixed cultural set-up (Blackburn 1988, 3; Vēlappaṉ 2000). Although European powers vied for this area as well from the seventeenth century onwards, it remained a part of Travancore, which was awarded the status of a princely state under British hegemony during the nineteenth and early twentieth centuries. Only in 1956, in the course of state reorganizations, which restructured state boundaries according to linguistic areas, was this region, where the majority of inhabitants speak Tamil, added to what is today Tamil Nadu state and named Kanyakumari.[13] Though the major population is and was Tamil, Blackburn (1988, 4) correctly writes that historically "for at least the past four hundred years, [Kanyakumari] has been a two-tiered society—a Tamil village culture under a Malayali court culture." Intense social ties between the people of these regions still mark out a unified cultural zone, which cuts across political divisions and the administrative borders of Kerala and Kanyakumari district of Tamil Nadu (Ram 2001b, 188; 2008, 137). This may explain why the largely geographically bounded practices of the vital spots, transcend the borders of contemporary Tamil Nadu and Kerala.

Social Setting

Varmakkalai is generally being connected to a specific caste group (Zysk 2008, 11), namely that of the Nadars (*nāṭār*). In the contemporary cities of Chennai, Madurai, or Tirunelveli numerous signboards reveal owners of shops as belonging to this caste and bear witness to the recent relative economic well-being of some portions of this group, especially in trade and businesses. Within Kanyakumari district, the importance of Nadars cannot be overestimated, especially with regard to their numerical dominance (Blackburn 1988, 9). This caste's social and political background has been depicted as a rags-to-riches story or as an example of "horizontal mobility" (Rudolph and Rudolph 1984, 36), since it managed to transform its politicoeconomic and ritual status alongside its name: from Shanar (*cāṇār*) to Nadar. Called "toddy-tappers," Shanars were known for climbing Palmyra trees to tap the sweet palm juice, which ferments to a mildly alcoholic beverage and which can be distilled into strong liquor, but it is a strenuous and disdained occupation. Nevertheless, as Hardgrave's seminal study (1968, 171) shows, this group was welded into a community with high degrees of self-consciousness and solidarity, which triggered economic and political ventures and successes.

Shanars argued they were descended from Tamil kings, adopted habits and rituals associated with higher castes,[14] and demanded to be collectively called Nadars. Many of the prolific Nadar authors to write on their

---

13. Kanyakumari district is named after the southernmost temple on landmass India, which is dedicated to the virgin goddess Kaṉṉiyākkumari.

14. Such pursuit of a higher social status has been termed "Sanskritization" by M. N. Srinivas (1966, 6).

community's royal and glorious past have focused on the role of *varmakkalai*. For those who emphasized the Nadar caste's royal and warrior heritage, the vital spots were not merely a precious sample of their martial tradition, but were argued to have been created and practiced exclusively by Nadars (Immanuel 2002; 2007). *Varmam* thus has not only played an important role in the Nadars' attempts for a higher social position, but has also become popularly identified with this caste group more than with others.

The few scholars who have commented on it generally emphasize the connection between the Nadars and vital spots. This connection is said to have

> evolved naturally from the fact that the men of this caste, while carrying out their task of climbing coconut and borassus trees to collect the fruits and sap . . . occasionally fell from great heights. In order to repair the injury or save the life of a fall-victim, skills of bone-setting and reviving an unconscious patient by massage developed among certain families within the caste, who have passed down their secret art from generation to generation by word of mouth. In the past, rulers employed members of this caste to cure injuries incurred in battle and to overpower their enemies by their knowledge of the Indian martial arts.
>
> (Zysk 2008, 11)

Indeed, climbing and tapping of Palmyra trees is not only a physically enduring and arduous labor, but also a dangerous one, which frequently causes injuries, and hence may induce the development of modes of curing them. Any fall from a Palmyra, often as high as 20 to 30 meters, might leave a climber dead or seriously injured. It must be stated that many Nadars today, for economic reasons and because the production of toddy in particular is prohibited by the government of Tamil Nadu, do not pursue the occupation of climbing and tapping trees. But for similar traditions of manual medicine it has been described that particular work groups and persons, men in particular, who experience traumatic injuries regularly, contribute the largest number of practitioners (Hinojosa 2002, 25). Thus, the occupational risk of falling off trees may be speculated to explain the development of *varmakkalai* among Nadars. This may be combined with the historical fact that some Nadar families were royal retainers and hence assigned to military service, which might account for vital spot martial concepts. Nadar practitioners relate this notion as well and connect to it a sense of community pride. To quote one of my Nadar practitioner informants, Manickam Nadar *ācāṉ*, practicing just outside Nagercoil town, in this regard: "Nadars have invented this art and you will find only Nadars practicing it. If you find people from other castes, they won't know the details, but only act as if they knew [the vital spots]."

Since Nadars comprise the largest social group in Kanyakumari district, with more than one-third of the overall population (Hardgrave 1969, 270), and with some villages being of exclusive Nadar composition (Nair, Sivanandan, and Retnam 1984), it may not be a surprise that my data also show that Nadars provide the largest single community to be employed in vital spot practices. However, *ācāṉ*s are found in all ranks of society, especially amongst the Sambavar (*cāmpavar*) caste (Zarrilli 1998, 28). This group is considered the equivalent caste of the Paraiyar in Kanyakumari, the "untouchable" South Indian caste par excellence, considered impure and of the lowest social position, and recognized as a Scheduled Caste (Nair, Sivanandan, and Retnam 1984). Several popular practitioners in Kanyakumari, including my main informant, Velayudhan *ācāṉ*, belong to this caste. Claims regarding the exclusive practice of vital spots on the part of Nadars, and the joining of *varmakkalai* with the Nadars' history hence have to be seen in the light of regional struggles over social positions, but also as characteristic of vital spots being a competitive healthcare practice in Kanyakumari district.

Although both Nadars (originally) and Sambavar (still) assume low- or middle-caste positions in the social stratification of Kanyakumari district, it cannot be readily concluded that vital spots are a low-caste occupation. Several higher castes are found to inherit the practice of *varmam* just as much, including Vellalars and Brahmins. However, some Brahmin exponents whom I interviewed were keen on linking their practice to ayurvedic sources rather than to siddha medicine, and in one case a practitioner preferred the term *marma cikitsā*, the name for related vital spot therapies in use in Kerala, where the practice has strong links with ayurveda (see also chapter 2). In any case, vital spot practices appear to intersect the caste structure of Kanyakumari, and most practitioners do not normally appear to reject or prefer patients on a caste basis.

Experiencing the Vital Spots, or How to Learn a Secret Practice

While I am greatly indebted to many *ācāṉ* informants as well as to their students, patients, and other persons related to my research in Kanyakumari district, I only mention them anonymously. This accords with the standard ethnographical procedure of protecting one's informants,[15] and respects the secrecy emphasized by practitioners. Moreover, many *ācāṉ*s offer medical services even though it is sometimes unclear, or contended, whether they are legally allowed to do so. I wish to avoid possible difficulties that practitioners might face due to revealing their identities or places of residence and practice. Many of the events described may not have appeared to convey delicate information at the time, but they may appear harmful or insulting at some time to some informants.

Regarding my most influential informant—I will call him Velayudhan here—I feel ill at ease to refer to him as merely an "informant." After arriving in Kanyakumari, I spent the first months surveying Nagercoil, the southernmost city on the Indian subcontinent, with regard to various vital spot practices. That is, I visited, interviewed, and observed *ācāṉ*s, intending to get an idea of the place and primary agents. I had planned to select one or several main informants, with whom I would stay and conduct participant observation, if allowed to do so. Despite their alleged and notoriously secretive behaviors, I found only very few *ācāṉ*s refused outright. One practitioner was particularly welcoming. I had spotted Velayudhan's dispensary by chance; several persons who obviously had just received a kind of medical treatment boarded the bus on which I was traveling one day. The scent of medicated oils and various types of bandages applied to different limbs were unmistakable signs. I learned that Velayudhan *ācāṉ* ran his dispensary close by in Chandrakavilai village in Agasteeswaram taluk, the southernmost taluk in the country's southernmost district of India, located just about 15 km. from the tip of the Subcontinent. This village is regionally reputed for being home to several successful *ācāṉ*s. When I arrived there the next day, I discovered within a village of about 300 households three thriving dispensaries devoted to vital spot ailments, which attract patients not just from surrounding villages, but from the entire district and even beyond. One amongst these is Velayudhan's dispensary, a buzzing practice, judged by the frequency and rush of patients, who gather in the front veranda of the *ācāṉ*'s house while waiting for a consultation. The dispensary consists of a room for consultation and diagnosis, and a back room for treatment. A second floor had recently been added, and serves as a small four-room ward for in-patients suffering from chronic or serious ailments. A garden full of coconut trees

15. See, however, May (2010) for critical views of anonymity and transparency in anthropology.

and a square-shaped, open space with sandy ground in the middle is Velayudhan's place for martial training.

As the *ācāṉ*, a man in his forties, was friendly and welcoming, I decided to ask him for permission to observe his practice. I had formulated my research questions in such a way that I would not get embroiled in ethical or epistemological dilemmas involving a possible breach of the system's code of secrecy—or so I thought. Naively, and contradictorily, I had planned to focus on the intricacies of knowledge transmission in a highly secretive, hereditary, lineage-based practice, and on its position within a pluralistic medical field, without necessarily having to wrench out delicate and secret information. I was therefore happy to discover that Velayudhan was teaching two students, Murugan and Manikandhan. I took care to communicate to the *ācāṉ* my respect for any potential secret and explain my somewhat naively planned nonintrusiveness. Indeed, although permitting me to be present at his dispensary, Velayudhan regularly excluded me from treatment sessions during the first two months. Nevertheless, I found myself absorbed imperceptibly into the daily routine, and in due course I was not only able to observe the production of medicine, but consultations of patients as well. A crucial moment occurred when I asked the *ācāṉ* for an explanation of pulse diagnosis. In response, Velayudhan reached out and placed my thumb over his wrist, saying that one had to learn pulse diagnosis through doing, and that it had to be experienced through feeling the pulse for oneself, but could not be adequately communicated through words. As I was to find out, this is true for most vital spot techniques: Most aspects are taught through practical demonstrations and physical directions, rather than through explication; they are experienced rather than discursively reflected.

Some three months into my research, I found myself learning *varmakkalai* in this way. Recognizing this, Velayudhan pointed out to me that, regardless of my own initial agenda, I had become a student of his, and would have to be treated accordingly. My further stay, and participation, he explained, would require a kind of initiation. Needless to say that I was thrilled with this prospect, and I expected this to provide insights into the particular mode of learning. This learning relationship, the *guru-śiṣya-paramparā*, or the teacher-learner tradition, is generally associated with strictness on the teacher's part coupled with unquestioning obedience on the student's part, but also implies a familial, almost parental relationship. In this new light, Velayudhan the *guru* had risen far above the level of an informant. He became my teacher. This development is reflected in and is based on the particularly close relationship which ideally evolves in this learning modality as in the nonverbal and experiential learning.

Despite acceptance and learning, I was unable to venture very deeply into the highly complex art of the vital spots during the comparatively short period of my stay in Kanyakumari. The main fieldwork for this study was carried out in Kanyakumari district from August 2008 to July 2009. A preliminary research study was conducted from November 2007 to March 2008, and a concluding field trip took place from October 2009 to January 2010. Palm-leaf manuscripts, however, stipulate the duration of a proper course of learning vital spots to be twelve years. Moreover, the teaching methodology, with its emphasis on hands-on learning and practice, and enclosed within its shell of secrecy, leaves little scope for verbalization, a process so vital in the framework of classical anthropology, which has difficulties doing justice to somatic experiences and sensory understanding in its discursive modes of explanation (Scarry 1985; Samudra 2008). For instance, description of a massage treatment fails to convey the physical contact between recipient and physician, the pressure of stimulation, the oily, warm feeling, or at least not all at once. A combat performance or exercise, when described by words, appears static and the often explosive, dynamic movement is lost. At times I was requested not to reveal a particular aspect or concept, and this further contributed to my difficulties in writing this account of my experiences. As a result, the *how* (as opposed to the *what*) of my learning experience provides the substance of most of this book. Importantly, it is not so much what I have learned, but how, that I want to stress within the following chapters. This aspect involves particularities of secrecy, on the one hand, and of experience and embodiment of sensory knowledge, on the other.

This book is therefore about *secrecy*, and less about *secrets*. This means that it is with the nature of concealment and the nature of that which is disclosed that I am involved. I am not going to reveal any secrets that I have been asked to keep. Sometimes, Velayudhan would advise me not to reveal to anyone a particular spot, its position, or ways of its stimulation. I have been complying with such requests most strictly while writing this book, and I will reveal neither what I have been asked to keep secret nor what I deem might be used in detrimental ways. In fact, this has not required any effort at all. Rather, it would have been more challenging to actually write about these, since most vital spot knowledge pertains to a category of information that can hardly be tackled in the form of a book like this, relying as it does on words, text, and description. It is a vital aspect of *varmakkalai*, and one of the core statements of this study, that *varmam* spots, alongside the related practices, pertain to a physical, embodied sphere and hence is not easily, if at all, revealed by words. It is experienced, and this experience is a somatic, sensory function. It is precisely this character of vital spot practices which defines for me most importantly the nature of its secrets. It is also here that the two focal points of secrecy and experience meet.

Experience and Fieldwork

The social sciences have come a long way in recognizing medicine as a field of studying India, from the end of the 1960s, when the sociology of medicine was largely neglected (Ahluwalia 1967), until today, with a growing corpus of publications, on various medical subjects, from scholars of indology, anthropology, sociology, and history. Nevertheless, ethnographic detail on Indian healing traditions is still sparse compared to textual analyses. Even anthropological studies have been mainly interested in ayurveda and other codified, textual medical systems of South Asia. It seems worthwhile to expound a little on fieldwork methods, experience, learning, and the senses.

Experience, although a key concept of the discipline (Kleinman and Kleinman 1991; Wikan 1991; Csordas 1994; Blake 2011), remains largely unexamined and taken for granted in anthropology (Throop 2003, 220). Moreover, experiences have been criticized as tools for research or for building hypotheses in anthropological and philosophical theorizing, for their nontransparency, subjectivity, and individuality. Experience has been condemned as "indeterminate, fluid, discontinuous, disjunctive, chaotic and/or fragmentary" (221). However, while my experiences and their outcome in the form of this study are highly subjective, the modes of attaining these experiences were not. I was taught what and how to experience; Velayudhan always guided me in undergoing sensory experiences. This is a mode of sensory coexperience, which characterizes the hereditary instruction in vital spot practices, and the same holds true even for therapies. Whatever deficits experience allegedly possesses as analytic tool, these do not alter the fact that it is the core of vital spot learning, and deserves to be acknowledged as such. It is thus the particular modality of knowledge transmission I feel equipped to describe, a form of experiential learning which relies heavily on the teacher's conveying of situations, techniques, and so on, through sensory, physical ways, while a student learns, begins to understand, and experiences in a similarly somatic, embodied way. It is in this sense that I use and understand "experience" as the applied learning of *varmakkalai*, and as a beneficial, if not necessary, medium for studying vital spot practices.[16]

Participant observation, the main accepted fieldwork method of social and cultural anthropologists since the second half of the nineteenth century, has been understood as "the conduct of an ethnologist who immerses her- or himself in a foreign social universe so as to observe an activity, a ritual, or a ceremony while, ideally, taking part in it" (Bourdieu 2003, 281). But more recent studies have remarked that this approach appears too cognitive especially with regard to physical, kinesthetic cultures or sensory practices. Exponents have demanded studies "not only of the body, in the sense of object, but also from the body, that is, deploying the body as tool of inquiry and vector of knowledge" (Wacquant 2004, viii; see also Jackson 1983). Various scholars in this vein have attempted to deepen the methodology of participant-observation, and have suggested concepts such as "thick participation" (Samudra 2008, instead of Geertz's [1973] "thick description"), "participant experience" (Hsu 2006), or "participatory experience" (Okely 2007, 76). Anthropologist Elisabeth Hsu, instead of observing and participating in the object of her inquiry, Chinese medicine and acupuncture, endeavored to go a step further and to acquire skills displayed by her informants herself. She spent considerable time learning acupuncture in China in what she calls "participant experience" (Hsu 1999, 5; 2006). This mode of inquiry allowed her to experience for herself fundamental intricacies of needling, such as the therapeutically relevant first healing successes of learners or the physicality and community-building character of pain shared between physician and patient—aspects which might elude an observer. An experientially involved research may indeed be a requirement when analyzing kinesthetic traditions, as is also instanced by the nature of secrecy, or the particular relationship involved in the transmission of the vital spots.

---

16. Victor Turner (Turner and Bruner 1986) and Clifford Geertz (1986), it should be noted, understood experience as shared, suprapersonal, external, and collective in nature (see Throop 2003; compare Kleinman and Fitz-Henry 2007, 53). This standpoint arguably involves the question of whether experience can be shared interculturally. I do not claim to have *correctly* understood or experienced all that I was taught. I regard it as more important to have grasped the crucial relevance of sensorial experience in *varmakkalai*, and it is this concept that I am analyzing.

Hsu had made a deliberate decision to study acupuncture herself in order to be able to understand the rationale of Chinese medicine. In my case, this was not so, and becoming a student of an *ācāṉ* did not happen by design, but in an unforeseen way. Still, this is not tantamount to providing for concise descriptions of what I have learned. Several scholars have described this very problem of writing about somatic experiences and bodily knowledge (Samudra 2008). Others have remarked that the lack of incorporation of sensory experiences and tactile aspects in anthropological work may be attributable to the textual and oral nature of anthropology alongside other academic disciplines (Herzfeld 2001, 240; Classen 2005, 5). Forming an anthropological text out of a researcher's sensory experiences entails a process of translation of feelings and tactile sensations into words and sentences. In the process, there lurks the possibility of the actual experiences being muted. All pleas for the incorporation of the body, and of the senses or experience (Csordas 1994; Turner and Bruner 1986; Howes 1991) into academic writing cannot fundamentally alter such an institutional discrepancy, which characterizes and constrains this account as well. Nevertheless, like other anthropologists who have conducted an apprentice-style method of research (such as most of the contributors to Marchand 2010), I was at the same time transformed into my own object of study, which forced me, or better yet allowed me, to contemplate learning and knowledge transmission and acquisition in a direct, reflexive way. As Esther Goody (1989, 254–256) put it, apprenticeship is an excellent way to learn a skill or craft or profession, an excellent way to learn about a skill or craft or profession, and an excellent way to learn about learning. By enriching classical ethnographic research methods by apprenticeship learning, we may indeed be able to broaden our horizons in order to cover the cognitive and anatomical processes involved in learning (Marchand 2010, 9–10).

Does the fact that it is a subjective, rather than an objective, description of the vital spots make this account less truthful? I feel that this is not the question at stake here. Referring to philosophers such as Gottfried Herder and his concept of *Einfühlung* ("feeling into the world"), to Martin Heidegger's *Gestimmtheit* ("attuning to the world"), to Wilhelm Dilthey's notion of *tonalité* ("adjusting to the pitch of the world"), and to Max Weber's concept of *Verstehen* ("knowing through emphatic attunement"), James Davies (2010, 4) convincingly argues that participation and detachment are two divergent methodological approaches, both of distinct value to social research. An even stronger statement in this regard is the thesis of George Devereux: he judged any attempt at objectivity to yield no more than pseudo-objectivity. Devereux therefore demanded of researchers who study human behavior to use "the subjectivity inherent in all observations as the royal road to an authentic, rather than fictitious, objectivity" (Devereux 1967, xxvii; see also Jackson 2010).[17] Many scholars have followed in this tradition to critique the possibility of objectivity. To mention just one example out of many possible, Donna Haraway (1988) has argued that the general understanding of objectivity is that of a disembodied, external point of view. However, she demonstrates that such is not possible, and that what generally passes as objectivity is the viewpoint of the powerful: white, male, and capitalist. If disembodied objectivity is not achievable, but only "situated knowledges," or embodied subjectivities, I am somewhat at ease, since I find an embodied, subjective account of a bodily practice a suitable one indeed.

Hsu (2006), despite intense periods of learning acupuncture, did not become an acupuncturist, nor did she ever feel at ease needling patients. Likewise, I do not claim to have learnt *varmakkalai* enough to practice it, even as I feel enabled to describe how I experienced learning it. Surprisingly enough, this in itself suffices to provide insights into both the transmission of knowledge and secrecy of the vital spots.

---

17. Similarly, Paul Stoller (1989) has argued that the incorporation of the ethnographers sensual experiences make an ethnographic account more scientific, rather than less so.

I

Vital Manifestations

MARMAN, MARMMAM, AND VARMAM SPOTS

WHILE ENGAGING WITH literature regarding vital spots, manual therapies, or related martial traditions, and in the exchanges with scholars working on similar aspects in South Asia, I was struck by the high degree of similarity discernible in these fields, regardless of the region of their practice. This chapter is an attempt to provide an introduction to, and a brief overview of, such "vital spots" in the Indian and South Asian context, and to explain the seeming relations between them. I suggest a framework for doing so here, one which would have a bearing also on wider categories of medicine, of the body, health, and well-being. The theory of vital spots and related manual techniques are conjectured to be expressions of a shared cultural concept. The described traditions would then be different manifestations of such expressions, or, to use the terminology of Sujatha, Aruna, and Balasubramanian (1991, 52), "orders" of mutually influencing knowledge and practice.

This chapter consists of an analysis of various textual and nonliterate[1] traditions and practices related to concepts of vital spots in India. Such vital spots include theories of the body and related manual techniques, which pervade numerous Indian cultural aspects. This includes the notions of vulnerable parts of the body and the accompanying semianatomical theory of *marman*, as reflected in Vedic, Upaniṣadic, and Purāṇic textual sources. The classical ayurvedic compendia describe vital spots by

1. I am consciously deploying the term "nonliterate," to denote those traditions which have not been textualized. They may be "oral," largely transmitted orally. They may also be "embodied," in cases where they are transmitted via, and are incorporated in, the body.

the same name, *marman*, which here comprise the theory of a medically relevant anatomical concept. Further, esoteric yoga traditions know of *marmasthānas*, "vital loci," which are given special importance in meditative exercises of yogic adepts. A still distinct set of *marmmam* spots is contemporarily used in Kerala, in martial arts practices called *kaḷarippayaṭṭu*, and also in related medical intervention techniques, termed *marmma cikitsā*, or "vital spot therapy." Similarly, Tamil palm-leaf manuscripts describe *varmam* vital spots, which are simultaneously the basis of healing and harming techniques. Such *varmam* spots, which will be the main concern of the rest of this book, are utilized in *varmakkalai*, "the art of the vital spots," for manual treatment modalities and combat activities by contemporary practitioners in the southern parts of Tamil Nadu. In short, there is a rich variety of traditions dealing with what I term "vital spots": vulnerable parts of the body of relevance to physical exercise, spiritual, esoteric techniques, anatomy, and medicine. Such traditions can be found on a pan-Indian level, as exhibited in various vernaculars and geographic regions. Even different marginalized practices such as midwifery or the medical lore, as found in household therapeutics, seem to know of vulnerable body loci and address their ailments in massage manipulations.

This abundance of practices has, however, hitherto not generated the attention and research the subject deserves.[2] What is more, there is an obvious affinity, as will become apparent, in all these vital spot traditions, transcending not only barriers of language, social groups, region, and time, but also of narrativity, medicine, martial arts, philosophy, astrology, and so on. This raises questions over *varmam* being treated as part of siddha medicine, and over the recent incorporation of siddha and ayurveda into the category of medical systems. Vital spots, in fact, elude the contemporary demarcations drawn between Indian medicines, as primarily exhibited in ayurveda and siddha medicine. Further, as even nonliterate practices of bodily manipulation and health in India might be incorporated into a broader picture of manifestations of the vital spots, the highly awkward, binary categorizations of "subaltern," "folk," or "oral" strands, in opposition to "learned," "classical," or "literate" cultural paradigms,

---

2. There are a few notable exceptions. Arion Roşu (1981) has given a brief overview of *marman* and its occurrence in ayurveda, yoga, and wrestling traditions. Mariana Fedorova (1990) has analyzed the *marman* as presented in ayurvedic literature, and Phillip Zarrilli (1998; 1992a; 1992b) has written on the vital spots of *kaḷarippayaṭṭu* and *varma aṭi* martial arts.

appear obsolete. Finally, vital spot practices also testify that demarcations between medicine, martial arts, astrology, yoga, and physical exercises are only a recent taxonomical construct.

The first part of this chapter is a survey of the different traditions, as gleaned from texts and prevailing practices, while its second part addresses the recently effected classification of siddha and ayurveda into medical systems, and a similar demarcation inflicted on the vital spot traditions. Just how recent and artificial such partitioning is will become clear from the analysis that follows.

Premodern Textual References and Classical Ayurveda

Vedic and Sanskrit Textual References

Textual references to vulnerable points in the body, called *marman*, can be found very early in Indian literature. For instance, passages in the *Ṛgveda*, the *Mahābhārata*, and the *Rāmāyaṇa*[3] all mention *marman* (Govindan 2005, 9). Contextually, these references are generally found within depictions of war and battle. The *Ṛgveda* thus extensively depicts the fight between god Indra and Vṛtra, a snake-demon, whom the former can defeat only by striking the latter's *marman* with his weapon, the *vajra*. According to the *Ṛgveda*, the demon can be killed only by severing this point, stating that "[Indra] found the *marman* of Vṛtra, who he thought was without [such] a mortal spot" (RV 1.61.6c).[4] The term *marman* here appears to mean "mortal or vulnerable spot," as this is the location or limb of the body to which a lethal blow can be executed. This seems to be the case both for divine beings and for mortals. The *Kauśikasūtra* of the *Atharvaveda*, according to Kenneth Zysk the first and principal source on medicine of the Vedic period,[5] contains instructions on how to ritually protect one's own *marman* when preparing for

3. Michaels (1998, 67–68) dates the *Ṛgveda* to roughly 1750–1200 BCE, the *Mahābhārata* and the *Rāmāyaṇa* to 200 BCE. Within the *Mahābhārata*, the sections of *Virāḍaparva* (31.12–15), *Bhīshmaparva* (95.47), *Droṇaparva* (125.17), *Karṇaparva* (19.31), and *Śalyaparva* (32.63) all mention *marman* (Mehra 2008, 1).

4. I am grateful to Jarrod Whitaker for pointing out and translating this scene. Other references to *marman* in the *Ṛgveda* include the following verses: 3.32.4c, 5.32.5a, 6.75.18a, 8.100.7c, and 10.87.15c.

5. Zysk (1991, 14) dates the *Kauśikasūtra* of the *Atharvaveda* to around the third century BCE.

battle, and how to afflict an enemy's *marman* spots by chanting *mantras*, spell-like incantations (Fedorova 1990, 8). Epics of later periods frequently mention the killing of demons by injuring their *marman* (8). Both the *Mahābhārata* and the *Rāmāyaṇa* repeatedly refer to *marman* spots, especially when malevolent beings are slain on the battlefield, as in the case of the demoness Siṃhikā, whose *marman* is torn apart by the monkey god Hanumān. One verse states: "Having cut through her [Siṃhikā's] *marman* with his sharp claws, the monkey [Hanumān] flew up with the rapidity of thought."[6] Within the *Rāmāyaṇa*, especially the *Yuddha Kāṇḍa* or "Book of War" contains numerous such references to *marman*. For instance, Lakṣmaṇa, the brother of Rāmā, the hero of this epic, is injured by an enemy's arrow: "He [Atikāya] hurled an arrow, which had the shape of a venomous snake toward Lakṣmaṇa. Struck by this arrow at a *marman*, the tormentor of his enemies [Lakṣmaṇa] fell unconscious for a moment" (6.71.98). Finally, even the villain of the *Rāmāyaṇa*—Rāvaṇa—is killed by Rāmā's arrow, which is said to possess the power to "pierce the *marman*" (6.108.16), at a very specific point located at the villain's belly.[7]

Considering the warlike context of the vital spots in Vedic and Sanskrit literature, Fedorova (1990, 8), Thatte (1983; 1988, 14), and Roşu (1978) have speculated that this theory might have developed from a kind of military medicine used in battlefield hospitals in ancient India. Indeed, instead of "vital spots," the Sanskrit word *marman* rather denotes "spots that kill." In its most literal sense, these are "lethal spots" or "mortal points," since the Sanskrit root of *marman* is *mṛ*, "to die; causing to die" (Rao 1987, 118).[8] The theory of *marman* might indeed have originated from knowing the anatomy and functions of the body intimately, and might have developed from martial practices and from battlefield surgeons, who gained their

6. From *Rāmāyaṇa* by Vālmīki, *Sundara Kāṇḍam*, 5.1.194 (Vālmīki 1927, 25). I am grateful to Harini Maranganti for translating this verse.

7. It may be interesting to note that Christian *varmakkalai* practitioners in Kanyakumari often draw upon biblical stories, such as the episode of David and Goliath, in order to give an example of vital spots. For instance, they may understand the point on Goliath's forehead, which David aims at with his slingshot, thus killing the giant, as *tilartakkālam*.

8. Fedorova (1990, 9) further explains that the term *marman* early on attained a metaphorical usage as describing problematic arguments or a possibly controversial theory. This metaphoric use betokens something essential, "the quick, the core of anything," according to the Monier-Williams *Sanskrit-English Dictionary* (1899, 791). Hence, the denomination "*vital* spots" appears as justified in this regard as well.

insights from emergency operations or from dissecting corpses (Roşu 1981, 417). A close relation to these textual *marman* can be recognized in vital spots as expounded in the classical ayurvedic compendia, called *marman* as well, which appear to share the development from military medicine.

Vital Spots in the Ayurvedic Treatises

Descriptions of a medically relevant *marman* concept are, according to Mariana Fedorova (1990, 15), not found until the time of the older Upaniṣads. In her dissertation in German, *Die Marmantheorie in der Klassischen Indischen Medizin*, devoted to analyzing these vital or mortal spots of ayurveda, Fedorova explains that *marman* may indicate any part of the body, which in case of a trauma will cause death or grave psychophysical damage. Ḍalhaṇa, a commentator on the ayurvedic compendium *Suśruta Saṃhitā*, in this vein notes that "*marman* [are the points which] kill" (Sanskrit *mārayantīti marmāṇyucyate*) (Roşu 1978, 417). Sāyaṇa, a commentator of the *Ṛgveda*, explains this lethal character by the circumstance of *marman* being points through which *prāṇa* departs from the body (Fedorova 1990, 7). *Prāṇa* is conceived as a most important aspect of life in much of ayurvedic theory. Life, it is assumed, is *prāṇa*. It must be considered as the life energy that is pervading every human being, conveying virility and prowess. Injury to *marman* spots causes maximum damage to a person's life, according to classical ayurvedic theory, precisely because such loci are intimately connected to *prāṇa*, since *marman* are spots of *prāṇa* concentration (Govindan 2005, 16).[9]

Of the authoritative canon of ayurveda, the three texts generally called the "great triad" (*bṛhattrayī*), namely, the *Caraka Saṃhitā*, the *Suśruta Saṃhitā*, and the *Aṣṭāṅgahṛdaya Saṃhitā*, all mention and describe vital spots to some varying extent. Although the *Caraka Saṃhitā*, for instance, mentions *marman* several times, and thereby seems to suggest that they were known to the reader, it does not analyze the loci extensively (Fedorova 1990, 15). Here, *marman*, in the most basic sense, are vital parts, including

---

9. The concept of *prāṇa* can also be found in most strands of Indian philosophy and yoga, and can be traced to very ancient origins (Zysk 1993). Like the vital spots, *prāṇa*, is a comprehensive pan-South Asian concept that links different abstract thought and practice systems (Tilak 2007).

the head (*mūrdha*) and organs such as the heart (*hṛdaya*) or the bladder (*basti*). A more detailed description and elaborate theory is found in the texts of *Suśruta Saṃhitā*,[10] *Aṣṭāṅgahṛdaya Saṃhitā*, and *Aṣṭāṅgasaṃgraha*,[11] all of which classify 107 *marman* points (Govindan 2005, 11). Measured in fingerbreadths (*aṅguli*), the size of these loci is here specified to range from one-half to five fingerbreadths.

The ayurvedic compendia further divide the vital spots into several classificatory systems, all of which are in agreement with the general logic of ayurveda. Of these, a "regional-anatomical" classification enumerates eleven *marman* found in each limb, twelve in the trunk, fourteen in the back, and thirty-seven vital spots in the region above the clavicle.[12] These 107 spots are known by forty-four names (Fedorova 1990, 18); due to the symmetric structure of the body and its limbs, some spots appear twice, or even four times, such as *kṣipra*, located on both hands and both feet. Further, in a kind of "systematic anatomy" (250), each *marman* is defined by a dominating body tissue, or *dhātu*. Thus there are eleven muscle spots (*māṃsamarmāṇi*), forty-one vascular spots (*sirāmarmāṇi*), twenty-seven tendon spots (*snāyumarmāṇi*), eight bone spots (*asthimarmāṇi*), and twenty joint spots (*sandhimarmāṇi*).[13] The *dhātus* are the physical locations of a *marman*, being present dominantly, yet not necessarily exclusively, in a particular vital spot. Indeed, the *Suśruta Saṃhitā* defines a *marman* as every junction of muscles, vessels, tendons, bones, and joints, in which *prāṇa* is present (*Suśruta Saṃhitā*, 3.6.15; Fedorova 1990, 251). As these spots are intimately connected to the *dhātus*, which, like any other structure or substance according to ayurvedic theory, comprise "five elements," or *pañcamahābhūta*, the vital loci contain, and are defined by, this category as well. Based on the five elements in varying proportions, a prognostic classification of *marman* emerges according to the dominance of one or the other of ether (*ākāśa*), air (*vāyu*), fire (*agni*), water (*āp*), and earth (*pṛthvī*) at a vital spot (Fedorova 1990, 287). Prognostically, or

---

10. Both the *Caraka* and the *Suśruta Saṃhitā* are generally dated to before 500 CE (Wujastyk 1998, 105).

11. Both the *Aṣṭāṅgahṛdaya Saṃhitā* and the *Aṣṭāṅgasaṃgraha* are dated to 600 BC (Meulenbeld 1974, 424; 2000). Both texts are believed to have been compiled by Vāgbhaṭa.

12. See, for instance, the *Aṣṭāṅgasaṃgraha, marma vibhāga* (classification of *marman*).

13. According to the *Suśruta Saṃhitā* (3.6.3). The classification given in the *Aṣṭāṅgahṛdaya Saṃhitā* in this regard deviates in allocating particular *marman* spots to a particular anatomical category (Wujastyk 1998, 290–291).

pathologically, *marman* are thus divided into five classes. These include those that "destroy *prāṇa* immediately" (*sadyaḥprāṇahara*). They are of the quality of fire (*āgneya*), and therefore bring death within seven days at the longest if the person is injured (Giri 2007, 158). Another category of *marman* "destroys *prāṇa* after some time" (*kālāntaraprāṇahara*), as these are both cool (*saumya*) and fiery (*āgneya*), a combination that is more stable than fire alone (which is blown out easily). Such a *marman* causes death within fifteen days to one month. The loci of a third category "kill due to [the removal of] a pointed object" (*viśalyaghna*), as these *marman* are constituted of wind (*vāyu*), which abandons the body as soon as a foreign object penetrating the body is removed. A further *marman* category "causes frailty" (*vaikalyakara*) because it is of a cool (*saumya*) quality, and its effect is limited to causing deformity or frailty in patients. Lastly, a fifth category contains those spots that are fiery (*āgneya*) but predominated by *vāyu*, and therefore merely "produce pain" (*rujākara*) (*Suśruta Saṃhitā*, 3,6,8; Thatte 1988, 15–16).[14]

To give an example of an ayurvedic vital spot: the *marman* called *adhipati*, located at the top of the head, occurs in only one place, its predominant body tissue is joint-based (*sandhi*), it causes instant death due to fire (*āgneyabhūta*) being present in it, and its size is that of half a fingerbreadth (*ardhāṅgula*) (Mishra 2005, 29; Fedorova 1990, 296).

Significantly, the authors[15] of the *Suśruta Saṃhitā* define *marman* as seats of *prāṇa* or as places where *prāṇa* is concentrated (*Śarīrasthāna*, 6/36). *Prāṇa* is a vital, life-endowing force, disturbance of which is said to cause disease or death. However, if afflicted, the *tridoṣa* composition gets disturbed. *Tridoṣa* are the three (*tri*) *doṣa*, the so-called humors, namely *vāta* ("wind"), *pitta* ("bile"), and *kapha* ("phlegm"). These three *doṣa* categories are in balance in a healthy being, but if in disequilibrium cause various ailments. An inflicted *marman* thus blocks *prāṇa*, which in turn disequilibrates the balance of the *doṣas*. This leads to diseases, possibly to lethal ones

14. The Sanskrit texts also assign different amounts of body tissues to these prognostic categories. Thus, at a *sadyaḥprāṇaharamarman*, all five *dhātus* are imagined to be present, contributing to its particularly high vulnerability. A *kālāntaraprāṇaharamarman*, in comparison, contains only four *dhātus*, a *viśalyaghnamarman* three, a *vaikalyakaramarman* contains two, and a *rujākaramarman* consists of only one *dhātu*, and is hence the least vulnerable category (Giri 2007, 160). The more *dhātus* present at a *marman*, the more lethal its injury.

15. As Wujastyk (1998, 104) has remarked, and as is the case with other Sanskrit compendia, such as the *Caraka Saṃhitā*, the *Suśruta Saṃhitā* is likely to be the composition of several authors.

(Thatte 1988, 5). Therefore *marman* are defined as "abiding place of life" (*jīvasthāna*), or as "that which sustains life" (*jīvadhāraṇī*) (Rao 1987, 118).

In ayurvedic theory, *marman* combine the physical, or gross (*sthūla*), structures and subtle (*sūkṣma*) aspects, as the same spots are seen as manifestations of bones or muscles, that is, of physical structures, and of transphysiological concepts such as *doṣa* and *prāṇa*. Furthermore, mental processes and characteristics are included as well. These are denoted by the *triguṇa* (the three *guṇa* "qualities," namely *sattva, rajas, tamas*)[16]

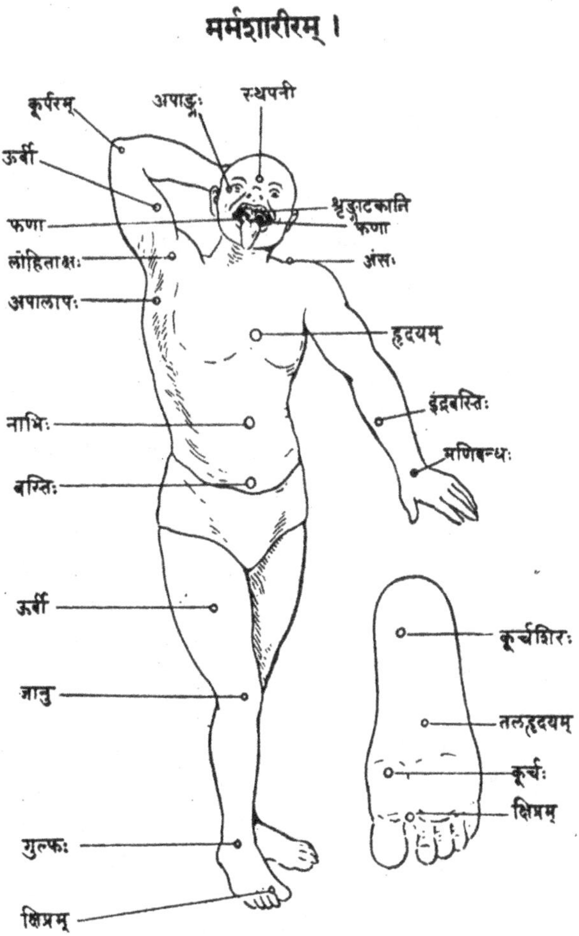

FIGURE 1.1 The *marman*. Illustration from a 1938 edition of *Aṣṭāṅgasaṃgraha*. Courtesy of Wellcome Library, London

16. For a stimulating discussion of the *guṇas*, see Daniel (1984a).

(Thakkur 1965, 33; Sharma 2002). Moreover, after observing these spots' lethal characteristics, ayurvedic physicians reasoned that the soul of a person, *ātman*, had to be present in vital spots as well (Fedorova 1990, 25). The *marman* can therefore be described as nodal points between the "gross body," the "subtle body," and the "causal body," or between *sthūlaśarīra*, which is the body of physical structures such as bones, muscles, and tendons, *sūkṣma śarīra*, which is the locus of *prāṇa*, and *kāraṇa śarīra*, which is the sphere of *ātman*. This is so, as not only physical, gross (*sthūla*) aspects—like bones and tendons (*dhātu*)—and transphysical, subtle (*sūkṣma*) concepts—such as *pañcamahābhūtas*, *doṣas*, and *prāṇa*—but also psychophysical (*kāraṇa*) characteristics of *guṇas* and *ātman* are present in a *marman*. Therefore, the *marman* are connecting points between all these levels—nodes linking the physical, the psychological, and the spiritual (figure 1.1).

Therapeutic Concepts of Marman Spots

The *Suśruta Saṃhitā* asserts that direct penetration of many loci is fatal, establishing a close connection between combat and medical intervention (Zarrilli 1989, 1294). The very word for surgery in Sanskrit, *śalya*, refers directly to foreign bodies such as weapons, and it has been argued that the authors of *Suśruta Saṃhitā* have gathered their anatomical knowledge and understanding of *marman* loci from dissecting corpses and in military hospitals near battlefields (Roşu 1978, 417; Krishna Rao 2007 [1937], ii). The *marman*-afflictions described in the ayurvedic compendia are indeed reminiscent of wounds and traumata caused by cutting and thrusting weapons. To quote from the *Aṣṭāṅgasaṃgraha* presenting two vital spots, *ūrvi* and *lohitākṣa*: "At the centre of the thighs is [the spot called] *ūrvi*; its injury causes emaciation of the thigh from loss of blood. Above the *ūrvi*, below the angle of the groin and at the root of the thigh is *lohitākṣa*; its injury causes hemiplegia from loss of blood" (Vāgbhaṭa 1999, 81). A trauma to a *marman* is mostly observed to cause manifold effects, often being incurable (*asādhya*), and/or lethal (Giri 2007, 158). Its symptoms seem to be largely caused by excessive bleeding, due to wounds inflicted by sharp weapons. A surgeon is thus advised to respond by amputating the affected part, such as a limb, above the concerned *marman*, in order to avoid further blood loss.

It is instructive to note that nowhere in ayurvedic literature is trauma to *marman* considered curable (*sādhya*). Rather, related inflictions are by definition incurable or untreatable (*asādhya*), and only considered manageable or mitigable (*yāpya*) in certain mild cases. Accordingly, no therapeutic value is accorded to *marman* loci in the ayurvedic compendia. Rather, the 107 spots are defined with regard to surgical intervention as being precisely those places that have to be avoided in surgery in order not to cause death or severe damage (Kutumbiah 1969, 33). *Marman* in classical ayurveda incorporates a certain prophylactic but no therapeutic value (Fedorova 1990, 340; Alter 2005a, 30). Acknowledging this, Dominik Wujastyk (1998, 244) writes that the *marman* theory "sits slightly oddly with the rest of ayurvedic doctrine ... it somehow speaks of a different milieu." This different milieu is likely to be the context of martial practices, and researchers have justifiably argued that the theory of *marman* may have been developed on the battlefields of ancient India (Roşu 1978; Fedorova 1990).

Unfortunately, apart from a few scattered references (Langford 2002, 212), there is not much literature addressing the contemporary medical use of *marman* in India. If there are specific utilizations of therapeutic *marman*, then their analysis is overdue. However, as early as 1937, Krishna Rao ([1937] 2007, iii), in a study on ayurvedic *marman*, lamented that its knowledge and practice had declined and "fallen long into oblivion, regarding its practical application" (see also Roşu 1978, 427; Mehra 2008, xxii). The neglect of vital spots—which are, as we have seen, a perfect blend of most ayurvedic principles—in contemporary (North) Indian medical practice, may be surprising. It may, however, be speculated that *marman* spots, alongside surgery, lost their medical and theoretical value with the much noted decline in invasive operations after about 400 CE, under the influence of Buddhist and orthodox Brahmanical ideologies (Zysk 1991, 5).[17]

Only in recent times have a number of publications, especially from esoteric and New Age healing circles, started to focus on *marma cikitsā*, vital spot therapy; these portray *marman* as locations for acupuncture-like stimulations by needles (Ros 1994) or by acupressure-like manipulation (Frawley, Ranade, and Lele 2005). The *Suśruta Saṃhitā*, however, explicitly cautions against the piercing, cutting, or cauterizing of *marman* loci, and therefore such recent publications display considerable innovative energy in (re)creating *marman* (Alter 2005b). With the influence derived

17. Surgery and anatomical knowledge in South Asia is argued to have developed from a recognized occupation to one looked upon with disdain, practiced only by low-caste practitioners (Zysk 1991).

from such innovative therapeutic New Age potpourri, forms of "ayurveda marma massage" or "marma yoga" are gaining increasing popularity, especially beyond India: in North America, Europe, and Australia, as gleaned from a growing presence of related information and advertisement on the Internet. On the other hand, within the curriculum of contemporary ayurveda colleges in India, students are not taught therapeutic concepts of vital spots, though different practitioners have argued for a revitalization of *marman* theory (e.g., Mehra 2008, xxiv).

Vital Spots in Yoga Traditions

While scholars have noted a striking difference of views of the body between ayurveda on the one side and tantric or yogic traditions on the other (Wujastyk 1998, 160), the vital spots must be noted as an exception in this regard. Some yoga scriptures incorporate a specific, partly distinct, yet obviously related theory of vital spots: *marmasthānas*, or *marmasthālas*. Among others, the Monier-Williams *Sanskrit-English Dictionary* translates *sthāna* as "place of standing or staying, any place, spot. . ., site," and *sthala* as especially applicable to prominent parts of the body. A *marmasthāna*/*-sthala* would then be the site of a vital spot. Jaggi (1979) has argued that a comparison of ayurvedic *marman* with yoga *marmasthānas* was not easily possible; the former related to physical, and the latter to transphysical spheres. However, not only do the obvious terminological analogies of both allow for recognizing a common ground, but so also does the fact that ayurvedic theory explicitly incorporates "transphysical" aspects, especially of *prāṇa*, as we have seen above. Despite all its esoteric "mystic physiology" (Eliade 1970, 239), I would therefore argue that yoga undeniably shares with ayurveda an important aspect in the concept of vital spots (see also Rao Siripuram 2009).

Yoga *marmasthānas* are eighteen in number, according to the *Yogayājñavalkya*, a manuscript dated to the thirteenth century CE (Eliade 1970, 480), as well as according to the *Triśikhibrāhmaṇopaniṣad* and the *Kśurikopaniṣad*, texts of even earlier periods (Rāya 1982, 228). These spots are largely congruous with eighteen among the 107 *marman*, yet partly labeled differently (Feuerstein 1990, 321). The eighteen *marmasthānas* are found at the big toe (*aṅguṣṭha*), ankle (*gulpha*), calf (*jaṅghā*), upper calf (*citi*), knee (*jānu*), thighs (*ūru*), anus (*pāyu*), coccyx (*deha*), genital area (*meḍhra*), umbilicus (*nābhi*), heart (*hṛdaya*), throat (*kaṇṭha*), palate (*tālu*), root of the nose (*nāsā*), eye (*akṣi*), in between the eyebrows (*bhrū*), forehead (*lalāṭa*), and the top of the head (*vyoman*) (Roşu 1978, 420; Mishra 2005, 24). These *marmasthāna* spots include the six *cakras*, which are important, transphysical centers in yogic theory, located at different positions along the spinal axis of the body.[18] The *cakras* are also an integral component of tantric and self-cultivation practices, and the *marmasthānas* and their application in yoga have much in common with a tantric understanding of the body. For instance, the *cakras* are connected to each other by a circuit system, called *nāḍī*, which transports the life-giving *prāṇa*, or vital energy. Of paramount importance among this system of *nāḍī* "channels" are three: *iḍā, piṅgalā,* and *suṣumṇā nāḍī. Suṣumṇānāḍī* is the central channel running along the axis of the body from the coccyx, or its root, *mūlādhāracakra*, up to the head, following the spinal cord. *Iḍānāḍī* starts in the big toe of the right foot, and ascends toward the left nostril, changing sides of the body along the way. *Piṅgalānāḍī*'s way describes the mirror reflection of *iḍā nāḍī*, and therefore both channels cross each other's paths in certain places, and change sides alternatingly. All three *nāḍīs* intertwine like snakes and are imagined to transport the *prāṇa* life force from the lowest *cakra*, the *mūlādhāracakra*, up toward the highest at the head region of a person, *ājñācakra*, thus passing all other *cakras*. Both *iḍā* and *piṅgalānāḍīs* are deployed in everyday usage, transporting *prāṇa*, but *suṣumṇanāḍī* has to be activated through yogic practices.

Activating *suṣumṇa* is to awaken the sleeping snake, or *kuṇḍalinī* (Eliade 1970, 246). To awaken this *kuṇḍalinī*, textual sources such as the *Yogakāṇḍa* of the *Vasiṣṭhasaṃhitā* (Roşu 1978, 419; Svātmārāma 2005) advise the *yogin* to make use of the *marmasthānas* in meditation (*dhyāna*). While inhaling, the yogic adept is to breathe into the *marmasthānas*, one after another. The *Kṣurikopaniṣad* directs the *yogin* to focus all attention on the vital spot of the big toe, then to proceed to the ankle and next to the calf, proceeding in this manner from the bottom of the body toward the top of the head.[19] The breath has to be retained in each vital spot respectively, an exercise which is called *pratyāhāra*, or "withdrawal," denoting the complete withdrawal from the world and from all sensory activities. This is conceived as not only assisting in meditation, but in activating *suṣumṇa nāḍī*, which

18. There is a seventh *cakra*, *sahasrāracakra*, considered of utmost importance in yoga. It is mostly perceived as a transcendental *cakra*, not located within the physical body (Rao Siripuram 2009).

19. *Kṣurikopaniṣad*, verses 12 and 13 (see also Feuerstein 2008, 81).

awakens the mentioned *kuṇḍalinī*. This in turn causes *amṛta*, "the nectar [of immortality]," to pass from one *marmasthāna* to the next one (Rao Siripuram 2009). The yoga vital spots therefore are a powerful yogic tool and held privileged in some meditation forms. These loci can furthermore be activated or influenced by specific root (*bīja*) *mantras*, which contain divine aspects (or manifestations of gods), and are connected to planets and thereby the whole universe. Therefore, *yogins* understand *marmasthānas* as a "cosmicization of the human body" (Eliade 1970, 240).

While classical, ayurvedic spots are reminiscent of the ancient South Asian battlefields and speak of wounds inflicted by cutting weapons and piercing arrows or spears and thus depict a quite graspable physical anatomy, the yogic *marmasthānas* speak of a more transcendent, transphysical anatomy of *nāḍī* and *prāṇa*, reflecting a more tantric tradition. As we will see, other, supposedly later vital spot traditions combine both physical and transphysical aspects closely, particularly the South Indian strands of *marmmam* and *varmam*, both aligned closely with martial practices.

Vital Spots, Manual Therapies, and the Martial Arts in South Asia

As already noted, the earliest textual references to *marman* are found in contexts of war. In many warlike combat practices in historical South Asia and in contemporary India we find martial practices that address specific parts of the body, perceived as particularly vulnerable. Furthermore, these are often paired with manual therapies and medical theories. Arion Roşu (1981) has explored the connections between *marman* spots and martial traditions of *mallavidyā* or *mallayudha* "wrestling," which have been and partly still are prevalent in many parts of India, especially in Gujarat and Karnataka. These traditions are described in different Sanskrit texts, such as the *Mallapurāṇa* or the *Mānasollāsa* (Wujastyk 1998, 244).[20] Several studies on North Indian wrestling practices agree on practitioners enjoying dual roles; wrestlers may administer massages and often offer other therapeutic treatments, such as setting of fractured bones, both to copractitioners and for patients (Alter 1989; 1992b; Lambert 1995; 2012). Johari (1984) maintains that *pahalwān* wrestlers

20. The *Mallapurāṇa* and the *Mānasollāsa* are dated to the fifteenth and seventeenth centuries CE respectively (Wujastyk 1998, 244).

of North India have a concise knowledge of the *marman* spots, which they deploy during massage as part of their training routine. In contemporary North India today, such wrestlers can also be observed offering their services or selling medical preparations on the streets; they set fractured bones and administer therapeutic massages (Lambert 1995, 93; Alter 1989).

Similar combinations of martial art forms and therapeutic applications can be described in *kaḷarippayaṭṭu*, practiced in the Southwest Indian state of Kerala, and the closely related *varmakkalai* of Tamil Nadu. Both comprise of medical and combat techniques and extensively deploy vital spots of the body, called *marmmam* and *varmam* respectively.

Vital Spots in Martial Arts and in Medical Treatment in Kerala

Marmmam, a derivative term of Sanskrit *marman*, in Malayalam has come to mean "knack of doing something" (Zarrilli 1998, 157) or "secret." *Marmmam* spot applications are found in contemporary Kerala, usually in martial arts practices called *kaḷarippayaṭṭu*, literally "training ground exercises." *Marmmam*, as described by Zarrilli in several publications (1989; 1992a; 1992b; 1998; 2005), are primarily utilized in combat situations. Medical applications are often connected to these, and thus *kaḷarippayaṭṭu* practitioners may administer massages to each other (Zarrilli 1995; Pati 2009). But knowledge and application of vital spots underlies the highest orders of secrecy within *kaḷarippayaṭṭu* practice. To cite Zarrilli (1989, 1295) in this regard: "The location of the vital points, the methods of attack and defense, and treatments for injuries [are] the highest forms of knowledge which masters traditionally confided only to their most trusted students." Some textual sources for such vital spots are in the possession of, and often jealously guarded by, martial practitioners. These may include oral commands (*vāyttāri*) for directing students in attacking and defending a particular vital spot. More often, though, *marmmam* knowledge exists primarily in the embodied practices of the master of a *kaḷari*, or training ground, and is passed on only to the most advanced and trustworthy students. Hence, different spots probably are known and utilized by different practitioners (Zarrilli 1998, 199), and endowed with an aura of secrecy.

Sreedharan Nair (1957, 12) argues that a distinct *marmmam* tradition of Kerala, as opposed to the *marman* tradition as found in classical ayurveda, is represented in texts and oral traditions of *kaḷarippayaṭṭu*.[21] While most practitioners seem to accept a total of 107 vital spots, as laid down by classical ayurveda, masters in Kerala recognize three distinct categories of loci, according to the effect of their application. They include the "great practical vital spots," or *kulabhyāsamarmmam*, direct penetration of which causes death or serious injuries. Further, *kaḷarippayaṭṭu* practitioners deploy "catch spots," or *koḻumarmmam*, which produce pain and are used to incapacitate an opponent, as well as "practice spots," or *abhyāsamarmmam*, the penetration of which is not as serious as that of the former two categories (Zarrilli 1989, 1295). Placing a greater importance on combat application, this tradition emphasizes the category of *kulabhyāsamarmmam*, deployed for attacking an opponent (Thatte 1988, 23). In total, these are sixty-four in number. The hands of a human contain twelve *kulabhyāsamarmmam*, the legs ten, the stomach three, the chest twelve, the back seven, the neck seven, and the head comprises thirteen such loci (Nair 1957, 10). These sixty-four points are known by thirty-seven names, which largely derive from Malayalam words (Thatte 1988, 29), such as *kaittaḷarppaṉmarmmam*, "the vital spot that weakens the hand [if injured]" (located above the elbow joint on both arms). Accordingly, there is considerable confusion about whether *marmmam* concur with the Sanskrit *marman* or not, as Nair (1957, 12) has pointed out. While some masters teach that the sixty-four *kulabhyāsamarmmam* are the most important of the 107 ayurvedic *marman*, others insist that at least half of these sixty-four are unique to *kaḷarippayaṭṭu* (Zarrilli 1998, 174–175). Though *kaḷarippayaṭṭu* specialists often utilize textual sources, which are derived from the ayurvedic compendia, such as the *Marmmanidāṇam*, more important are "much less Sanskritized texts like *Marmmayogam*, which are the kalarippayattu practitioner's handbook of empty-hand practical fighting applications and emergency revivals for the 64 'most vital' . . . spots" (164), and which considerably deviate from the ayurvedic compendia. Thus, other than in the classical ayurvedic compendia, which recognize five *dhātu* body tissues to be present in *marman* spots, the *marmmam* are classified structurally into six different types, according to six different body tissues, including muscle (*māṁsa*),

21. I am grateful to Harilal Madhavan for translating passages from Nair's *Marmmadarppaṇam* (1957).

arteries (*sirā*), veins (*dhamaṇī*), ligaments and nerves (*snāyu*), bones (*asthi*), and joints (*sandhi*) (Nair 1957, 12).[22]

Typically, the name of a particular *kulabhyāsamarmmam* signifies a point's prognostic or symptomatic quality, such as in the case of *svāsamaṭappaṉ*, literally "[the *marmmam* that] arrests the breath [if injured]." This spot is located on the chest and, if hit, causes the body to get hot, the eyes to pop outwards, and the stomach to swell up (Nair 1957, 16). *Malamarmmam* literally is the "excretion [blocking] vital spot." It is situated four finger-breadths below the navel and, if affected, arrests defecation. *Triśaṅgupuṣpam*, "three-conch-flower," is a popularly known vital spot, and is frequently featured in popular Malayalam cinema and its fight scenes.[23] It is located on the breast in between the nipples, and, if struck, the eyes are said to pop out, while the victim, screaming unknowingly, spits blood (Nair 1957, 22).

Such symptoms appear as more likely to be caused in unarmed combat or by blunt objects, rather than by swords and arrows, which would cause excessive bleeding as described in the ayurvedic compendia. Indeed, to effectively attack an opponent's vital spots, *kaḷarippayaṭṭu* practitioners have to bear in mind the location of a *marmmam* and the way of penetration (Luijendijk 2007, 111). Therefore, either the weapon deployed has to have a particular size, or, in unarmed combat, particular hand postures (*mudrās*) are utilized, of varying numbers and forms to hit a particular vital spot. Thus, the *kaḷarippayaṭṭu* vital spots are rather pressure points which are best penetrated by hand or small clubs or sticks (Zarrilli 1998, 180). Whereas the *Suśruta Saṃhitā*, for example, speaks of cuts and wounds at a *marman* causing endless bleeding, *kaḷarippayaṭṭu* texts deal with vital spots threatened by blows and kicks, rather than by weapons.

While Roşu (1978, 427) has remarked on the virtual disappearance of *marman*-based ayurvedic practices—this may or may not be true for North India—ayurveda in Kerala makes extensive use of them. Apart from administering massages to their students to provide flexibility and a supple physique for martial exercises, these practitioners may offer various

22. It must be stated, however, that the *Aṣṭāṅgasaṃgraha Saṃhitā* does enumerate six *dhātu* classifications as well (Fedorova 1990). *Marmmam* theory thus appears greatly influenced by the *Aṣṭāṅgahṛdaya Saṃhitā*. This textual preference, as opposed to other ayurvedic compendia, has been remarked on with regard to ayurveda practiced in Kerala in general (see Zimmermann 1978).

23. I am grateful to Harilal Madhavan for bringing this information to my attention.

therapeutic services to patients. Hence martial "[a]pplication (prayogam) and treatment (cikitsa) are inseparably linked and always taught in tandem," as Zarrilli (1992a, 1295) has asserted, and numerous physicians in Kerala offering *marmma cikitsā* are also *kaḷarippayaṭṭu* martial arts masters (Pati 2009; 2010). They are frequently approached to address effects of physical traumata, such as bone fractures, sprained muscles, and *marmmam* afflictions requiring emergency treatment. Therapies offered by *kaḷarippayaṭṭu* masters range from massages, deploying hands, feet, or other body parts of the practitioner's body, to manipulations, tractions, and countertractions for the setting of fractured bones, to bandaging or plastering, prescription of medications, and dietary restrictions.

Marmmam therapy shares the notion of bodily equilibrium as a foundation of health. If a vital spot is injured, the three *doṣa*s or "humors" of the body are said to become unbalanced, thus causing diseases by deterring the bodily equilibrium. *Vāta*, *pitta*, and *kaphadoṣa* will be unbalanced according to the part of the body afflicted or according to the spot impacted. Not only are the *doṣa*s unsettled by a vital spot accident, *prāṇa*, "life-energy," also becomes obstructed at the site of injury. This weakens the entire system of *nāḍī*s, the channels which transport *prāṇa* through the body. As Zarrilli (1989, 1296) points out, when a *marmmam* is penetrated, the entire physical structure may be in danger of collapsing and ultimately lead to death. Hence, counterapplications have to be administered within a prescribed period of time to restore structural balance and health. This emergency treatment is called *maṟukai*, "opposite hand" (Zarrilli 1998, 174), or *maṟutaṭṭu*, "opposite stroke" (Nair 1957, 13). Usually such therapy consists of a strong slap with the palm of the physician's hand on the side directly opposite to the affected spot. Afterwards, the entire body or specific body parts of the patient are massaged, twisted, pulled, or jerked at *marmmam* junctures. This emergency treatment has been noted to countershock the *nāḍī*s, activate *prāṇa* energy, and restore the structural balance of a patient (Zarrilli 1998, 174). Apart from manual techniques, recipes for internal medication are known and utilized in the form of pills (*guṭika*) or decoctions (*kaśāya*), which are conceived of as controlling the disrupted *dōṣa* and as releasing the obstructed *prāṇa* in a patient (Thatte 1988, 32). Medicated oils (*thailam*) of similar qualities are further used in massage methods.

The *marmmam* tradition thus features certain distinctive aspects, including an elaborate set of therapeutic techniques—*marmma cikitsā*—which the Sanskrit compendia lack. The same holds true for the distinct set of points called *kulabhyāsamarmmam*, deployed in *kaḷarippayaṭṭu* martial practices. Similar observations can be made about the *varmam* spots, as found in Kerala's neighboring state of Tamil Nadu.

The Vital Spots in Tamil South India

Since the *varmam* loci and related practices constitute the main focus of this book, and will be described in detail throughout the following chapters, I provide only a brief introduction and overview here, in order to allow for a comparison with the traditions discussed so far. References to vital spots in Sanskrit epics mention a type of body armor called *varman* to protect the *marman* points (Fedorova 1990, 8; Govindan 2005, 9). From this *varman*, the term *varmam* might well have developed.[24] While some Tamil scholars have held that *varmam* is a corrupted form of the Tamil word *vaṉmam*, "malice, grudge, spite, or force," thereby providing a Dravidian etymology for *varmam*, most practitioners whom I met expressed the view of an association of *varmam* with *marmam*, meaning "secret" in Tamil, and of a close relationship to the ayurvedic *marman* loci.

Medically and martially inclined practices, which revolve around *varmam* vital spots, are generally clubbed together under the term *varmakkalai*, "the art of the vital spots." Therapeutic techniques are individually referred to as *varma maruttuvam*, or *varma vaittiyam*, "*varmam* medicine." Martial practices are called *varma aṭi*, which literally means "hitting the vital spots." The medical techniques are considered a subbranch or specialization (*ciṟappu maruttuvam*) of siddha medicine, the codified indigenous medicine of Tamil South India. Siddha medicine, like ayurveda, enjoys state support and the instruction of professionalized siddha practitioners according to a standardized curriculum in siddha medical colleges. Yet the siddha medical colleges do not provide comprehensive instruction on the vital spots and the majority of *varmam* practitioners are not institutionally trained. They have received their education in hereditary lineages of knowledge transmission from an experienced teacher, or *guru*. Accomplished practitioners of the combined martial and therapeutic application of vital spots are called *ācāṉ*, teacher, esteemed person or *varmāṇi*, the one who deals with the vital spots. Though spread

24. *Varmam* has also been spelt *vaṟmam* in some Tamil palm-leaf manuscripts (Irājēntiraṉ 2006, 50).

over all rungs of society, such practitioners, to a large extent, are primarily found in formerly lower castes, such as Shanar, now Nadar, and in very low castes, such as Sambavar.

Numerous Tamil palm-leaf manuscripts (*ōlaiccuvaṭi*) bear witness to *varmam*, specifying names, locations, and characteristics of loci, and both treatment and combat modalities, all in poetic verses (figure 1.2). The *varmam* textual corpus is considerable, and some practitioners have estimated it to contain up to 200 different manuscripts of various lengths and coverage (Irājēntiraṉ 2006, 10; Vasanthakumar 2004, 41; Aleksāṇṭar Ācāṉ 1998, 10). Practitioners often possess several such texts, or handwritten copies of them. Like siddha manuscripts in general, these are actually poetic songs (*pāṭal*), intended for chanting. It has been argued that they use a coded, at times deeply ambiguous language, "a language in which words are on purpose semantically polyvalent" (Zvelebil 1973, 21). This characteristic is mirrored in an emphasis on concealment of knowledge and practices, due to *varmam* loci being potentially dangerous, possibly causing death if injured, according to practitioners. *Varmam* combat practices are designed to either directly address a vital spot, with a view to quickly incapacitating an opponent, or to shield one's own vital spots.

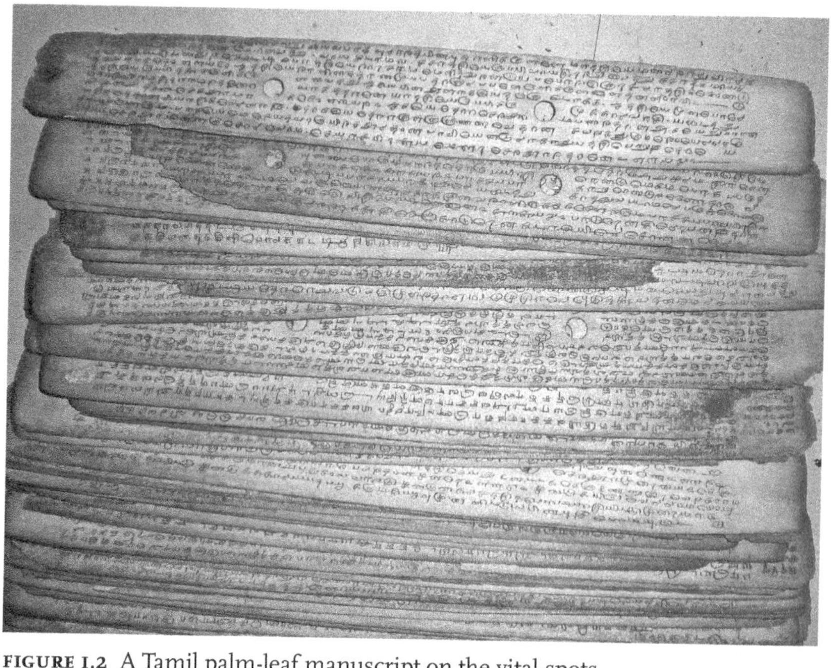

FIGURE 1.2 A Tamil palm-leaf manuscript on the vital spots

These tasks are accomplished with the use of a practitioner's hands and sometimes with weapons, but generally the knowledge of the methods employed is zealously guarded, and released only to the most trusted among an *ācāṉ*'s students, as is done in *kaḷarippayaṭṭu* martial training. Also, though practitioners stress the importance of their manuscripts, they give ultimate preeminence to hands-on and experience-based instruction (see also chapter 6).

Similar to *marmma cikitsā*, practitioners deploy vital spot therapy to treat fractures (*muṟivu*), nerve-related problems (*narampu nōy*), including hemiplegia (*pakkavātam*) and many other ailments. They frequently deliver emergency treatments for severe vital spot injuries, or resuscitate unconscious patients by stimulating *varmam* loci. When stimulating a *varmam*, *pirāṇam* (Skt. *prāṇa*, life force) is perceived to be activated in its circulating flow through the *nāṭi* (Skt. *nāḍī*) channels of the body (Vasanthakumar 2004, 35). *Varmam* are hence important body loci, vulnerable but also of therapeutic relevance, and therefore critical for maintaining health and life. Patients sometimes describe *varmam* stimulations as a slightly painful, tingling sensation, or like an "electric current." This current, according to *ācāṉs*, is *pirāṇam* when forced to flow through the *nāṭis* during vital spot manipulations. This eliminates the blockages caused by a *varmam* injury and restores the body's structural balance. Indeed, like *marman* in the ayurvedic compendia, the *varmam* spots are described as locations that house *pirāṇam* (Irācāmaṇi 1996, 26; Irājēntiraṉ 2006, 41; chapter 4). As *pirāṇam* is considered a most vital force of life, it is generally equated with life (*uyir*) itself. Logically, the *varmam* loci are also called "seats of life" (*uyir taṅkumiṭam*) (Subramaniam 1994, 3). This explains their vulnerability, as *varmam* are points where life is concentrated.

According to the presence of *pirāṇam*, the *varmam* spots can be classified prognostically, and especially the categories of *paṭuvarmam* and *toṭuvarmam* have to be mentioned in this regard.[25] A *varmam* which directly concurs (*paṭu-ttal*) with *pirāṇam* and its circulation is a *paṭuvarmam*, a "severe" or "lethal spot," which, if affected, is said to cause immediate unconsciousness (*mayakkam, mūrccai*). This means that a particular *paṭuvarmam* is located directly on a *nāṭi* channel, and any damage to such a spot will have direct, detrimental effects to *pirāṇam* circulation. If

25. Irājēntiraṉ (2006, 71) calls this classificatory system "*kuṟikuṇavakaippāṭu*," or "prognostic sign system."

receiving a blow of a certain force, a *paṭuvarmam* may even cause death (Kēcavappiḷḷai 1983, 30). A *varmam* which only touches (*toṭu-ttal*) upon *pirāṇam* is called a *toṭuvarmam*. *Toṭuvarmam* spots are less serious loci, injury of which nonetheless can cause various ailments. Altogether there are twelve *paṭuvarmam* and ninety-six *toṭuvarmam*, bringing the total number of *varmam* spots to 108 (Irājēntiraṉ 2006, 41); this is a point of contrast with the stated 107 loci of both *marman* and *marmmam*.

Practitioners consider *varmam* to be nodal points between the three bodies of human beings. These three include the "gross body" or *tūlacarīram* (Skt. *sthūla śarīra*), the body of physical structures. Further, the "subtle body" or *cūṭcumacarīram* (Skt. *sūkṣmā śarīra*), is the body of *pirāṇam* and the *nāṭi* system. Finally, the "causal body," *kāraṇacarīram* (Skt. *kāraṇa śarīra*), is the encapsulation of *karma*, acquired through deeds of previous lives, and it also contains *ātmaṉ*, the soul of a being. Thus an affliction of a *varmam* can cause repercussions upon all these bodies or levels of life, including their physical and mental aspects, ranging from bone fractures, to fainting, to memory loss, or to sudden death (see also chapters 3 and 4).

In *varmakkalai*, a separate set of points called *aṭaṅkal*, "relief spots," is endowed with therapeutic importance, and is subject to manual stimulations in most treatments. *Aṭaṅkal* loci are deployed in setting of fractured bones, administration of massages, and direct attention to specific ailments. This includes spot stimulation for countering unconsciousness, treatment of immediate ailments, such as headache, or therapies for chronic suffering, including various nerve-related problems (Maṇiyaṉ 2012, 143). Even hemiplegia cases (*pakkavātam*), often resulting from a stroke, are frequently treated by manipulations of relief spots. In case of an acute affliction of a *varmam* due to a physical impact, such therapeutic spots may be slapped, pulled, twitched, pinched, turned, or otherwise stimulated in a kind of emergency treatment (*iḷakkumuṟai*), similar to those performed by masters of *kaḷaris* in Kerala. Above taking care of all nerve-related ailments (*narampuviyāti*), such as *vātarōkam* (often translated as rheumatism), *ācāṉs* thus take pride in claiming skills to reanimate unconscious patients. Next to manipulations, practitioners apply bandages and medicated oils (*eṇṇey* or *tailam*) to speed up recovery (*Varmakkaṇṇāṭi*, verses 327–502; Mariyajōcap n.d., 168–254; chapter 4).

Having to bear in mind such aspects as time, timing, and force, *ācāṉs* stress the need to know a great deal about astrology (*cōciyam*), but also about yoga and meditation (*dhyāna*), apart from mere medicine and martial arts, in order to become accomplished. The theoretical concepts of *varmam* also show a close affinity with the yogic *marmasthānas*, and *ācāṉs* learn to focus on their own vital spots and to control *pirāṇam* within the body, which is said to have beneficial effects on both therapeutic techniques and martial exercises. The following chapters will provide a more detailed description of underlying theoretical concepts (chapter 2) and of martial (chapter 3) and therapeutic practices (chapter 4), making up the core part of this book.

Vital Spots and the Relationship between Siddha Medicine and Ayurveda

Some of the traditions that we have seen are allocated to different, clearly demarcated medical systems. *Marmma cikitsā* is today perceived as pertaining to ayurveda, and *varmam* to siddha medicine. Though possibly cognate, *varmam* and *marmmam* are thus clearly distinguished from each other, just as ayurveda and siddha medicine are discerned and administered as distinct medical systems. This is an outcome of the institutionalization, professionalization, and standardization of Indian medicines, processes which commenced in the colonial period (Muraleedharan 1992; Brass 1972). Despite that fact that initially, after the setting up of Indian medical colleges in the twentieth century, ayurveda and siddha medicine were taught together (Sébastia 2010), and although different scholars have tried to argue for a mutual relationship of both ayurveda and siddha—mostly by stating the derivation of the latter from the former (Scharfe 1999)—most siddha practitioners today claim a uniqueness and antiquity for their medical system, refuting a derivation from ayurveda (Narayanaswami 1975; Sambasivam Pillai 1993, 11). On the other hand, a brief analysis of siddha medical history and its relation to ayurveda helps to show that clear demarcations between ayurveda and siddha as "medical systems" are but recent constructs. This is further stressed by the case of the vital spots—*marman*, *marmmam*, and *varmam*—in particular. Such vital spot traditions, transcending regional borders, historical periods, and forms of practice and theory, speak a different language than the contemporary delineations of clearly defined, neatly demarcated medical systems of India.

Siddha Medicine and the Siddhars

Siddha medicine is alleged to go back to a group of mythical sages, the Siddhars, who are said to have lived in parts of South India which today comprise Tamil Nadu. The term Siddhar is derived from the Sanskrit root *sidh,* meaning "to be accomplished."[26] The Siddhars' accomplishments included both physical and spiritual achievements, even an alleged immortality, which was striven for by various methods: alchemical transmutations of substances, transformations of body and mind through yogic exercises, and elixirs credited with panacea-like powers. In this regard, they are close to other esoteric traditions of mystics in South Asia, such as the *Nāth Siddhas* (White 1996), and it therefore has been correctly argued that the Tamil Siddhars cannot be considered as "an isolated and unique body of freethinkers, but [rather are] an integral part of a pan-Indian tradition" (Zvelebil 1973, 25). Those Siddhars who are associated by modern-day siddha practitioners with having founded siddha medicine are known almost exclusively in Tamil South India, however (Weiss 2009, 47). Though always referred to as eighteen in number—the term "eighteen Siddhars" (*patiṉēṇ cittarkaḷ*) is deployed as a uniform appellation—sources disagree on who belongs to this group. Accordingly, various, divergent lists exist, each enumerating eighteen different names.[27]

The Siddhars' legacy, and with it the compendium of siddha medicine, is said to have been preserved for posterity in the form of palm-leaf manuscripts, which were copied down time and again by their students. An analysis of this corpus, however, reveals a high degree of heterogeneity; it contains medical theories, philosophy, poetry, astrology, and alchemical recipes (Little 2006, 13). While some of these writings might date back to the eighth century, others cannot be older than a hundred years,[28] and this is true for many of the manuscripts dealing with *varmam* spots.

---

26. See Monier-Williams *Sanskrit-English Dictionary*. The precise Tamil spelling and transliteration of Siddhar would be *cittar*. However, I deliberately use "Siddhar," the Anglicized version of a Tamilized Sanskrit root-term, and, similarly, "siddha medicine." Not only does siddha/Siddhar constitute the more commonly known term, which is used in popular, administrative, and scholarly accounts, but also, as Weiss (2009, 47) points out, it importantly conveys the high degree of linguistic (and cultural) hybridity, which has formed these terms.

27. See, for instance, the list provided by the Central Research Institute for Siddha: http://www.crisiddha.tn.nic.in/siddhars.html, which deviates from the lists of Zvelebil (1973), Venkatraman (1990), and Shanmuga Velan (1992), who all stress that the number of Siddhars was much higher than eighteen. See also V. R. Madhavan (1984, 19–26), who presents no fewer than eighteen different lists of eighteen Siddhars.

28. Narayanaswami (1975, 3) emphasizes that many manuscripts appear as rather recent in language and content: "the language of some of the siddha literature is so modern that it cannot be the work of any sage of the hoary past but that of comparatively modern authors who have attributed it to Agasthya." Krishnamurthy and Chandra Mouli (1984, 45) state that a linguistic analysis suggests that most siddha texts have to be dated to after the thirteenth century CE. Some *varmam* texts have been dated to the seventeenth century (Jēms 2010, 59–60).

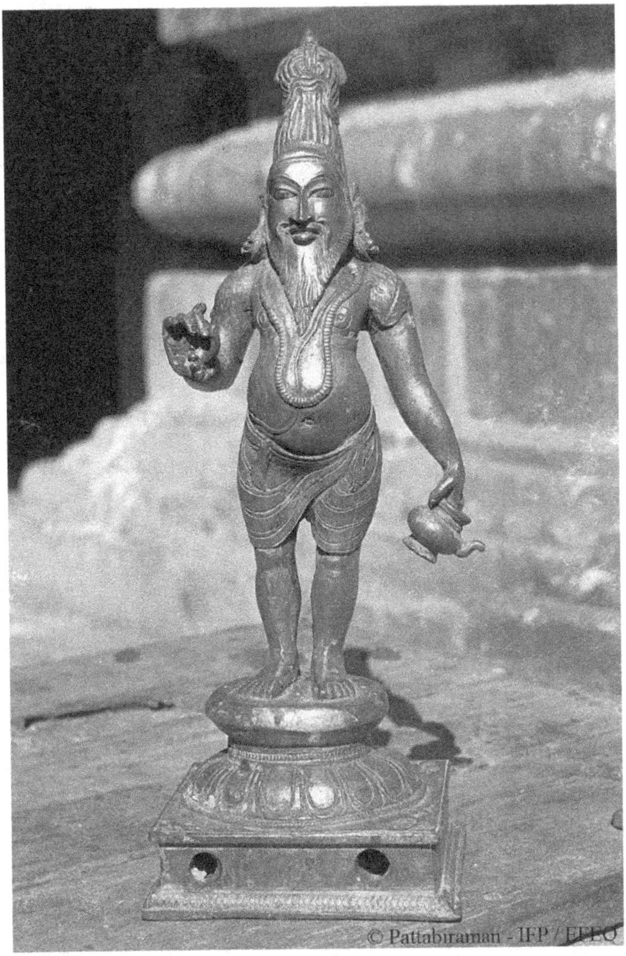

FIGURE 1.3 Bronze statue of Siddhar Agasthiyar. Courtesy Institut Français de Pondichéry and École Française d'Extrême-Orient

Especially Agasthiyar (figure 1.3),[29] revered as first and foremost amongst the Siddhars, has numerous such manuscripts to his credit, too numerous and too varied in terms of topics and language, to be the products of a single author. Rather, such texts have to be accredited to a lineage of writers, instead of to the authorship of one, individual author, an aspect typical of South Asian literary traditions (Michaels 1998, 123; Wujastyk 1998, 104). "Siddhar" thus must be seen as a generic term which depicts

29. In Tamil, the name of this Siddhar is generally written as *Akastiyar* or *Akattiyar*.

a heterogeneous group of persons, including poets, philosophers, bards, mystics or tantrics, alchemists, and physicians; they belonged to various periods of time, roughly from the eighth to the twentieth centuries (Krishnamurthy and Chandra Mouli 1984), and are not easily reducible to a common denominator (Venkatraman 1990, 74; Zvelebil 1973, 17–18).

Some scholars have characterized the Siddhars as "heretics who challenged the religious orthodoxy in the Tamil region" (Sujatha 2009, 78). Zvelebil (1973, 113) in this respect writes: "Siddha non-conformism is often expressed in the external appearances and attitudes. They resembled madmen, roaming about at will, scantily clad, and eating whatever they were given." Unorthodox in their ideas, the Siddhars were presumably outcasts rather than holy men from the point of view of orthodox Hindus, a notion represented by Srinivasa Iyangar in 1914, who describes them as "plagiarists and impostors . . . being eaters of opium and dwellers in the land of dreams their conceit knew no bounds" (Little 2006, 14). Their language has been called "enigmatic diction, mysterious, hidden, full of ambiguous symbols and double meanings, but the language the text employs in its syntax and lexicon is more often than not almost vulgar [and] simple colloquial idiom, close to the speech of the masses" (Zvelebil 1973, 21). Siddhars did not use the classical, refined, or literary language of Tamil, but that spoken by the "common man," adopting a kind of "folk-song" style (Meenakshi 2001, 112). Still, a kind of "intentional language," *paripāṣai* (Skt. *paribhāṣā*, also *sandhābhāṣa*), a codified, technical, but also deeply esoteric language, characterizes most of the siddha works, allegedly designed to conceal secrets they had discovered on diverse subjects (Trawick 1983, 939). With such "ciphered songs" (Eliade 1970, 251), the Siddhars supposedly also demarcated themselves from a larger group, which they wanted to prevent from understanding their secrets (Little 2006, 13).

Moreover, the writings of the Siddhars did not always enjoy the place of respect they enjoy today. During the late nineteenth and early twentieth centuries, street hawkers sold many texts of the siddha compendium together with cheap and popular publications on crossroad markets. Only later were some of these ballads and popular forms of literature "sanitized," edited, and integrated into the canon of classic Tamil literature, in the form of *ciṟṟilakkiyam* or "minor literature," as Venkatachalapathy (2012, 139, 166) shows in an analysis of book production in colonial Tamil South India. The Dravidian Movement at the turn of the century furthermore provided a kind of rehabilitation and legitimization to the Siddhars' writings and thought, since some members of the Dravidian Movement, such as E. V. Periyar, regarded the siddha movement as nonbrahmin Dravidian in outlook and as a social revolt directed against the caste system (Steever 1994, 365n8). As Steever states, the "Siddha verses against the temple cult and the caste system became slogans of [the Dravidian] movement" (366n13). Any reconstruction or analysis of siddha theory must be cautious of these later influences of Tamil language revivalism and of the Dravidian Movement.

Furthermore, the Siddhar treatises make clear that their métier was far from narrowly limited to medicine—whatever this category entails. Rather, they incorporated philosophy, alchemy, nature observations, tantric rituals, astrology, and insights on yogic exercises. Also, though today largely portrayed as rational scientists by many siddha practitioners (Narayanaswami 1975, 5; Sambasivam Pillai 1993, 28) and some Tamil scholars (Ganapathy 1993; 2008; Sarma 2007), the mystic Siddhars deployed considerably unorthodox methods by both modern and contemporary standards. Zvelebil (1973) in particular provides numerous descriptions of esoteric tantric rituals—including having sex with virgin representatives of the divine power (*cakti*)—utilized by different strands of historic Siddhars. Sujatha (2009, 83) is thus right in asserting that "siddha medicine today is by no means identical to the viewpoint of the early siddhars." Despite such apparent heterogeneity, unorthodoxy, and eclectic approaches, many contemporary Tamil practitioners are quick to assert their Siddhar lineage and the antiquity of their siddha system (Ramalingam and Veluchamy 1983, 44). Such a perception is a recent one, however, and has been shaped partly vis-à-vis other medical systems, such as ayurveda and biomedicine.[30] It is therefore important to briefly reflect on the emergence of contemporary siddha medicine.

The Emergence of Siddha Medicine

Richard Weiss (2009, 7–8) has fittingly placed the modern promotion of siddha medicine squarely in the realm of Tamil revivalism, emphasizing in this regard the importance of the Dravidian nationalism of the

30. Different terms are in vogue for addressing the dominant medical system of Euro-American origin, and for distinguishing it from other medical practices, including "regular," "allopathic," "scientific," "modern," and "cosmopolitan medicine" (Leslie 1976; Dunn 1976). I follow Hahn and Kleinman (1983) in adopting the term "biomedicine," since much of its practices focus primarily on a human pathophysiology (Pordié 2007, 10), often to the extent of reducing disease to biological factors alone (Baer et al. 2003, 11).

late nineteenth and early twentieth centuries. This Tamil revivalism was impelled largely by sociopolitical circumstances in postindependence India (Ramaswamy 1997). In Tamil South India, the Tamil language, in competition with Hindi in a bid for supremacy, was promoted and supported by the "movement for pure Tamil" (*taṉittamiḻ iyakkam*). The leaders of this movement argued for the use of Tamil in a pure form, uncorrupted by English, Sanskrit, and Hindi loan words.[31] Tamil revivalist leaders, feeling sidelined by North Indian politics and power, demanded "labor" for Tamil (*tamiḻpaṟṟu, tamiḻcēvai*) to effect a consequent cleansing of the language (Ramaswamy 1997, 20). The Tamil language, it was argued, had to assert itself against the Hindi that was becoming the national language of a united and independent India, and which, it was feared, might oust Tamil even in its homeland (Katre 1969; Ekbote 2007). One of the main aims of the demanded labor hence was to cleanse and thereby save Tamil from the oppression and assumed defilement of alien languages, which were supposed to be degraded and crude, as against the refined and "sweet" Tamil. Tamil became personified and even deified as "mother Tamil," *tamiḻttāy*, and the primary symbol of Tamil nationalism and pride.

A similar development can be observed in the case of the promotion of medicine in South India, which shares much with the broader Tamil revivalist movement. Tamil and siddha medicine thus became intertwined, and "siddha" and "Tamil medicine" interchangeable, as the following quotation shows:

> This tr[a]ditionally contained Tamil Medical Science, the outcome from the ancient superb Tamil language was neglected for a long time. And now, under the present Government rule, the siddha medicine has regained its world worthy status with the enterprising uplift by Tamil enthusiasts.
>
> (Ramalingam and Veluchamy 1983, 44)

Just as Tamil began to be referred to as *tāy*—"mother"—some practitioners of siddha medicine likewise started both to claim antiquity for their medical system and to label it as *tāy vaittiyam*, "mother medicine" (Manu

31. I am fully aware of the brevity of this account, which disregards Western Indological and missionary contributions and the influences of Tamil classicistic and religious movements. These have been forces in the emergence of Tamil revivalism which have to be taken seriously as well. For an excellent description of the Tamil revivalist movements, see Ramaswamy (1997).

Vaidyar 2007, 61). In parallel with the feared linguistic hegemony of the North, physicians of Tamil South India saw their occupations threatened by North Indian ayurveda and biomedical practitioners. Many *vaittiyars*, that is siddha physicians, argued that their medicine was indigenous to Tamil Nadu and unrelated to the North Indian—aryan—ayurveda, which was of a more recent origin, as they claimed (Sampath 1983, 5; Geetha 1983, 133; V. R. Madhavan 1986, 123).[32] Siddha medicine thus gradually came to be regarded as "Tamil medicine," described as a distinct medical system, and as distinct from medicines of North India in particular. Siddha became denoted as "Dravidian," "non-*aryan*," South Indian, and most of all "Tamil" (Ganapathy 1993; 2008; Sarma 2007).

Parallel to Tamil-language valorization, promotion of siddha can be seen to have been accelerated under feelings of being sidelined both academically and administratively, especially with regard to ayurveda (Weiss 2008). Often denoted as "pan-Indian," or as *the* Indian medical system (Wujastyk and Smith 2008, 1; Pordié 2007, 1), ayurveda has been assigned utmost importance and attention both in scholarly writing and in government policies. A large number of studies were therefore published from the 1960s onwards by siddha practitioners with the objective of "highlighting the special features of the Siddha System ... [with the] task of justifying the indigenous individuality of the ancient Siddha System of the South" (Narayanaswami 1975, iii–iv), arguing for a separate identity of siddha medicine.

However, unlike present-day scholars or practitioners, none of the ancient Siddhars in their treatises had used the term "siddha medicine" (*citta maruttuvam* or *citta vaittiyam*) (Krishnamurthy and Chandra Mouli 1984, 46). Instead, therapeutic recipes are sometimes described as *āyurvētam*, or *āyuḷvētam*. Siddhar Yukimuṇi even notes that he created his work after examining the Sanskrit literature of *āyurvētam* to explain it in Tamil (46). A passage of Agasthiyar's *Paripūraṇam* reads: "this (subject of) ayurveda is told in four sections" (46). Even Tamil *vaittiyars* in the early twentieth century did not unanimously refer to their medicine as "siddha," nor did they clearly differentiate themselves from other South Asian practitioners of medicine, as has been remarked by Hausman (1996, 238) in a historical analysis of the institutionalization of medicine in South India.

32. Ramalingam and Veluchamy (1983, 53) write: "[the] siddha system of medicine was flourishing in various parts of Tamil Nadu in ancient days also and it has not generated from any other system of medicines as some perverted people opine."

The Muslim practitioner Hakim Abdullah Sahib of Madras, for instance, writing in 1888 on the enhancement of procreation and semen, characterizes his medical practice as derived from the *cittars*, but as ayurvedic and as yunani at the same time, often listing all these denominations in succession (Aptullā Cāyapu 1888, 10, 13). For medical practitioners of preindependence India, it might therefore be argued, it was more important that what they practiced was medicine (*vaittiyam, maruttuvam*) than a specific medical system called siddha.

As Weiss (2009, 80) points out, while Hindu-Muslim religious tensions are reflected in ayurveda-yunani formulations, an emergent Tamil revivalism has characterized siddha medicine as distinct from ayurveda. Thus, viewing siddha and ayurveda as strictly separate is a rather recent development:

> In asserting a distinct historical trajectory for their knowledge, siddha practitioners overwrite a past in which the lines between two discrete medical systems called ayurveda and siddha were not clearly, and rarely even faintly, drawn. Scholars, practitioners, and patients today too often assume the durability of these lines that have come to distinguish South Asian medical systems.
>
> (Weiss 2009, 80–81)

This circumstance is probably nowhere better exemplified than in the case of the vital spots, which not only transcend the taxonomical category of "medicine" (I will come back to this point in chapter 3), but which also transcend the demarcations between ayurveda and siddha medicine as drawn today.

Conclusion

I have outlined several theories and applications of vital spots in India in this chapter. These include the Vedic and Sanskrit *marman* of ritual scriptures and epics, and their later development into a full-fledged medical theory, as gleaned from the ayurvedic compendia. Esoteric yogic theory further details a distinct set of spots, *marmasthānas*, utilized for meditative purposes to attain a higher consciousness or salvation. Traditions of vital spots in South India, of both therapeutic and martial applications, incorporate both the more physical aspects of ayurvedic *marman* and the transphysical, transcendent concept of yogic *marmasthāna*. In Kerala, *marmmam*, of *kaḷarippayaṭṭu* martial traditions and *marmma cikitsā* therapy, are utilized in combat applications and in various medical treatments offered by persons who are fighters and physicians at the same time. *Varmam*, the loci of *varmakkalai*, are closely related, also combining therapeutic and martial uses. Further, it may be speculated that related aspects of knowledge of the body and health are found in less visible traditions—the medical lore, in the family and the household—and exhibited by so-called lay practitioners, such as midwives.

Interestingly, though, while both *marman* and *marmmam* are regarded as being part of ayurveda, *varmam* is described as pertaining to siddha medicine, and these vital spot traditions receive a clear demarcation in contemporary parlance and in their institutionalized promotion. Yet an analysis of Indian vital spots should desist from clearly demarcating such medical "systems," or from perceiving their contemporary divisions as historically backed facts. Sujatha (2009, 78) captures this by stating:

> The difference between ayurveda and siddha may be discerned in terms of philosophical orientation, history, spatial spread and language of expression. But their conceptual framework for medicine is the same. ... The pharmacological preparations in ayurveda and siddha follow similar principles as applied to plant, animal and mineral ingredients.

One should not forget that medical systems tend to be tied to, and to be perceived as closely connected with, a particular nation-state in contemporary societies. This is true for ayurveda, being understood as uniquely Indian—"*the* traditional Indian medicine"—though it may just as well have partly evolved in what is today Afghanistan, Bangladesh, Nepal, or Pakistan, and no doubt has been shaped by trade and other over-regional contacts (Alter 2005a, 2). Notwithstanding an administrative, scholarly, and general discourse on medical systems, which confines them to the borders of particular nation-states or regions, medical systems always have and will crosscut political boundaries. It has been documented by historical sources, and becomes clear when analyzing the perception of siddha medicine since the twentieth century, that the emergence of "medical systems" in South Asia is a rather recent phenomenon, which can be largely traced back to nationalism and the hegemony of biomedicine. A comparative analysis of the vital spot traditions shows that this indeed is true. With regard to the relationship between siddha medicine and ayurveda—a recurring and intensely debated topic—most scholars are today arguing for a relationship of dependence of one upon the other (Scharfe 1999). In fact, the relatedness is quite apparent, and becomes even more so in most comparisons of the vital spots. Still, it should be acknowledged that neither enjoys an antiquity or preeminence over the other. Rather, instead of emphasizing systematicity with regard to South Asian medical practices, fluidity must be stressed, and in this, I follow Høg and Hsu (2002, 209), who have demonstrated "how arbitrary it is to draw boundaries between the various medical traditions." As Sujatha, Aruna, and Balasubramanian (1991, 52) have argued, indigenous medicine in India is an "elaborate and complex system in which many levels and layers of medical knowledge and practice coexist and function simultaneously"; several, mutually interacting layers of medical knowledge and practice with varying degrees of professionalization and institutionalization.

Following this, and by contrastively analyzing the medical knowledge, or the medical lore, of the household, of nonprofessionalized practitioners such as bonesetters or midwives, and professionalized doctors of, say, siddha medicine, one might thus argue that all are but nodal points in a broader network of health; orders or manifestations of a broader concept. This study of the vital points and the current manual therapies considers the seamless merging of the orders—the textual and the oral or nonliterate, the standardized and the nonstandardized, and the "classical" and the popular folk traditions. The binary distinctions already mentioned can be in part attributed to Robert Redfield's concept of "great traditions" and "little traditions" within a society and culture. For Redfield (1956, 67), great and little traditions described "the separation of culture into hierarchic and lay traditions, the appearance of an elite with secular and sacred power and including specialized cultivators of the intellectual life, and the conversion of tribal peoples into peasantry." But, if anything, the binary concepts of "folk" and "classical," "minor or subaltern," "major or supra-altern," and "great or little" practices, are at best grounded on social factors and literacy (Ram 2001a, 70), yet are not functional tools to analyze medical practices. A current and largely accepted discourse would be to assume the development, codification, and practice of medicine of complex societies as an achievement of the literate elite. In the case of South Asia, at least, more popular forms of medicine kept on influencing these learned strata and vice versa (Balasubramaniam 2004, 73).[33] The same case might be argued for many Asian medicines today. It is argued thus that, parallel to the evolution of epics and stories in India (Hiltebeitel 1999), medical practices have been and presumably still are informed by so-called folk and textual traditions alike, and aspects of both therefore are seen as mutually integrated.

Furthermore, in the introduction to his edited volume *Asian Medicine and Globalization*, Joseph Alter (2005a, 3) cautions that the term "medicine" itself might be not only misleading but also a distorting analytical concept in the case of therapeutic concepts in South Asia. Indeed, the vital spots, and their diverse theories, which incorporate not only aspects of healing, but also of apparently nontherapeutic facets, such as yoga, astrology, philosophy, and so on, underscore this challenge. In this regard Laurent Pordié (2007, 9) seems justified in demanding that with regard to anthropological theory in South Asia, a "culture of healing must be distinguished from *medicine*, not only from biomedicine but from medicine as a category."

I have tried to suggest that the vital spots are part of a comprehensive pan-Indian concept, which links different abstract thought systems and practical applications. The vital spots are part of a cultural current—of a shared knowledge about the body, health, and well-being. Different vital spot theories and practices as traced over different parts of South Asia can be seen as different manifestations of this knowledge. Its branches are seen in the past and the present, in literary evidence as old as 3000 years, but also in contemporary, inexpensive pamphlets and in scholarly publications. Vital spots are being integrated into the contemporary codified medical systems, while at the same time being practiced by noninstitutionalized healthcare providers and presumably even in households. To perceive such expressions as manifestations of a concept, or as "variants in medical practice," in the words of Francis Zimmermann (1978, 97), allows for a more dynamic exploration of the spread and incorporation of knowledge than dualist notions of "oral" or "folk" on the one side and

33. Similarly, McKim Marriott has argued for a two-way influence of so-called "great traditions" and "little traditions," meaning the Sanskritic, textual tradition and ritual on the one hand, and religious manifestations at the rural village level on the other (Redfield 1956; Miller 1966). For Marriott, processes of "universalization" and "parochialization" described the mutual influencing of both. Universalization is the process of local practices being introduced into standard Sanskrit traditions. Parochialization in contrast describes how the Sanskrit canon influences local adaptations of ritual practices (Marriott 1955).

"literate" or "classical" traditions on the other. Further, as the example of the vital spots in India shows, academic and taxonomical demarcations between medicine, (martial) arts, yoga, and astrology are likely to be but recent constructs. *Marman, marmmam,* and *varmam* loci blur today's observed boundaries between healing, harming, physical exercise, spiritual achievement, and so on. Clear-cut demarcations of such concepts may be insignificant for past as well as present vital spot practitioners. This is true for the hereditary practitioners of *varmakkalai*, "the art of the vital spots" in Kanyakumari.

2

The Vital Spots

HETEROGENEOUS THEORIES, CONSISTENT TRADITIONS

Within a living being, that, which is encased by life,
drifting and vibrating all about,
in spontaneous circulations of transcendental supremeness,
that is a vital spot.

Varma cūṭcā cūṭcam, verse 5

I will tell [you about] the combined rule of the three kings
within the house built of ninety-six principles.
I will name the twelve lethal spots,
and the ninety-six graceful vital spots.
I will elucidate even the inner spots,
and the relief spots, two times six.
Here, vātam, pittam, and kapam, the three kings,
jointly reign over this body.

Varmakkaṇṇāṭi, verse 23 (Mariyajōcap n.d., 12)

THIS CHAPTER PROVIDES an account of the theoretical underpinnings of vital spots, which will allow for an understanding of their practical applications by hereditary physicians and martial art exponents in South India. Drawing on diverse data and material including original palm-leaf manuscripts and published versions, comparatively recent publications, and informant's explications, little-known details of these vital spots can be depicted, which clarify their relations to more general Indian traditions of the body, health, and well-being, as well as to esoteric yoga and astrology.

Importantly, however, there is no single theory of vital spots, but rather a polyphony of ideas and heterogeneous aspects. While conducting research in Kanyakumari, I interviewed various informants and read source texts and more recent studies on vital spots in Tamil. All along, I found it problematic to meld these different voices into one coherent, meaningful theory. While one approach made sense for itself, it was contradicted by the explanations of another practitioner or manuscript. What was even more challenging, vital spots themselves appeared too numerous and confusing to be studied in detail, and *ācāṉ*s as well as published accounts seemed to draw in part on different loci. This is exemplified by the existence of innumerable synonyms and varying locations. In what follows, I do not attempt to synthesize a consistent theory of *varmam*. Rather, I depict accounts of the vital spots and their underlying theories as multiple and diverse as I have found them to be. I have no doubt that there are *ācāṉ*s who exhibit ideas different from, and conflicting with, what I present here, and this would merely serve to underscore the conclusion of this chapter: *varmakkalai*, as found in the practices of contemporary *ācāṉ*s, in manuscripts, in publications, and recent textbooks, reveals a high degree of heterogeneity, ambiguity, and at times even mutual inconsistency.[1]

Reasons for such diversity, inherent and crucial to all aspects of the vital spots, as will become apparent in the subsequent chapters, can be identified in two central and partly interrelated circumstances. First, *varmakkalai* is not just a partly oral tradition but also a decidedly embodied one. This means that its intricacies are found more in the incorporated practices of *ācāṉ*s than in textual sources, and are therefore subject to individual interpretations and practices. Secondly, *varmakkalai* is an esoteric tradition, which is characterized by secrecy and deliberate nondisclosure of related information. These circumstances have led to the development of knowledge and techniques through individual practice and its transmission within closed lineages, and serve to explain a decisive nonstandardized character of *varmakkalai* today.

1. Textual material deployed to achieve this includes: *Caracūkṣattiṟavukōl* (Key to the garland of subtlety), as published by Irājēntiraṉ (n.d.); *Varma Cūttiram* (Treatise on the vital spots), as published by Subramaniam (1994); *Varma Cūṭcāmaṇi Pañcīkaraṇa Piṉṉal* (Garland [of songs on the] creation of the precious vital spots), as published by Nicivilcaṉ (2004); *Varma Cūṭcā Cūṭcam* (The supreme subtlety of vital spots); *Varmak kaṇṇāṭi* (Mirror of vital spots), as published by Mariyajōcap (n.d.); *Varma viti* (Vital spot conduct), as published by Aruḷmiku paḻaṉi taṇṭāyutapāṇi cuvāmi tirukkōyil (The Murukan Temple of Palani) (1976); as well as *Varmapīraṅki* (The vital spot cannon), *Varmapīraṅki Cūttiram* (Treatise on the vital spot cannon), *Varmapīraṅki Tiṟavukōl* (Key to the vital spot cannon), all published by Nicivilcaṉ (2003), and *Varma Oṭimuṟivu Cara Cūttiram* (Treatise on vital spot fractures and breakages), as edited and published by Jēms (2010). These texts are edited, printed, and published versions of original Tamil palm-leaf manuscripts on vital spots.

Siddha Theory and the Vital Spots

Despite the existence of multiple views on *varmam*, a kind of entry point into our topic can be made out, which is compatible with most practitioners' understanding of vital spots and with a general siddha medical view of the human body. This is epitomized in the concept of *pirāṇam* (Skt. *prāṇa*),[2] which in siddha as well as ayurvedic theory is perceived as a crucial aspect of life and well-being, as vital in nourishing the physiological structure of human beings and as present in all *varmam* spots.

The human body, according to the text *Varma Cūṭcāmaṇi Pañcīkaraṇa Piṉṉal* (Garland of songs on the creation of the precious vital spots), is a physical structure made up of bones, the framework of all vertebrates, which is held together by flesh, muscles, and tendons (Nicivilcaṉ 2004, 3–4). But the actual life (*uyir; jīvaṉ*), the vitality of this structure, is only represented by *pirāṇam*, a vital energy which pervades the body, and which bestows animation and existence. *Pirāṇam* is described as life itself by most siddha physicians, who affirm that where *pirāṇam* is, there is life, *uyir*, and vice versa (Sujatha 2009, 80), or who simply equate *pirāṇam* with *uyir* (Jekatā 2005, 24). Emphasizing the importance of *pirāṇam* even further is the fact that the vital spots are potentially deadly loci, which can cause maximum damage to a person, precisely because they are closely connected to *pirāṇam* and hence with life itself. Thus, the vital spot theory follows siddha and ayurveda in perceiving *pirāṇam* as a crucial factor of health and well-being. However, although Alter (2005a, 32) holds that *prāṇa* is not of great significance for therapy in ayurveda, it is of central importance for *varmam* in both its martial art and treatments modalities.

Ayurveda and siddha medicine further share an idea which might be termed holistic, as every substance and every being is always seen in relation to other, larger processes and connections. Every individual body is thus understood to be connected with its environment and indeed with the whole universe. This is reflected by Siddhar Caṭṭamuṇi's oft-cited verse, which states the universe is contained within the body and vice versa.[3] The same substances and processes that constitute the

---

2. It must be stated that siddha medicine shares many concepts and terms with ayurveda, and generally deploys Tamilized versions of Sanskrit words. I use Tamil terms where they deviate in spelling from Sanskrit loan words, but provide the Sanskrit (Skt.) original in brackets upon first occurrence.

3. In Tamil: *aṇṭattil uḷḷatē piṇṭam—piṇṭattil uḷḷatē aṇṭam.* See also Sambasivam Pillai (1993, 12).

universe are regarded as composing a person and his or her state of well-being. Foremost amongst such substances are the "five elements," *pañcamakāpūtam* (Skt. *pañcamahābhūta*). These are: earth or solid matter (*maṇ*), water or fluid matter (*nīr*), fire or radiant matter (*tī*), wind or gaseous matter (*kāṟṟu*), and ethereal matter (*akācam*) (Narayanaswami 1975, 9). These elements are present inside each body, and form, in different combinations, further refined substances, such as the *tātu* (Skt. *dhātu*), body tissues, and give rise to physiological processes called *tōcam* (Skt. *doṣa*). *Tātu* body tissues are seven: lymph (*iracam*), blood (*irattam*), muscle (*tacai*), fat tissue (*koḻuppu*), bone (*elumpu*), marrow (*majjai*), and venereal fluids (*cukkilam*).

Tōcam is a category of great importance, which in most publications has been translated as "humors,"[4] but more literally means "blemish, fault, or disease." The *tōcam* are three and describe different functions or processes in the body: *vātam* is connected to the functions of the nervous system, *pittam* is responsible for the metabolic activity, and *kapam* provides for the adhesiveness of physical structures and fluid substances. As an abstraction, one could therefore say that *vātam* designates all gaseous or pneumatic processes, *pittam* the acidic processes, and *kapam* the unctuous processes of the body. The prominence of these physiological processes exemplifies that it is not so much the organs themselves as their functions that are important in siddha medicine. It may therefore be recognized as merely consequential that siddha allows for a conception of the body which includes the mind by definition: mental processes are constituted as much by food and external or internal influences such as lifestyle and bodily tissues, and vice versa, as all these are characterized and influenced by *tōcam* (Sujatha 2009, 79).

The state of the *tōcam* regarding the balance or disequilibrium of *vātam*, *pittam*, and *kapam* vis-à-vis each other is of crucial importance; a specific balance is pivotal for health, whereas disequilibrium in the *tōcam* categories is likely to precipitate disease. *Tātu* and *tōcam* moreover are interrelated, as one particular *tōcam* predominates in a specific body tissue, and both categories influence each other, as a dysfunction or imbalance in one

---

4. The term "humors" derives from European medical history and, having a distinct history of its own, is bound to distort meanings of *tōcam*/*doṣa*. The same applies to the terms *vātam*, *pittam*, and *kapam*, which are often routinely translated as "wind," "bile," and "phlegm." From my understanding, the *tōcam* are rather processes or functions than substances. In order to avoid distortions, I prefer to use the original terms to translations.

affects the other. For instance, *vātam* primarily acts in the lower part of the body, such as in the legs, and often *ācāṉ*s hold it to predominate in bones. *Pittam* is active in the center of a person and in muscles, and *kapam* is found concentrated in the upper part of the trunk, in the brain and the lungs, but is also said to predominate in nerves (Citamparatāṇuppiḷḷai 1991, 42). Hence, in the case of *tōcam* disorders, *tātu*s will be affected accordingly (Narayanaswami 1975, 7). An increase or a decrease in a *tōcam* will generate a corresponding change in a body tissue, the effect of which may be observed as symptoms of an ailment.

As the underlying substances of the human body are present everywhere in the universe, the remedies for an illness consequently are chosen for their innate qualities. As each substance consists of the five elements in different proportions, they increase or decrease a particular *tōcam* when ingested. Following this logic, physicians of siddha medicine rely heavily on dietary prescriptions (*pattiyam*) for treatment, and most drugs are used to establish equilibrium amongst the three *tōcam*.[5] Therefore, the character of the drug being administered complements that of whatever is causing the ailment at hand.[6] If, for instance, *pittam* is aggravated in a patient, a therapy will aim at administering substances that suppress *pittam*.

Vital spots are interconnected with both *tōcam* and *tātu*, and can both influence and be influenced by them. A physical trauma to a vital spot causes a blockage of *pirāṇam*. Deviations of *tōcam* result, starting with a vitiation or aggravation of *vātam*. Conversely, even an unbalancing of one of the *tōcam* categories can cause a vital spot ailment, by causing a blockage of *pirāṇam* at a particular spot. *Pirāṇam* circulates through the body in a kind of channel system, *nāṭi*. The *Varmakkaṇṇāṭi* (Mirror of vital spots) describes *nāṭi*s as "pervading the human body like the veins that pervade the luffa sponge gourd [*pēyppīrkku*]" (verses 55–56; Mariyajōcap n.d., 27–28). The luffa gourd—popular in its dried form as a natural bathing sponge, or loofah—consists of innumerable fibers, which crisscross, and hence make an ideal metaphor for the system of *nāṭi* channels, which transport *pirāṇam* throughout the whole body. Narayanaswami

5. For this reason, medicine and food are not viewed as two distinct categories in Tamil South India. One popular saying of siddha practitioners is: *maruntē uṇavu—uṇavē maruntu*, which translates as "food is medicine and medicine is food."

6. Accordingly, albeit risking over-simplification, one might say that this approach is contrary to homoeopathy, or "Treating with the same," but close to the term (!) allopathy, or "Treating with the opposite" (see Pordié 2007, 10).

(1975, 9) writes that *pirāṇam* "is the vital representative of the centripetal movement in matter. This is instanced in inspiration, in swallowing food, drink, etc." The *nāṭis*, moreover, are important with regard to *varmam*, as vital spots are placed on different locations along them. Basically, vital spots are precisely those places of the body where *pirāṇam* occurs in a concentrated form, and therefore the circulation process of *pirāṇam* is intimately related to vital spots. Manuscripts and practitioners corroborate this view, stating that vital spots are locations which "house" *pirāṇam* (Irācāmaṇi 1996, 26; Irājēntiraṉ 2006, 41). As *pirāṇam* is considered the most vital force of life, or as life itself, the *varmam* are called "seats of life" (Subramaniam 1994, 3).[7]

One *ācāṉ*, while actually demonstrating his explanations by touching various parts of my body, elucidated the intimate connection between vital spots, *pirāṇam*, and life as follows:

> If I press this point on your body—*kurunāṭivarmam* [located near the radial artery on the forearm]—you will quickly feel giddy and faint. [This is so, because] it contains *pirāṇam*. If there is an injury, *pirāṇam* circulation is diminished [*curukkamāyirukkum*], and the capacity of legs and hands perishes. Once unconsciousness sets in, and if the patient does not receive treatment quickly, death is certain.

At this point I had to ask the practitioner to stop his demonstration, as I did indeed feel very dizzy! If *pirāṇam* circulation is interrupted by a trauma to vital spots, death or a variety of ailments are caused. As an instance, *ācāṉs* explain an illness called *pakkavātam*, generally identified as paralysis or hemiplegia, to be caused by an injury to a *varmam*. *Pakkavātam* is said to result from the blockage of *pirāṇam* circulation at one or several vital spots, which hinders the flow of the life energy through the *nāṭi* channels, and thus causes deviations of *tōcam* functions and *tātu* tissues. Depending on the specific spot afflicted, such a blockage can cause mild ailments or lead to severe damage.

This also implies that only if *pirāṇam* circulation is present in a particular point is that point a vital spot. Hence, a particular location in

7. Also, one of the manifold synonyms for *varmam* spots as listed by Cukumāraṉ (2006, 55) is *pirāṇaṉ*, a masculinized form of neuter *pirāṇam*, which equates *pirāṇam* with *varmam*.

the human body is not a *varmam*, unless *pirāṇam* is concentrated at it (Caṇmukam 2006). Furthermore, given that life force circulates within the body, and its ebb and flow may vary from one instant to another, time becomes an important element in the assessment of a patient's vulnerability or in combat.[8] According to an increasing or abating of *pirāṇam* at a specific *varmam*, the concerned spot is more or less vulnerable at a given point of time.

The *Nāṭi* System

The *nāṭi* system is made up of numerous channels; most sources mention the number 72,000 (*Caracūkṣa Tiṟavukōl*, 3; Eliade 1970, 231). Three amongst these are important for the present analysis. They are *cuḻumuṉai* (Skt. *suṣumṇā*), *piṅkalai* (*piṅgalā*), and *iṭakalai* (*iḍā*). Apart from being important in esoteric yogic theory and most medical traditions in South Asia, these channels are crucial to an understanding of the concept of *pirāṇam* life force and the vital spots. *Nāṭi* channels transport life force throughout the body, supplying every organ and limb. While doing so, *cuḻumuṉai*, *piṅkalai*, and *iṭakalai* pervade the body and cross each other in several places, thus "intertwining like the aerial roots of a banyan tree" (*Varmakkaṇṇāṭi*, 126; Mariyajōcap n.d., 59–60). *Iṭakalai* takes its beginning in the big toe of the right foot and reaches the pelvic region, from where it alternates sides and travels on the left side of the spine, toward the left nostril, from where it finally moves downward into the arm, ending in the tip of the left hand's middle finger. The path of *piṅkalai* is situated on the opposite side to that of *iṭakalai*, originating in the left foot, passing through the right nostril and terminating in the tip of the right hand's middle finger. *Iṭakalai* and *piṅkalai* thus cross paths several times (Mariyajōcap n.d., 29–30). Velayudhan described the way of life force within these two as "scissor-" like:

VELAYUDHAN: This circulation works like a scissors. It transports *pirāṇam* from left to right and from right to left. It also means that if I strike this side, there will be an effect on the opposite side. I will show you. Stretch

8. On the importance of time and seasonal contexts in ayurvedic texts, see Zimmermann (1980).

out your hands (*he flips his index finger lightly against the knuckle of my extended right hand's middle finger, and then has me wait for a few seconds*).

ROMAN: Now there is a strange feeling in the middle finger of my *left* hand!

VELAYUDHAN: Yes! But I have tapped against the *right* hand! Does it feel cold?

ROMAN: Yes, it feels somehow cold.

VELAYUDHAN: How come you feel a difference in the opposite hand? It's the *nāṭi*'s scissors structure [*kattari amaippu*]! I have tapped against a vital spot in your right hand and the effect can be felt in your left, because life force circulates from left to right, and vice versa.

This goes to show how intimately the vital spots are connected to *pirāṇam*, to its circulation, and to the channels of its circulation, the *nāṭis*.

Unlike *piṅkalai* and *iṭakalai*, *cuḻumuṉai* is located along the central axis of the human body and travels from the area close to the coccyx upwards through the body to the forehead. *Cuḻumuṉai* thereby repeatedly crosses the paths of both *iṭakalai* and *piṅkalai*.[9] The points of intersection of all three are places where *pirāṇam* life force exists in an increased degree, and hence they are especially important and vulnerable at the same time. Along the center of a human body, there are six such intersecting points which are of utmost importance. Yogic theory knows these as *cakras*, important transphysical centers of a human being, as body parts on which yogic adepts direct their meditative concentration (Eliade 1970, 70). Most *ācāṉs* recognize these *cakras*, generally called *ātāram* in Tamil, as vital spots. The six *ātārams* are: *mūlātāram*, near the coccyx; *cuvatiṭṭāṉam*, located in the umbilical region; *maṇipūrakam*, near the pit of the stomach (epigastrium); *aṉākattam*, at the solar plexus; *vicutti*, on the throat; and *ākkiṉai*, situated between the frontal sinuses (*Varmakkaṇṇāṭi*, 79–93; Mariyajōcap n.d., 38–43) (figure 2.1).[10] If *ātārams* are in any way vitiated, they cause ailments, but such spots may be deployed for

9. In tantric yoga, this central (*suṣumṇā*) *nāḍī* is generally described as inactive unless activated by a practicing *yogin* (Eliade 1970, 238). It must be noted that the notions of *nāṭi*/*nāḍī* and *pirāṇam*/*prāṇa* are important ideas in several theories in South Asia, despite deviations. Here, I focus on the important aspects for *varmam*, without assessing differences in approach of ayurvedic or yogic traditions.

10. The respective Sanskrit terms are *mūlādhāracakra*, *svādhiṭṭhānacakra*, *maṇipūracakra*, *anāhatacakra*, *viśuddhacakra*, and *ājñākhyacakra*. There are more *cakras*, notably a seventh, *sahasrāracakra*, which is supposed to be located at the top of the head. It is, however, not considered as one of the six *cakras*, which play a role in this account (Eliade 1970, 240).

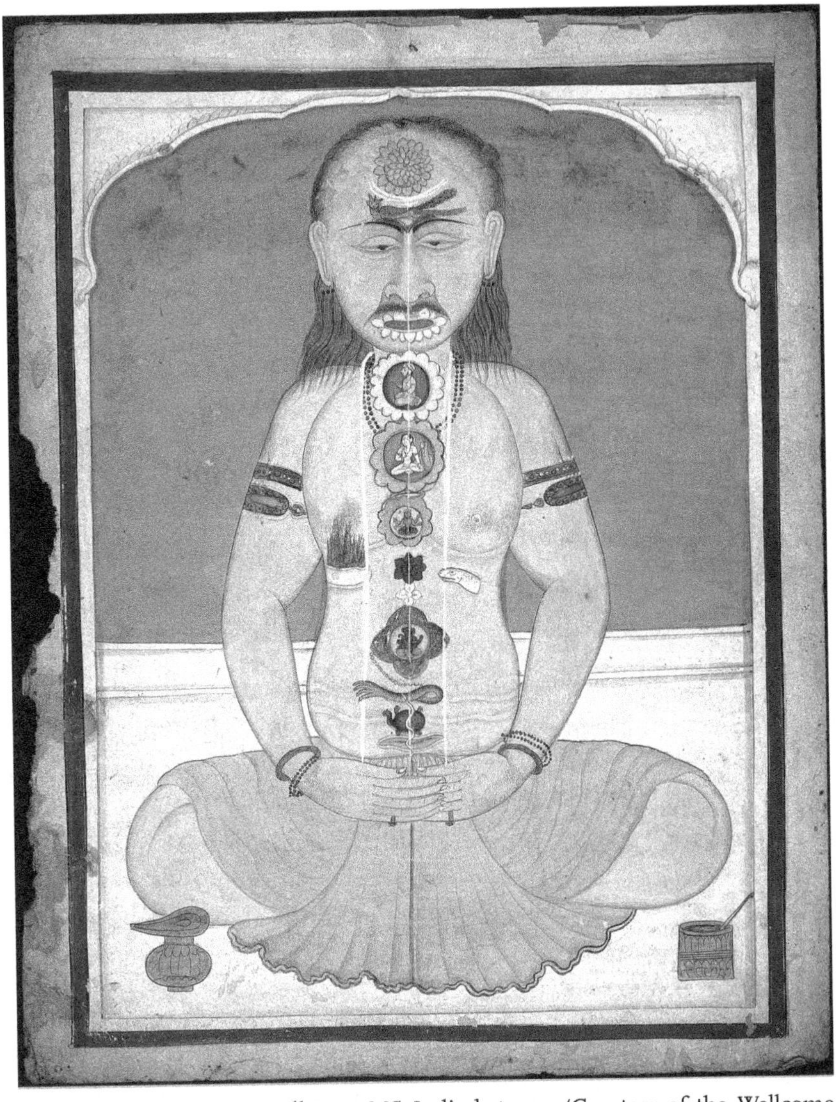

FIGURE 2.1 The *cakras*. Wellcome MS Indic beta 511. (Courtesy of the Wellcome Library, London)

treatment purposes as well. The area of the spinal cord is thus especially important with regard to the health and life of a person and to treatment of various diseases.

Most *ācāṉ*s accept these centers as prototypes of vital spots, since they comprise a high degree of life force and are located at the confluences of three *nāṭi* channels. However, not all practitioners acknowledge the *ātāram* as *varmam* loci (Govindan 2005, 22). For some, each *ātāram* should rather be visualized as an important compartment of the body, which governs the nature (*kuṇam*) and energy (*cakti*) of the areas adjacent to them. Each *ātāram* in this regard *houses* several vital spots, which are governed by and themselves influence a corresponding *ātāram* (Kaṇṇaṉ Rājārām 2007b, 74). Those loci adjacent to a particular *ātāram* are related to the latter and therefore, in the case of *mūlātāram*, three vital spots, namely *kaṅkalaṅkivarmam, vittuvarmam*, and *taṇṭuvarmam*, can be considered as *mūlātāram* spots, that is, *mūlātāravarmam* (75, 257). In other words, some practitioners recognize particular vital spots as *cakra*-related loci—such as the three mentioned *mūlātāram* spots—but do not recognize the *cakras* per se as *varmam* spots.

In general siddha theory, only ten *nāṭi* channels (*tacanāṭi*) are pointed out as being of special importance. In contrast, a total of twelve *nāṭis*, including *cuḻumuṉai, iṭakalai*, and *piṅkalai*, are crucial with regard to vital spots (Caṇmukam 2010, 6). One *varmam* locus spot is directly connected or coincides with one of these twelve channels (Kaṇṇaṉ Rājārām 2007b, 250). These twelve are referred to as "severe" or "lethal spots," *paṭuvarmam*. Each of these twelve *nāṭis* is further related to eight vital spots, called "touch" or "connect-spots," *toṭuvarmam*, numbering ninety-six in total. The difference between these two categories of spots is that while a *paṭuvarmam* directly coincides with, or "strikes" (*paṭu-ttal*), a particular *nāṭi* channel, and hence *pirāṇam*, a *toṭuvarmam* merely comes into contact with, or "touches" upon (*toṭu-ttal*), a *nāṭi* channel and its *pirāṇam* life force (Aleksāṇṭar Ācāṉ 1998, 161–163; Kaṇṇaṉ Rājārām 2007b, 251). However, deviating from this categorization, Maṇiyaṉ (2012, 96) states that *paṭuvarmam* spots are part of bones, while *toṭuvarmam* are part of nerves. According to either understanding, *toṭuvarmam* spots are vulnerable and can cause severe ailments if injured. *Paṭuvarmam* spots on the other hand are considerably more dangerous loci and their afflictions are often known to cause instant death. *Cuḻumuṉai* channel, following this logic, houses one "lethal spot, called *tilartakkālam*, located in the middle of a person's forehead,[11] and is furthermore connected with eight touch spots, namely: *koṇṭaikollivarmam, cīṟuṅkollivarmam, pālavarmam, cūṇṭikkālam, caṅkutirikkālam, kaṇṇāṭikkālam, oṭṭuvarmam*, and *carutivarmam*" (Aleksāṇṭar Ācāṉ 1998, 161; see figure 2.2). As each of the twelve *nāṭi* channels contains one lethal spot and eight ancillary touch spots, the overall number of vital spots is 108.

11. *Tilartakkālam* is located at the spot on a person's forehead which people of Hindu faiths anoint by applying sacred ash in ritual expression and to signify different social or religious aspects (*tilaka*).

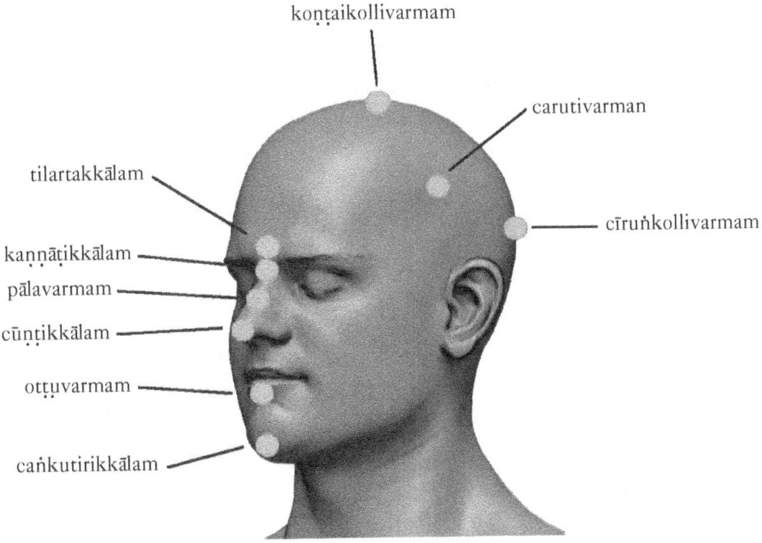

FIGURE 2.2 *Paṭu-* and *toṭuvarmam* associated with *cuḻumuṉai nāṭi*

The Three Bodies and Their Five Sheaths

Practitioners emphasize that vital spots both protect and endanger a person's body, mind, and life, due to their intimate connection with all three such aspects (Caṇmukam 2006). Valentine Daniel (1984a, 278) describes how human bodies in South India (and beyond) are thought to consist of three different body categories (*carīram*; Skt. *śarīra*), which correspond to five sheaths, or layers (*kōcam*; Skt. *kośa*). First, the *tūlacarīram* (Skt. *sthūla śarīra*), translated as "gross body," is described as having "weight and form" (279). It is the body of a human being as perceived by the eye, made up of skin, bone, and flesh, and nourished by food. It covers a more "subtle body," or *cūṭcumacarīram* (Skt. *sūkṣma śarīra*), which is the seat of emotions such as love and hate, and the realm of *pirāṇam*. A dead body, therefore, merely is a *tūlacarīram*, from which the life force has departed. The third body category is indestructible and imperceptible by the senses. It is called *kāraṇacarīram* (Skt. *kāraṇa śarīra*), or "causal body," and is encompassed by both *tūla-* and *cūṭcumacarīram*. Being weight- and formless, the *kāraṇacarīram* "encases the soul and moves with it from one place to another inside and outside the sūkṣma śarīra" (284). This concept of the human body as "psychophysical continuum encompassing both gross physical constituents and subtle psychic faculties" (Holdrege

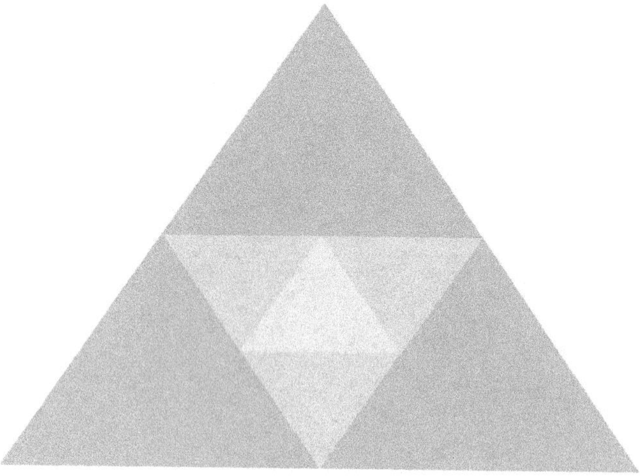

FIGURE 2.3 The three bodies or a schematic depiction of a vital spot

1998, 346) has its roots in the Upaniṣads and has been elaborated in *Sāṁkhyā* philosophy (347).[12] Velayudhan, in an attempt to clarify some notions regarding the vital spots, composed a schematic drawing for me, which depicted the gross, subtle, and causal body. All three bodies, he explained, are not only interrelated, but encompass another (see figure 2.3). The grossest body, visible and palpable, is the outermost form, schematically depicted by the outermost triangle in Velayudhan's drawing. The subtle body is represented by the triangle placed upside down inside the gross body, and itself encompasses the causal body, the innermost in the layering of bodies, and the innermost triangle in the drawing. Yet there are connecting nodes between all three; in Velayudhan's depiction, this is represented by one triangle touching the other triangle's sides. These junctures are especially endangered by injury, which could potentially affect all three bodies. To be sure, there are more junctures in a body as displayed in the *ācāṉ*'s schematic drawing. Importantly, all three bodies are joined in every vital spot, which means that within every *varmam*, *tūlacarīram*, *cūṭcumacarīram*, and *kāraṇacarīram* are present and joined. This also means that

12. As Holdrege (1998) points out, the mind-body dichotomy that has preoccupied Western philosophy does not appear to be a central concern in Hindu philosophical traditions, where the mind, along with other psychic faculties, is a subtle aspect of the body. Hence, according to the theory of the three bodies, the mind, just like the physical body, is a type of matter—albeit a subtler one than the physical body.

Velayudhan's drawing can be considered a schematic depiction of a vital spot, combining within itself the three bodies or aspects of life.

The three bodies are further divisible into five shells or sheaths, *pañcamayakōcam* (Skt. *pañcamayakośam*). The *tūlacarīram* corresponds to *aṉṉamayakōcam*, the sheath of food, since this gross body has to be nourished by food. *Cūṭcumacarīram* coincides with *pirāṇamayakōcam*, or the "sheath of *pirāṇam*." The third body, *kāraṇacarīram*, comprises three shells. *Maṉōmayakōcam*, or sheath of mind, is the site of intellectual faculties: mind (*maṉam*), intellect (*putti*), determination (*cittam*), and conception of individuality (*akaṅkāram*). Second, the *viññāṉamayakōcam*, or the shell of intelligence, is, amongst others, the site of time (*kālam*) and *karma*, the results of deeds done in former births (*viṉai*, *niyati*). Last, and innermost, *āṉantamayakōcam*, the "sheath of bliss," is the seat of knowledge (*vidyā*) (*Varmakkaṇṇāṭi*, 76; Mariyajōcap n.d., 36–37; E. V. Daniel 1984a, 281). Vital spots penetrate all these five sheaths of the body, like nodal points which connect all layers and spheres of life and existence. Accordingly, due to the fact that within a *varmam* all aspects of existence are present, vital spot ailments not only have lifelong reverberations (Ram 2001b, 192), but any injury to a vital spot may affect a person's physical body (*uṭal*), mind (*maṉam*), and nonphysical, transcendental, or *karmic* aspects (*uyir*). Jaggi (1979) has argued that while *cakras* are of a transphysiological nature, the ayurvedic *marman* vital spots are concrete, tangible, and physically manifest. However, such a proposition is not tenable in the case of *varmam* spots, which connect both physical and transphysical categories by being intersecting points of all three bodies and their five sheaths.

A *varmam* affliction, therefore, can cause many conditions that are not obviously related to human physical anatomy alone. A vital spot injury is understood to possibly result in unconsciousness, or cause mental problems and even initiate repercussions with regard to afterlives, since vital spots affect body, mind, and life of a person. In an inferential conclusion, it can simultaneously be argued that diseases pertaining to these three aspects of being can also be treated by vital spot therapies, an aspect to which I will return with ethnographic detail in chapter 4.

Clearly, *ācāṉ*s have to incorporate various aspects into their day-to-day practices. As one practitioner said, "If you want to practice this medicine, you have to know astrology [*cōciyam*] as well. This is not just about preparing medicines and administering massage!"

Vital Spots, Time, and Astrological Concepts

For Velayudhan the triad of *caram, iṭam, kālam*, or "circulation, location, time," describes the system of vital spots in a nutshell. As shown above, the circulation of *pirāṇam* life force provides for particular locations to be vital spots at specific times. Concepts of time are a crucial consideration for *ācāṉ*s, who repeatedly told me that being an "astrologer," *cōciyar*, was part of their job (compare Zarrilli 1998, 168), emphasizing a relationship between vital spots and astrology (*cōciyam*) or time (*kālam*), in temporal, periodical, and seasonal cycles. Analyzing this, I will move from the micro to the macro levels of temporal cycles.

"If You Want to Be an *Ācāṉ*, You Need to Know Astrology as Well"

Amongst others, such a close relation to temporal factors and concepts means that differences in the qualities of weekdays (*kiḻamai*) affect the efficacy of treatment and of medicine production. In siddha medicine in general, Sundays, Mondays, and Wednesdays are considered inauspicious for starting treatment, but as excellent days for preparing medicines and collecting medicinal plants. Commencing treatment is thought to be more effective on Tuesdays, Thursdays, Fridays, and Saturdays. Still, most practitioners start diagnosis and treatment irrespective of the day of the week. This does not mean, however, that *ācāṉ*s are not conscious of such intricacies. Velayudhan held that while it did take a longer time for an overall treatment process to be effective, to the extent that a cure might be delayed or less satisfactory, treatment generally had to be commenced irrespective of the day, especially in emergency cases. Starting therapies on Tuesdays, Thursdays, Fridays, or Saturdays, on the other hand, was especially auspicious, although this was not normally known by, or communicated to, patients.

As seen above, a *varmam* is not necessarily one particular point or another, but more properly a system. A vital spot is found where *pirāṇam* life force exists in a concentrated way, and only if *pirāṇam* is present in a particular place is it a *varmam*. In the absence of *pirāṇam*, it may be just another physical spot, and does not have any special vulnerability.[13] Life force circulates through the body, increasing and decreasing its fluctuating presence in

13. Canmukam (2006) has described this by saying: "[T]he spot which holds the vital force is a *varmam*. A spot [in itself] is not a *varmam*. The force is *varmam* [*Iṭam varmam ākātu. Āṟṟaltāṉ varmam*]."

particular loci. Vital spots are accordingly more or less vulnerable at different times, and *ācāṉs* refer to *kālam*, "time," to describe such periodic undulations. The term *kālam* itself denotes a category of vital spots, which bear the suffix *-kālam* in their names. This is the case with *tilartak-kālam*. This spot is most vulnerable during a particular period of time because of the heightened presence of *pirāṇam*, and hence, during this period, it is called *tilartakkālam*, or *tilartakkālavarmam*. Since practitioners believe that *uyir*, "life," is present in its most concentrated form during such a moment, death is certain if a vital spot is injured during an unfavorable part of the day (Irājēntiraṉ 2006, 135). Knowing at any given moment in time where *pirāṇam* is accumulated inside a body—whether this be the body of a patient, an opponent, or even one's own body—therefore becomes a crucial concern for *ācāṉs*.

The vital spots in many ways depend on natural, seasonal processes, and thus there are body loci that are influenced by the waxing and waning of the moon, since *pirāṇam* is constantly circulating throughout the body in conjunction with the periodic moon cycles. For each position of the thirty days from new moon to new moon, there is a corresponding location of the highest *pirāṇam* concentration within the body. Each lunar month according to the Tamil calendar is made up of a "bright" fortnight, or *cukkilapakṣam* (Skt. *śuklapakṣa*), which ends at full moon, and the "dark" fortnight, or *kirusṇapakṣam* (Skt. *krṣṇapakṣa*), which ends at new moon. Both fortnights consist of fifteen *titis* or "lunar days."[14] Vital spot practitioners connect this cycle with the concept of *amirtanilai*, the "seat of life" or, more literally, "state of ambrosia" (Narayanaswami 1975, 43; Chidambarathanu Pillai 1995b, 42). In men, according to Velayudhan, during the first day after a new moon and the beginning of the cycle, called *piratamaititi*, the *amirtam* or concentrated *pirāṇam* life force is localized in the big toe of the left foot. This spot is therefore on this particular day a "seat of life," since it is the location of concentrated life force and hence a potentially lethal body part on this day. For the duration of its housing *amirtam*, it is known as *piratamaitivarmam*, the "vital spot of the lunar day [called] *piratamai*."

Moving with the waxing of the moon, *amirtam* is found in a different location every day, ascending in the body's left half. In the heel of the left

14. The fifteen *titis* (*tithi*) of both fortnights are called: *piratamai, tuvitiyai, tiritiyai, caturtti, pañcami, ṣaṣṭi, captami, aṣṭami, navami, tacami, ekātaci, tuvātaci, tiriyotaci, caturttaci,* and *paurṇami* (full moon), or *amāvācai* (new moon) (Fuller 1980, 55). The influence of the moon is observed in many South Asian traditions, and especially in (Hindu) ritual practices; timings and dates for festivals may be stipulated according to the moon and many people observe fasts during certain *titis* (Chidambarathanu Pillai 1996, 17).

foot on the second day, on the third day in the ankle, on the fourth day in the thigh, on the fifth day in the generative system, in the navel on the sixth day, in the left side of the chest on the seventh day, in the left armpit on the eighth day, in the throat on the ninth day, in the mouth on the tenth day, in the left ear on the eleventh day, in the left nostril on the twelfth day, in the left eye on the thirteenth day, in the left eyebrow on the fourteenth day, and in the third eye, or the pineal gland on the fifteenth or full-moon day. In this way *pirāṇam* travels through one side of the body during a fortnight. The pineal gland remains the seat of life on the first day after the full moon as well. Subsequently, *pirāṇam* descends in the body's right half in the reverse order. After the new moon, this cycle starts again as described. This, at least, is the case in males. In females, the circulation happens contrariwise: starting in the big toe of the right leg. A descending (*ēṟuvatu*) and ascending (*iṟaṅkuvatu*) of *pirāṇam* can thus be observed according to the moon cycle, and for every lunar day one spot is especially vulnerable and hence called *titivarmam*, "lunar day vital spot." Injuries to a location while it is the seat of life are described as lethal by practitioners. While *ācāṉ*s agree on the importance of *amirtanilai*, there is much divergence of opinion as to which spot is a *titivarmam* on which day. Therefore it should not be a surprise that the account of Velayudhan, which I have depicted above, conflicts with other opinions in many respects (compare Nicivilcaṉ 2004, 68; Chidambarathanu Pillai 1995b, 42; Kaṇṇaṉ Rājārām 2007b, 230; Maṇiyaṉ 2012, 47, 98–99).

The *amirtanilai* system is not the only element of the vital spots on which time has an influence. For instance, *naṭcattiram* (Skt. *nakṣatra*), commonly translated as "star," is an important category, to be considered in this regard as well. There are in all twenty-seven *naṭcattiram* stars in Hindu astrology. Aybin Raj (2008) stresses that these twenty-seven stars are closely connected to, and have an effect on, twenty-seven respective spots, which are therefore called "star vital spots," *naṭcattiravarmam* (Kaṇṇaṉ Rājārām, 2007c, 104–105). The twelve signs of the zodiac, or *rāci*, of Hindu astrology, likewise relate to twelve spots. Both the stars and the zodiacs of the Indian system have an influence on specific loci, and during the zenithal phase of a specific zodiac and star, the spots labeled *naṭcattiravarmam* and *rācivarmam* are especially vulnerable (Zysk 2008, 4). The same is true for the times during which treatment is delivered, which is also influenced by both zodiacs and stars: these can have adverse effects on the healing of corresponding body parts. *Naṭcattirams*, for instance, include categories of stars during the influence of which vital spot ailments are said to be difficult to cure (*tiruvātirai, catayam*), and during the ascent of which chronic ailments may be caused more frequently (*acuvati, mākam, mūlam*), and those stars during the influence of which incurable injuries may be increased (*paraṇi, āyiliyam, pūram, cōti, kēṭṭai, ōṇam,* and *aviṭṭam*) (Vasanthakumar 2004, 147). A similar relationship obtains between the influences of the nine planets of Hindu astronomy, *navakirakam,* and of the severity of vital spot impacts, on the one hand, and of the efficacy of therapy, on the other. The nine planets of Hindu mythology in Tamil are: *niyāyaṉ* (Sun), *tiṅkaḷ* (Moon), *cevvāy* (Mars), *putaṉ* (Mercury), *viyāḻaṉ* (Jupiter), *veḷḷi* (Venus), *caṉi* (Saturn), and *irāku* and *kētu* (*rāhu* and *ketu*).[15] These, in general astrology and ritual, are perceived as having a strong influence on persons (Sambasivam Pillai 1993, 13). This is so, as they influence the circulation of life force and therefore the state of the vital spots as well.

Vital spot practitioners frequently told me that only by being mindful of the astral and planetary influences, benefic or malign, could one hope to become an effective practitioner of *varmakkalai*. Velayudhan explained: "If people have body pains, they will not bother to go to an oracle. They know we can cope with such issues and they think it is a twisted nerve or a sprained ankle and come directly to us. They will never think it may be due to a planetary problem [*kirakakkōḷāṟu*]." As a result *ācāṉ*s have to be intimately familiar with different concepts of time and astrology for their practices, medical and martial.

On the macro level, most practitioners even hold vital spots to be influenced by previous lives. Many practitioners state that those who die of an incurable ailment do so because of their bad deeds of previous lives, *viṉai* (Jeyrāj 1999, 28). *Viṉai*, literally "deed," corresponds to the concept of *karma*: the accumulated result of actions of former births, and its effect on subsequent lives (S. B. Daniel 1983, 28). This can be of the character of *tīviṉai*, sinful or morally reprehensible deeds, and *nalviṉai*, good deeds, both having an influence on the afterlives of an individual, and *ācāṉ*s may trace an affliction of vital spots to "bad deeds." Such might cause *varmam* ailments in successive lives, as any accident, or any trauma to a specific point, might be the result of accumulated reprehensible deeds. Moreover, a person's "deeds," or *karma* influence both the severity of ailments and

15. *Irāku* and *kētu* are described as chasing the sun and moon respectively, and as occasionally swallowing up these two celestial bodies—phenomena viewed as solar and lunar eclipses according to Western astronomy.

their healing chances. Indeed, as we have seen above, vital spots are intimately connected even with this aspect of life.

The Vital Spots: Classification and Confusion

Whereas it is possible to describe a more or less coherent theory of *varmam*, the listing, naming, and classification of spots pose a considerable challenge. There are innumerable names and synonyms, and different practitioners point out different categories of spots. Some of these categories relate to functions of vital spots, others relate to their relevance to either therapeutic or combat techniques. This is combined with a multiplicity of names and an ambiguity with regard to locations and the actual number of vital spots. I want to draw attention in the following paragraphs to the nonstandardized nature of theories and practices of *varmakkalai*. While every practitioner knows and utilizes a particular set of vital spots, and classifies these into different categories, neither categories nor, it appears, the loci themselves are established, fixed concepts accepted by all. This underscores the heterogeneous nature of vital spot practices, which are characterized by differing individual approaches rather than by commonly accepted standards. In order to highlight this, I analyze different methods of classification, which have been described in textual sources on *varmam*.

Anatomico-Regional Classification

Vital spots can be classified according to the regions of the body in which a particular spot is located. The standard classification in such an anatomico-regional framework is to divide spots into those found in the head and neck, between neck and navel, between navel and anus, of the arms and hands, and in the legs and feet.[16] Several manuscripts (*Varmakkaṇṇāṭi*, 137; Mariyajōcap n.d., 64–65) and practitioners express this idea. As the body is here zoned into five sections, this system is generally called *kaṇṭam aintu*, the "five sections." According to the *Varmakkaṇṇāṭi*, twenty-five loci are found in the region above the neck, forty-five between neck and navel, nine between navel and base, fourteen in arms and hands, and fifteen spots in the legs of a human being

16. Irājēntiraṉ (2006, 71) calls this classificatory system "anatomical system," *uṭaṟkūṟu vakaippāṭu*.

Table 2.1 Anatomico-regional classifications of vital spots according to Balasubramaniam (1991, 13), Kēcavappiḷḷai (1983, 35), *Varmakkaṇṇāṭi* (139–149; Mariyajōcap n.d., 66–71)

	Anatomical Region	Number of Spots
1	above the neck	25
2	neck to navel	45
3	navel to base	9
4	arms and hands	14
5	legs and feet	15
Total		108

Table 2.2 Anatomico-regional classifications of vital spots according to Irājēntiraṉ (2006, 72), citing *Varma kurunūl*, verse 56

	Anatomical Region	Number of Spots
1	head	25
2	neck	9
3	neck to navel	28
4	back	13
5	navel to base	10
6	arms and hands	11
7	legs and feet	12
Total		108

(Balasubramaniam and Dharmalingam 1991, 13). The total number of *varmam* hence is 108 (table 2.1).

However, we also find a system of dividing the body into seven parts instead of five. The *Varma Kurunūl* (Book of the vital spot teacher), for instance, recognizes seven such body parts, enumerating the vital spots located in each accordingly (Irājēntiraṉ 2006, 72). The body is here divided into the following regions: head, navel, neck to navel, back, navel to base, arms and hands, and legs and feet (table 2.2). These parts contain twenty-five, nine, twenty-eight, thirteen, ten, eleven, twelve vital spots respectively, adding up to a total of 108. Yet classifying the body differently is not the only deviation encountered here. Whereas the *Varmakkaṇṇāṭi*, having divided the body into five parts, recognizes fourteen *varmam* on the arms and hands, and fifteen on legs and feet, the *Varma Kurunūl* mentions eleven and twelve vital spots in these regions, respectively, yet points out other vital spots in other categories, which are not given by the *Varmakkaṇṇāṭi*. Thus, although both versions recognize a total of 108 spots, the loci listed appear as partly deviating. Moreover, these are only two possible interpretations and it seems likely that there exist numerous others, both in manuscripts and with practitioners.

Humoral Classification

Another way to differentiate vital spots might be called the "humoral classificatory system," as it relates to the influence of one of the three "humors," or *tōcam*, that is, the psychophysical processes of the body, in a particular spot: *vātam*, the pneumatic processes; *pittam*, the acidic, metabolic processes; and *kapam*, the adhesive, unctuous processes.[17] One informant, Bal *ācāṉ*, explained this as follows:

BAL: *Vātam, pittam*, and *kapam*; all diseases originate from these. If a particular spot is impacted, inside of it *caḷi* [phlegm] may form. In that case we call this a *caḷi*-spot or *kapavarmam*.

ROMAN: A *kapavarmam*? Are there also *vātavarmam* and *pittavarmam*, then?

BAL: There are. But *pittavarmam* are rare. Close to the gallbladder [*pittappai*], there is a *pittavarmam*; if injured, it causes nonstop vomiting. Most spots are *kapavarmam*, some are *vātavarmam*.

Like Bal, most practitioners closely associate a particular *tōcam* with an individual *varmam*. The predominance of *vātam, pittam*, or *kapam* at a vital spot can be observed in the effects of an injury. As *vātam* is "the windy humor of the body," according to the Madras *Tamil Lexicon*, and its characteristics include coldness, a *vātavarmam* causes the place of injury to feel cold to touch immediately after an injury, and the whole body to suffer from coldness and stiffness after a certain time. A *pittavarmam* causes excessive heat and fever or vomiting in a patient, as this *tōcam* is seen as the expression of *tī*, or "fire" in the body, causing heat and sourness (*Varmakkaṇṇāṭi*, 33; Mariyajōcap n.d., 17–18). At a *kapavarmam*, phlegm (*caḷi*) is produced, and the site of injury feels sweaty and cold to the touch. In the course of a disease, body coldness (*cītaḷam*) prevails alongside

17. Irājēntiraṉ (2006, 71) uses the term "humoral system," *tōcaviyal vakaippāṭu*, for this classification.

kapam-related disorders. Thus, vital spots can be divided according to the dominance of one of the three *tōcam* into *vātavarmam, pittavarmam*, and *kapavarmam*.

However, there seems to be considerable confusion both in manuscripts and amongst practitioners regarding which spots correspond to which *tōcam*. I will briefly provide just two differing humoral classifications. The *Varmakkaṇṇāṭi* (309; Mariyajōcap n.d., 159) and the *Varma Cūttiram* (Subramaniam 1994, 148; Chidambarathanu Pillai 1995a, 85) both state the number of loci related to *vātam* and *kapam* as sixty-four and six respectively (tables 2.3 and 2.4). The accounts, however, differ by two spots regarding the classification of *pittavarmam*; one account lists twenty-four, the other twenty-six *pittavarmam*:

Maṇiyaṉ (2012, 163) asserts that there are sixty-four *vāta*- and twenty-six *pittam*- vital spots, thus confirming the former group of practitioners. However, he categorizes all remaining spots among the total of 108 as *kapavarmams*, thus proclaiming this latter category to number eighteen, and thereby deviating from all other accounts in this point. Further, not all loci

Table 2.3 Vital spot categories according to Chidambarathanu Pillai (1995a, 85) and Vasanthakumar (2004, 39)

	Category of Spots	Number of Spots
1	*vātavarmam*	64
2	*pittavarmam*	24
3	*kapavarmam*	6
4	*uḷvarmam*	6
5	*taṭṭuvarmam*	6
Total		108

Table 2.4 Vital spot categories according to Subramaniam (1994, 148) and Jekatā (2005, 10)

	Category of Spots	Number of Spots
1	*vātavarmam*	64
2	*pittavarmam*	26
3	*kapavarmam*	6
4	*uḷvarmam*	12
Total		108

can be unambiguously assigned to one of the humoral categories. There are other *varmam*, which do not fall into any of the three *tōcam* groups, namely *uḷvarmam*, "inner vital spot," and *taṭṭuvarmam*, "tapping spot," categories to which I will come back shortly. And not only do we find differing numbers for *pittavarmam*, but whereas one pair of accounts lists six inner vital spots and eight tapping spots as excluded from the humoral framework (Subramaniam 1994, 148; Jekatā 2005), another recognizes twelve inner vital spots but no tapping spot at all (Chidambarathanu Pillai 1995a, 85; Vasanthakumar 2004, 39). Further, both notions regard *vātavarmam* as the category containing the most spots by far, while *kapavarmam* comprises only six spots. This strongly conflicts with the notion of Bal *ācāṉ*, cited above. For him, *kapavarmam* are the most numerous vital spots, thus contradicting the accounts mentioned earlier. Furthermore, while the *Varmakkaṇṇāṭi* (309; Mariyajōcap n.d., 159) describes all ailments of *vāta-* and *pittavarmam* as curable, while it emphasizes that an injury of a *kapavarmam* is incurable (see also Chidambarathanu Pillai 1995a, 85), this conflicts even more with Bal *ācāṉ*'s notion, which considers *kapavarmam* as the most commonly found and most easily cured category of vital spots. This is all the more interesting as the *Varmakkaṇṇāṭi* is a text in the possession of Bal, even if it contradicts his own ideas in this regard. I will come back to such discrepancies between text and practice in chapter 6.

Admitting the varying accounts of vital spot classification, Jekatā (2005), in a publication on *varmam*, asserts that although at first glance it might appear that practitioners and manuscripts disagree on some aspects, these differences were limited to the body's region-wise classification or to the categorizations of disease and impact. Such deviations, Jekatā notes, dissolve in the light of the overall 108 spots consisting of twelve "lethal spots," *paṭuvarmam*, and ninety-six "touch spots," *toṭuvarmam*, on which all practitioners unanimously agree.

Prognostic Classification

The categories of *toṭuvarmam* and *paṭuvarmam* describe different vital spots with regard to their respective pathological natures in case of injuries and are therefore part of a prognostic classificatory system of *varmam*.[18] As frequently noted by textual sources and routinely stated by

18. Irājēntiraṉ (2006, 71) calls this kind of classification *kuṟikuṇa vakaippāṭu*, "prognostic sign system," or "pathological classification."

practitioners, these two categories are made up of twelve *paṭuvarmam* and ninety-six *toṭuvarmam*, and, therefore, we arrive at a total of 108 spots. An impact measuring a certain amount of force on a *paṭuvarmam* is described as causing immediate unconsciousness. In excess of that measure, it is believed to kill. Their extreme vulnerability might be a reason to label the *paṭuvarmam* as "lethal" or "seriously dangerous" loci. The verb *paṭu-ttal* can translate as "to kill," and *paṭu*, as an adjectival intensifier, denotes "cruelty, seriousness," as in *paṭukolai*, "cruel murder." Injury to a *toṭuvarmam*, on the other hand, might be deadly as well, but this category is less dangerous in comparison, and impacts generally cause pain and manageable ailments (Kēcavappiḷḷai 1983, 30). This is so, because a *paṭuvarmam*, or "lethal spot," coincides with a *nāṭi* channel, and hence with *pirāṇam*, which a *toṭuvarmam*, or "touch spot," only touches upon.

Although lethal spots are invariably stated to be twelve, and touch spots ninety-six, different practitioners and textual sources appear to include different loci as belonging to these categories. For instance, two authors, Chidambarathanu Pillai (1994c, 45) and Kaṇṇaṉ Rājārām (2007b, 211), demonstrate substantial variations in respect of the lethal spot category. Comparing lists, as few as three loci can be seen to be featured in both; even these three spots, however, are labeled differently. Only one lethal spot, namely *tilartakkālam*, is identical in both accounts regarding both name and location, while as many as nine spots are clearly incongruent. This cannot be explained away as merely a matter of semantics. Such is confirmed by the fact that spots counted as *paṭuvarmam* in one account are found described as *toṭuvarmam* in the other. This is also true when we compare the publications of Nicivilcaṉ (2004, 26) and Irājēntiraṉ (2006, 280) in the case of a vital spot called *tūmmikālam*. For the former, *tūmmikālam* is a lethal spot located in the larynx. Irājēntiraṉ lists *tūmmikālam* as a touch spot, and includes *ciṟiyatticurukkivarmam* as a lethal spot in *tūmmikālam*'s stead, which is a touch spot in Nicivilcaṉ's account.[19] Another case in point is *aṭappavarmam*, located on both sides of the ribcage. It is given as an important *paṭuvarmam* by various writers (Kaṇṇaṉ Rājārām 2007b, 211; Nicivilcaṉ 2004, 27), but is not counted as such by others (Chidambarathanu Pillai 1994c; Irājēntiraṉ 2006). *Atticurukkivarmam* is acknowledged by most practitioners as a lethal spot and as consisting

19. According to Irājēntiraṉ (2006, 253), a vital spot with the name *tummikālam* has a different location in each of three different manuscripts.

of two very closely located, but distinct spots. Hence, some count *atticurukkivarmam* as two actual spots within the same category of twelve *paṭuvarmam* (Chidambarathanu Pillai 1994c, 49), whereas others count the spots as one (Kaṇṇan Rājārām 2007b, 211).

This understandably leads not only to different lists of spots, but also to varying numbers. Whereas all the textual sources that I have taken into consideration agree on the total number of lethal spots as twelve, the practitioner Irājēntiraṉ, in a publication entitled *Varmamum Taṭavumuṟai Aṟiviyalum* (The vital spots and massage method), shows that there are manuscripts which list up to eighteen spots as *paṭuvarmam* (2006, 80). Still, this circumstance might be accounted for by the fact that some lethal spots are so-called double spots, *iraṭṭaivarmam*, being found on both sides of the body, due to the body's symmetry.[20] Such points may be counted either as double or single. However, Irājēntiraṉ (2006, 80) also shows that some manuscripts suppose *paṭuvarmam* to comprise twelve loci, but when detailing these, list thirteen individual spots instead. Another author has attempted to compare seven different manuscripts, including different editions of one and the same text, with regard to the lethal spots. He was astonished to find as many as twenty-five clearly separate spots in total (Subramaniam 1994, 97–98). Of these seven different manuscripts, four detailed thirteen spots as being of the *paṭuvarmam* category, and only three pointed out twelve spots.[21] One *ācāṉ*, whom I interviewed, admitted that lethal spots, though generally stated as twelve, under critical examination turned out to be twenty; according to him, a fact known only to very few practitioners.

Similar disagreements among practitioners, published accounts, and manuscripts are innumerable, and recording them would be an unending task. To summarize, it appears that *ācāṉ*s, scholars, and manuscripts are agreed on only very few vital spots regarding their nature, location, and name.

---

20. Vital spots found in only one location are called *oṭṭai*, "single [spots]," those that appear in two places on the body, *iraṭṭai*, "double [spots]." Some vital spots exist in even more locations, such as in both hands and feet. Further creating confusion are chains of spots, such as *eṭṭelumpuvarmam*, or "eight bones vital spot," consisting of eight individual locations, situated in one row over the chest, which are known under one common name, but recognized as one spot by some, and as eight loci by others (Irājēntiraṉ 2006, 86–87).

21. The manuscripts under scrutiny here are: *Paṭuvarma Tiraṭṭu*, two different versions of *Varma Cūṭcam*, two different versions of *Varma Cūttiram*, *Varmakkaṇṇāṭi*, and *Varma Kaṇṭi* (Subramaniam 1994, 98).

Numbers, Names, and Discrepancies

The point here is not to question whether there really are 108 spots or twelve lethal spots, but to highlight that vital spot practices are far from possessing a determined, fixed, or shared standard among *ācāṉ*s. Rather, *varmakkalai* appears to be a highly individualized practice. Different practitioners subcategorize vital spots into various classifications, some of which include *taṭṭuvarmam* (tapping spot?), *uḷvarmam* (inner spot), *pūtavarmam* or *peypūtavarmam* (spirit spot?), *nakkuvarmam* (tongue spot or lick spot?), *nōkkuvarmam* (gaze spot), *taṭavuvarmam* (massage spot), *meytīṇṭākkālam* (invisible spot or spot that does not touch the body?), *carvāṅkavarmam* (whole body spot), *tūṇṭuvarmam* (arousal spot?), *kuṭōrivarmam* (slit spot?), or *tantiravarmam* (cunning spot?) (see Irājēntiraṉ 2006, 70; Balasubramaniam 1991, 14; Irācāmaṇi 1996, 94; Chidambarathanu Pillai 1995a, 120; 1994a, 33). It is unclear, however, what functions loci of these categories perform or how they can be distinguished from each other. This means that most practitioners deploy their own sets of categories of vital spots, and it is difficult to assess if different denominations specify the same entity, or if the same appellation has different meanings for different practitioners. Being unable to explain all the categories listed above, since textual sources and practitioners seldom elucidate them, I will briefly use only the categories of *taṭṭuvarmam, nōkkuvarmam*, and *nakkuvarmam* to explain this problem.

Taṭṭuvarmam, literally "tapping spot," is mentioned by most *ācāṉ*s as an important vital spot category, and generally enumerated as including eight loci. Intriguingly, two opposing ideas about what this category constitutes can be found. According to Maṇiyaṉ (2012, 96), this category of spots is characterized by its joining with fleshy portions of the body. Slightly in conflict with this notion is Irācāmaṇi (1996, 21), who cautions that any affliction of one of the eight *taṭṭuvarmam*, all of which according to him are located along the spinal cord, is especially difficult to cure. Some of the names which Irācāmaṇi gives figure in other accounts as *toṭuvarmam*, others as *paṭuvarmam*, and thus his *taṭṭuvarmam*s are found within the fold of the overall 108 vital spots. The practitioner Vasanthakumar (2004, 40) states, in another published account, that eight among the twelve lethal spots are *taṭṭuvarmam*; hence the latter's high vulnerability (see also Citamparatāṇuppiḷḷai 1991). Velayudhan referred to *taṭṭuvarmam* as a secret category, known to only the best of *ācāṉ*s and not to be revealed to anyone else. *Taṭṭuvarmam* according to him are the most deadly loci.

Once injured, these cause serious health conditions, and hence are synonymously termed *ācāṉvarmam*, the "*ācāṉ*'s spots," to be entrusted to and handled by only an experienced practitioner. The author Caravaṇakaṇēṣ (2009, 27) points out these loci's combat value, etymologically explaining *taṭṭuvarmam* as derived from *taṭṭu-tal*, "striking, beating." Such "strike spots," he writes, are spots which "very easily produce an effect in your opponent's body without him feeling any pain, by only using one finger to strike." On the other hand, I have found practitioners who viewed *taṭṭuvarmam* rather as points of therapeutic value, especially for giving massage. For them, this category consisted of spots which are to be "patted," palpitated—another possible translation of *taṭṭu-tal*. The notions presented here are not all compatible: after I had recounted these different opinions to Velayudhan, he was appalled by both the ideas of using this category as therapeutic or combat spots, due to their—according to his view—dangerous nature.

Another disputed vital spot category is that of *nōkkuvarmam*. It is supposed to be accessible both for healing and for harming purposes by means of a practitioner's gaze alone, and many *ācāṉ*s claim to be able to injure or cure vital spots by a mere look. Most practitioners thus explain *nōkkuvarmam* as a category of loci, which are penetrated by the power of an experienced *ācāṉ*'s glance alone (*nōkku*: gaze, sight), and not by touch. However, there is disagreement on whether this category comprises a single spot or several spots, whether it is of medical or martial relevance or both, and whether a *nōkkuvarmam* is a separate category of vital spots, which can be penetrated exclusively by sight or is penetrable by touch as well. Chidambarathanu Pillai (1995b, 37) seems to interpret *meytīṇṭākkālam*, which he states to be synonymous with *nōkkuvarmam*, as "spot which cannot be seen," and describes it as a particular *varmam* located "where the eyes meet the nose," that is, high on the bridge of the nose (compare Maṇiyaṉ 2012, 80). Some practitioners hold that *nōkkuvarmam* is not a category of vital spots at all, but that the term describes the manner of penetration, in this case by gaze (see also chapter 5).

A final case in point is *nakkuvarmam*. I was told by one *ācāṉ* that *nakkuvarmam* was a spot present only in women, which had to be addressed by a practitioner's tongue by way of licking, *nakku-tal*, and was considered useful in bringing about cures in certain maladies, and when licked produced great pleasures in the female patient. At this point, the *ācāṉ* showed some embarrassment, hinting that the site he was referring to was analogous to or contiguous with the clitoris. Another *ācāṉ* contrastingly stated *nakkuvarmam* to be located on the tongue, *nākku*, of a person. Both ideas conflict with Rājēntiraṉ's notion (2008, 46), according to which *nakkuvarmam* describes a category of spots which can be utilized both for therapeutic and for combat applications, and which, when stimulated, cause a licking (*nakku-tal*) sensation in a patient or opponent.

Healing Spots

Similar ambiguities are encountered with regard to a particularly important set of spots, utilized in therapeutic applications: *aṭaṅkal*, a kind of "relief spots." A mythological account of the origin of vital spots is found in the *Varma Oṭimuṟivu Cara Cūttiram*. According to it, Pārvatī, the wife of god Śiva, once saw a hunter falling from a tree and losing consciousness. Feeling pity for him, she asked her divine husband to revive the hunter. In order to comply with his wife's wish, Śiva created both *varmam* and *aṭaṅkal* spots, by taking a stick and writing with it on the hunter's body the letters *hari* and *śrī*, and thus revived him. Hence it is stated, that *Hari*, a name of Śiva, and *Śrī*, a name of Pārvatī[22] entered the body of the hunter, and with it of all human beings, and became *varmam* and *aṭaṅkal* spots respectively: vulnerable spots in which Śiva is present, and therapeutic spots in which Pārvatī is present (Subramaniam 1994, 87; Irājēntiraṉ 2006, 4).[23]

One informant referred to these therapeutic spots as "switch[es]." *Aṭaṅkal*, according to him, are loci which must be stimulated after a vital

22. Albeit both are more common names of the gods Viṣṇu and Lakṣmī, respectively.

23. The myth as found in the *Varma Oṭimuṟivu Cara Cūttiram* (Treatise on vital spot fractures) goes thus: Śiva [Aruṇār] and Pārvatī [Umaiyavaḷ] were wandering through the forests on Civakirāyām Mountain during the inauspicious time of the day. At this same time, a gifted hunter fell unconscious, as he had fallen from a tree, into which he had climbed. He had fainted and was unconsciousness; not a soul in sight, he was lying there on the ground. As soon as Śiva spotted the hunter, he quickly turned away as though otherwise occupied. But Pārvatī invoked him with the words: "Oh golden Lord, do not act that way." Śiva, who had walked away from the hunter, listened to what she had said, stopped, and turned to declare: "Those two, which are called *varmam* and *aṭaṅkal*, are among the evils and sins of humans: behold their peculiarities." He took a golden bamboo stick which he had kept clasped under his arm and with it wrote the letter "Śrī" on the hunter's body. The hunter's unconsciousness was repelled, his health restored, and he got up to receive water from the hands of Pārvatī. Śiva and Pārvatī then left to continue their walk. Since that day, *varmam* has been known in the world. Translated from Jēms (2010, 13); there are a number of similar myths regarding the origin of *varmam* (see Irājēntiraṉ 2006, 4–9).

spot injury. Deploying a metaphor of electricity and currents, he elucidated that a vital spot trauma caused a "current cut," which gradually shut down the body's power. This had to be countered by activating a "main switch" as fast as possible. In *varmam* treatment, the concept of *aṭaṅkal* relates to particular therapeutic spots for administering relief measures, especially in cases of emergencies; such as in reviving an unconscious patient. Etymologically, *aṭaṅkal* means (amongst other things) "submitting, being included; abiding place," according to the Madras *Tamil Lexicon*, and the related verb *aṭakku-tal*, means: "to subordinate, detain, or tame." Similarly, Velayudhan explained *aṭaṅkal* spots to me as "those places which have the ability to subdue [*aṭaṅkiyirukkak kūṭiya iṭaṅkaḷnā aṭaṅkal*]. This means, a place which will give relief after a particular *varmam* has been hit is an *aṭaṅkal*." These are therapeutic devices, which in the case of an injury to a vital spot have to be stimulated to save a patient from immediate dangers. What *aṭaṅkal*s affect is a countering of a *varmam* affliction by slackening the injured spot (*varmattai iḷakku-tal*). Stimulating these relief spots is a crucial part of *iḷakkumuṟai*, literally meaning "slackening, relaxing method, or revitalization treatment." Since an injury to a vital spot disturbs the whole system due to the blockage of life force, the *Varmakkaṇṇāṭi* (129; Mariyajōcap n.d., 61) speaks of *aṭaṅkal* as "that which calms [*aṭakkamatu*] by activating the circulation of life force," and thus relaxing the affected vital spot.

*Aṭaṅkal*s are also called "keys," *tiṟavukōl* (Balasubramaniam and Dharmalingam 1991, 49).[24] In Tamil *tiṟavu* means "opening" and *kōl* denotes a rod, or a stick-like instrument. Thus, a *tiṟavukōl* is an opening device, or, simply, a key. In fact, practitioners speak of "opening" (*tiṟa-ttal*) vital spots, with which they describe the particular penetration of a spot in order to produce an effect. This includes both injuries or deliberate attacks and therapeutic measures. If a particular *varmam* has been opened in the course of a physical trauma, a particular *aṭaṅkal* has to be opened as a countermeasure. The therapeutic spots used for such stimulations are often points on the opposite side of the injured *varmam*, and hence are called *māṟṟu varmam* (*māṟṟu*: "relieve, change"), and the accordant methods of stimulation are termed "vital spot relief method" (*māṟṟu varma muṟai*).[25] For every vital spot being afflicted, manuscripts point out one

24. *Tiṟavukōl* is also a pseudonym given to some manuscripts, which deal with *aṭaṅkal* spots and related emergency techniques, such as *Varmapīraṅki Tiṟavukōl*.

25. In this sense, *aṭaṅkal* comes close, and probably corresponds, to the *kulabhyāsamarmmam* of *marmma cikitsā* as practiced in Kerala (Zarrilli 1998, 164). Used in medical emergencies as well, they are said to number sixty-four (Thatte 1988).

or several such "relief spots," which have to be opened within a stipulated time if a patient is to be saved from impending death.

However, regarding which loci actually are relief spots, there seems to be considerable controversy. The *Varmakkaṇṇāṭi* enumerates twelve *aṭaṅkal* (306–307; Mariyajōcap n.d., 157–158; see also Chidambarathanu Pillai 1995a). Conflicting with this number is, for instance, practitioner Dharmalingam (Balasubramaniam and Dharmalingam 1991, 49), who adamantly considers relief spots to be sixteen. Velayudhan held that there were thirty-two regularly deployed *aṭaṅkal*s, out of which eight enjoyed a most prominent status. The *Varma Cūttiram* expounds fifty-three relief spots (see also Subramaniam 1994, 113). The practitioner Aleksāṇṭar Ācāṉ (1998, 52–53) states that this category consists of fifty-six individual spots, as does Vasanthakumar (2004, 143), who, however, concedes that only twelve out of these fifty-six are important spots. Moreover, it is not clear from most accounts if *aṭaṅkal*s correspond to *varmam* spots, or if they constitute an altogether different category and set of spots. One faction of practitioners holds that relief spots are included in the total category of the 108 *varmam*, while another repudiates such a notion, treating *aṭaṅkal*s only as a separate category of spots. Still, for Velayudhan, each and every vital spot is a potential relief spot and any vital spot becomes an *aṭaṅkal* in case of injury of a particular other, related spot.

Relief spots and their applications appear to be a matter of individual *ācāṉ*s' practices. According to Velayudhan, the most effective relief spot is *carvāṅka aṭaṅkal*, or "the whole body relief spot," able to stimulate all vital spots at once, when opened or stimulated. Located in the tip of the middle finger, it has to be jerked sharply to be opened. Aleksāṇṭar Ācāṉ (1998, 53), on the other hand, has stated that a *carvāṅka aṭaṅkal* is located beneath the edge of the *mūlātāram*, that is, near the coccyx. Again another *carvāṅka aṭaṅkal* is described in the manuscript *Varma Kuṟavañci* as consisting of three spots: one located on each side of the sacro-iliac region, a further spot near the ankles, and another spot behind the ears, all of which, when stimulated, are said to revive unconscious patients (Chidambarathanu Pillai, 1994b, 37). I would therefore suggest that *carvāṅka aṭaṅkal* be seen as a generic term which *ācāṉ*s deploy for one or more therapeutic spots or even for distinct sets of healing techniques.

This is accentuated by the fact that whereas *aṭaṅkal* is commonly understood as a particular set of therapeutic spots, for some practitioners the same term more closely describes a set of remedial techniques. Subramaniam (1994, 113) states that *aṭaṅkal*s are "methods which enable the patient to sit up and regain consciousness," and Mohana Rao, in a preface to an edited version of the *Varmakkaṇṇāṭi* (Mariyajōcap n.d., v), describes *aṭaṅkal* as a "specialised type of physiotherapy." Similarly, for Vasanthakumar (2004, 35), *aṭaṅkal* is a technique in which "a particular spot or point of the body is stimulated for curing . . . symptoms . . . or varma hurts." The description of thirteen relief spots by Maṇiyaṉ (2012, 180–186) details techniques and courses of actions in cases of severe vital spot injuries, often complete with a particular medical preparation, not necessarily specific loci. Thus, we see there is considerable disagreement as to what exactly *aṭaṅkal* means, whether the word denotes techniques or particular spots, whether these spots fall into the category of *varmam* or constitute a separate entity, and with regard to their numbers.

What's in a Name (and Number)?

As pointed out above, most practitioners and textual sources agree that there are twelve *paṭuvarmam* lethal spots and ninety-six *toṭuvarmam* touch spots, and hence a total of 108 *varmam* (*Varmakkaṇṇāṭi*, 149; Mariyajōcap n.d., 71). The number of 108 spots in particular can be viewed as one of the most commonly communicated aspects of *varmakkalai*. The number 108 is a highly meaningful one in various regards, many of which are of a ritual or religious nature and found in abundance all over South Asia. In the Hindu tradition, the most important gods, such as Śiva, are known by 108 (or, as an augmentation, 1008) names, which are said to confer prosperity on devotees when recited. In Bhāratanāṭyam, an Indian form of dance that originates from South India, 108 dance postures (*karaṇas*) are described by Bhārata in the *Nāṭyaśāstra*, a compendium of theatrical matters, and depicted in several temples throughout Tamil Nadu (Subrahmanyam 2003; Purecha 2003). The rejuvenative category of siddha drugs which allegedly bestow immortality is said to consist of 108 substances (Geetha 1983, 135).[26]

However, even the number 108 is not free from ambiguity with regard to enumerating vital spots. Though the *Varma Cūṭcāmaṇi Pañcīkaraṇa Piṉṉal* (13; Nicivilcaṉ 2004) explicitly mentions that there are 108 *varmam*, the editor of a published version of the manuscript has appended a series

26. For more instances of the number 108 in meaningful contexts with regard to *varmakkalai*, see Immanuel (2007, 67). In contrast, it might be asked why the ayurvedic *marman* spots consist of only 107 points.

of charts depicting the spots mentioned by this text as including 124 loci (Nicivilcaṉ 2004, 10–12). Similarly, Aleksāṇṭar Ācāṉ (1998, 33–39), after stating the total number as 108, gives a list of 123 individual spots, including descriptions of their respective locations. It is not only the case that contemporary practitioners have drawn attention to discrepancies of this type, but one can see them for oneself when one compares edited versions of manuscripts themselves. Kaṇṇaṉ Rājārām, a lecturer at the ATSVS Siddha College in Muṉciṟai, Kanyakumari, has conducted painstaking research, in which he compared different textual sources in order to gather information on the vital spots. He elucidates that a point called *puruvavarmam* is accorded seven synonyms in seven different manuscripts (Kaṇṇaṉ Rājārām 2007c, 85). Similarly, the practitioner Irājēntiraṉ (2006, 275–276) manages to show that different manuscript sources allow for interpreting numerous loci differently. *Maṇipantavarmam*, for instance, is pointed out to be a spot near the wrist of one's hands by many; some *ācāṉ*s however maintain that it is situated at the forearm closer to the elbow joint than to one's wrist (Caravaṇakaṇēṣ 2009, 55; Rācā [1997] 2002, 26). Even more dramatically, *teṭcaṇaikkālam* is a spot that has been interpreted in five different ways and at five different locations (Irājēntiraṉ 2006, 275–276). Varying names, synonyms, numbers, and locations give rise to confusion if one tries to take account of the available manuscripts and practitioners' viewpoints on the vital spots. The spot *naṭcattiravarmam*, for instance, is known by different names in four different manuscripts; five different manuscripts name five completely different characteristics of this spot's symptoms (*kuṟikuṇam*) if afflicted; two differing time frames for treatment can be found, and three different treatment methods (Kaṇṇaṉ Rājārām 2007a, 31–34).

Another point of differing views on the vital spots is gender-related. Practitioners often represent a male-centered view of the human body, describing the 108 vital spots present in men, while women are stated to possess only 107 points (Jēms 2010, 175–176). I have been repeatedly told by *ācāṉ*s that men's 108th spot, called *pītaikkālam*, is located in the penis (Irācāmaṇi 1996, 5). In contrast, Velayudhan adamantly expressed his view that men indeed possessed 108 *varmam*, while holding that females even had a 109th spot, *cūlvarmam*, "pregnancy vital spot," located at the uterus (*karuppai*). This idea is supported by Kaṇṇaṉ Rājārām (2007a, 267), who describes a *karppavarmam*, or "womb vital spot," which men lacked. If this *varmam* was affected, a woman faced difficulties during childbirth, abortion of an embryo, or a disability of the infant. Irājēntiraṉ (2006, 234), on the other hand, names three vital spots which are said to be different in the two sexes. While men possessed *tātuvākivarmam*, "spot of creation of tissues"; *vittuvarmam*, "semen vital spot"; and *pījakālam*, also "semen vital spot"; women had *allivarmam*, "water lily spot"; *aṇṭavarmam*, "ovum spot"; and *pūvalvarmam*, "flower spot." These are apparently different loci due to the distinct anatomies of the sexes. Again, contrastingly, one *ācāṉ* maintained that women had six *yōṉivarmam* or "vaginal vital spots," inside the genital organ. However, he added that females missed *kalliṭaikkālam*, a lethal spot located on the penis, and thus women had only eleven such *paṭuvarmam*as against twelve in men (see also Chidambarathanu Pillai 1994a, 33).

Kaṇṇaṉ Rājārām, after an admirable attempt to collect and map all vital spots as gathered from four manuscripts, concludes that differences between his sources are vast, and that although all maintain that the total number of spots was 108, a close comparison of the given locations and names shows that the total number of individual spots exceeds 300 (2007b, 231–249). In a similar attempt, Subramaniam (1994, 392–402) compared six different manuscripts and came up with a list of 295 loci. Due to the multiplicity of some loci, the total number of such spots spread over the whole body may well exceed even 400. It would thus appear that 108 is not necessarily to be accepted at face value as the number of actual loci involved. Rather, being an auspicious number, 108 can be understood to suggest a perceived importance, but also a wholeness or completeness of the vital spots.

Indeed, sometimes *ācāṉ*s, despite normally adamantly maintaining that *varmam* consist of 108 loci, concede the existence of more such spots. N. Shanmugom, who has founded a research institution devoted to the vital spots in Coimbatore, claims to have in his possession manuscripts which mention as many as 8000 different points, out of which he himself has been able to discover the exact locations of 2000 vital spots.[27] One of my informants in Kanyakumari quickly ascertained that the 108 spots were like "main railway junctions," and that these spots were of comparably greater importance as compared to minor ones. He conspiratorially leaned toward me, whispering that the actual number of *varmam* loci was 1008. *Tilartakkālam* for instance, this practitioner went on, thus was made

27. N. Shunmugom: Introductory Speech to Nursing Students from San Diego State University, Arts Research Institute, June 10, 2010; http://www.ari.org.in/news/Visit-by-Nursing-Student-from-San-Diego-State.

up of 115 minor spots, although most *ācāṉ*s did not know this. Conversely, it is of course also imaginable that a practitioner might maintain that there are a total of 108 vital spots, while he or she knows only a smaller number. This is important, since the affirmation to know all the 108 loci implies knowledge of the whole system of *varmakkalai*.

Acknowledging such divergent views on *varmam*, and that accounts on the vital spots widely vary, Subramaniam (1994, 146) laments that "the thorough study and understanding of this science" is inhibited, as "[t]here are variations in the total number of varmas, their names, locations, their qualities, the signs and symptoms of an injury, the time limits for revival methods, etc." (149). Hausman (1996, 54) shows that it is possible to interpret one and the same text differently. In his dissertation on siddha medicine, he relates that he obtained a copy of the manuscript called *Varma Oṭimuṟivucāri*, and asked different practitioners for elucidations. One *ācāṉ* pointed out a particular spot to be "the only important point of the text," while a second did not even mention the same point in his explanation of the same text (47).

A single concise catalog of points therefore does not exist, and different practitioners apparently know and use different points for different outcomes. Why is this inference important for our investigation and for what follows? It is related to, and serves to underscore, some of the key features of *varmakkalai* practices and therefore of the main interests of this present study. First, the vital spots in Kanyakumari are subjected to a considerable degree of secrecy and concealment, and this characterizes the practice alongside the related knowledge and its transmission. When Hausman, cited above, obtained the manuscript mentioned, he was told that neither possession, nor elucidations would help him to understand it, if it was "authentic" at all:

> The primary attitude of "traditional" *vaittiyar*s [physicians] seemed to be that should any outsider happen to obtain a medical text, it would not be authentic; even if it were somewhat authentic, one would need a good commentary to explicate it; and even if it had a commentary, one could not comprehend it without practical experience.
>
> (Hausman *1996, 48*)

Vital spots are treated as subject to secrecy and kept concealed by *ācāṉ*s. Instruction of *varmakkalai* ideally happens only within lineages (*paramparai*) of medical and martial practice, and knowledge is passed on to initiated, selected individuals. Vital spots are not normally or openly exchanged, and this indeed serves to explain to a large part for the described heterogeneous, at times ambiguous and nonstandardized character of *varmakkalai* theory and practice. It is therefore quite possible that informants have been dishonest with me, and that I was deliberately provided with misleading information. But even this would only serve to highlight that the vital spots are not systematized or in any way part of a standardized practice.

Further, as Zarrilli, in his study of the *kaḷarippayaṭṭu* martial arts traditions in Kerala, has observed, the embodied practice of a master is the only authentic account of combat practices, especially with regard to the vital spots. While different lineages complete with their own techniques have always existed, "the authoritative text in the living tradition is the master's embodied practice," as Zarrilli (1989, 1291) notes. This is of a vital importance for *varmakkalai* as well. From the perspective of a practitioner, who has been instructed according a particular lineage of knowledge transmission, having learned from a particular *ācāṉ*, the personal practice possesses its own internal logic and coherence. This is the case, even if such logic and coherence contradicts that of another lineage (compare Zarrilli 1998, 159).

Internal logic, efficacy, and coherence therefore appear to arise foremost or exclusively from the successful practice of one norm—one localized, individual practice—and therefore *varmakkalai* becomes perpetuated in its character of being highly related to the locality, the lineage, and of course the person practicing. Considering the inscription of theory and practice within individuals, lineages of transmission, different and sometimes conflicting logics, which present themselves as contradictory versions of vital spots, are indeed prone to evolve. *Varmakkalai* is therefore highly heterogeneous, and, for different reasons, highly individualistic as well. To cite Velayudhan in this regard: "to the one who knows *varmam*, every place is a vital spot."

Conclusion: Ambiguity and Heterogeneity of Varmakkalai

Informants' voices, edited versions of palm-leaf manuscripts, scholarly studies, and publications by practitioners of *varmakkalai* all attest to an intriguing, complex theory of health, the body, and the vital spots. However, there is no single concise theory of *varmakkalai* to be found, nor a standard, accepted set of spots. Rather, different *ācāṉs* draw in part on vastly different ideas and utilize immensely varying practices. While it is therefore vain to attempt a concise account of vital spot theory, the fact that even *ācāṉs* are often at a loss for exhaustive explanations may provide solace in that regard. Velayudhan in fact held that this precisely was the reason for the name the system bears, *varmam* or, alternatively *marmam*—meaning "secret," or "hidden, unseen." *Varmam* in this regard is like a riddle or mystery—never entirely fathomable and hard to detect—and therefore remains a mystery, no matter how hard one tries to explain or explore it.

This is not to suggest that vital spots are devoid of theoretical underpinnings—quite the contrary. Much of the described theory is close to the esoteric ideas of yoga, such as are exhibited in the concepts of *pirāṇam, nāṭi, ātāram*, the three bodies and their five sheaths, and so on. As such, it must be seen as closely related to the broader esoteric, tantric traditions of South Asia. Given that nature, its likely tantric roots, and its emphasis on concealment and restricted transmission of its knowledge, variation found in the perception and interpretation of *varmakkalai* theory and praxis should not surprise anyone.

Analyzing and highlighting the theoretical and practical heterogeneity of *varmakkalai* is in several ways important for the remainder of this study. On the one hand, such a variety in the range of theoretical explanation poses certain difficulties for attempts at curricular integration of vital spot practices into medical colleges in Tamil Nadu, and is likely to affect the selection and standardization of teaching material and methods at the higher centers of learning. On the other hand, the differing views are in several ways closely related to "secrecy," as *ācāṉs* describe it. *Varmam*, in the words of the practitioners, is not only that which is kept hidden, but also that which cannot be comprehended. Being concealed means, in this sense, being ungraspable, because vital spots are partly beyond the intellectual and discursive grasp of a human being. But *varmakkalai* is also deliberately restricted, and this, understandably, gives rise to differing notions as well. As has been described for other manual therapies, practices often vary greatly among practitioners, who reveal highly individualized approaches to their patients, the ailments they treat, and how they treat them (Hinojosa 2002)—an aspect which might be seen as due to the bodily, nonverbal, or nonverbalized nature of the practice (Walkley 2004; Oths and Hinojosa 2004). The fact that textual sources, palm-leaf manuscripts, and the accounts of informants reveal a high degree of disagreement does not mean that one version is always superior to another. Rather, the conflicting views convey a sense of the heterogeneity and the diversity which can be found in contemporary *varmakkalai* and highlights that knowledge of the vital spots is an ongoing, flowing, fluid activity, inseparable from its practice, as there is no standard, no standardized canon.

3

Dispensary and Training Ground

MEDICINE AND MARTIAL ARTS INTERTWINED

VARMAKKALAI IS "THE art [*kalai*] of the vital spots [*varmam*]," and it combines therapeutic and combative techniques in a mutually enhancing, complementary fashion. This is so as vital spots are vulnerable points in the body, which can be used for therapy as well as for incapacitating an opponent. "Western" thought and taxonomy, however, do not normally recognize such an intersection of medicine and martial practices. This is exemplified by academic classifications and educational models, which tend to segregate the aspects neatly, labeling one as "arts" or "sports," and the other as "science." However, *ācāṉ*s, the hereditary practitioners of *varmakkalai* in Kanyakumari, maintain that this very intersection is crucial in their practice, each complementing and supporting the other. This chapter takes a close look at the symbiotic relationship between two apparently antithetical systems: healing and fighting. It also calls into question the rigid distinction between martial arts and medicine (a version of that between arts and sciences), which is found in contemporary Indian education. For *ācāṉ*s, such a dichotomy is not meaningful. On the contrary, the combination of both martial and medical aspects defines their very practice.

Medically and martially relevant aspects are mutually supportive and required for *varmakkalai* in general and particularly for a hereditary or "traditional" form of instruction. This is illustrated by observing how most aspects of vital spots figure prominently and simultaneously in the *kaḷari*, the training ground of martial practices, where combat techniques called *varma aṭi* ("hitting the vital spots") are taught, and inside the *vaittiyacālai*, the dispensary for *varma maruttuvam* or vital spot treatments. All practices related to the settings of both training ground and dispensary enhance an *ācāṉ*'s or an apprentice's overall skills, and the progress in one can be gauged by progress in the other. The therapeutic and martial aspects are further closely related as injuries incurred in the training ground are addressed with therapeutic techniques in the dispensary. Furthermore, anatomical insights gained by students or practitioners in one setting may be constructively applied in the other. The transmission of vital spot knowledge includes yoga and meditative exercises, which are explained as augmenting mental strength, needed to effectively and safely heal patients, on the one hand, and to confidently confront opponents, on the other. Moreover, physical strength is required for both combat and medical practices. Blows, kicks, blocks, and handling of weapons require physical stamina, but the same is true for administering massage and manipulations of vital spots, which are physically challenging as well. In the course of the training and practice of *varmakkalai*, physical strength and prowess, and the mental progression of students are crucial, and in a combined way develop a kind of psychosomatic intuition. This intuition is the medical or martial competence of *ācāṉ* practitioners; it allows for confidently detecting and penetrating *varmam* loci—for both combat and healing purposes. All this underscores the assertions of practitioners that *varmakkalai* must consist of both medicine and martial practices.

Dispensary and Training Ground: Interrelated Spheres

The spheres in which *varmam* finds an expression—the *kaḷari* training ground and the *vaittiyacālai* dispensary—are in several respects in close proximity. They are generally interlinked spatially and with regard to the main actors. Similar ritual and hierarchical behavior characterizes life in the *kaḷari* and in the *vaittiyacālai*, and, importantly, the vital spots figure prominently in both. In what follows, I will analyze some of these commonalities in detail.

Inside the Vital Spot Dispensary

A *varma vaittiyacālai*, or "vital spot dispensary," is the place where *varmam* ailments are therapeutically addressed by healthcare specialists called *ācāṉ* or—more specifically, thanks to the medical procedures they specialize in—*varma vaittiyar*, "vital spot doctors" (figure 3.1). They offer a wide

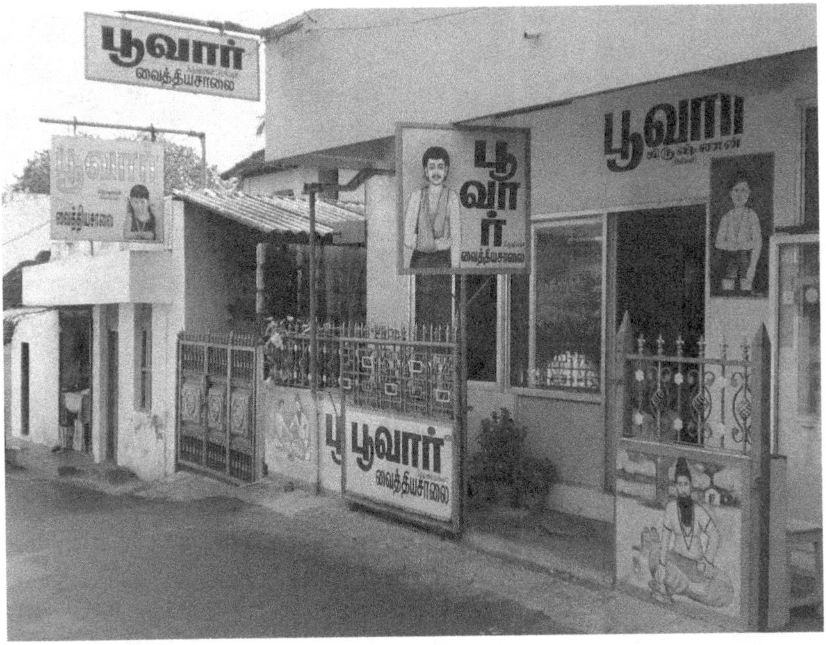

FIGURE 3.1 A vital spot dispensary

range of treatments which often directly stimulate *varmam* loci, by administering manual techniques, such as massages or manipulation of limbs. One of the most striking features of a typical vital spot dispensary is a provision to ensure secluded treatment procedures. Many *vaittiyacālai*s have a back room for separating the activities inside from the observing gaze of bystanders and uninvolved persons. At a minimum, a curtain in small dispensaries achieves a similar effect of seclusion. In contrast to the procedure in most South Asian doctor-patient encounters, where relatives are generally present throughout diagnosis and treatment (Halliburton 2002, 1127), *ācāṉ*s normally avoid conducting their therapies observably. Vital spot dispensaries are thus spatially set up in such a way as to guarantee the concealment of treatment, an observance prescribed by manuscripts on *varmam*. The *Varmakkaṇṇāṭi* (7; Mariyajōcap n.d., 4) notes that an *ācāṉ* should attempt to revive an unconscious person only after sending everyone else away, and to treat him or her under cover of a screen or inside a separate room. Many dispensaries consist of a veranda, where arriving patients are received and wait to see the *ācāṉ*. It is either here or in a room inside that diagnosis is carried out, within sight of the accompanying relatives and others. On the other hand, in most cases the actual treatment is conducted either in a separate room or behind a drawn curtain or screen, where frequently patients' relatives and others are not permitted to enter.

Within their dispensary, *ācāṉ*s enjoy considerable respect. It is not only patients who accord this respect, but also, if present, the students, who, as a prerequisite to receiving instruction, acknowledge their *gurus*' authority. No task within the dispensary is done without the *ācāṉ*'s permission or order. But even experienced practitioners regard their devotion toward their own *guru*(s) as a vital part of their practices, and as even important with regard to therapeutic efficacy. *Ācāṉ*s do not start their day, nor do they commence treating patients, without contemplating their past preceptors. In most dispensaries, thus, the picture of a former *guru* is installed in a prominent place, often overseeing the physician. In some cases, a whole doorway or hall might be furnished with pictures showing successive generations of *gurus* of an *ācāṉ*'s lineage, the *paramparai*. These pictures are regularly adorned with flowers and in the morning receive the first attention of the practitioner, alongside idols of gods of Hindu or Christian practitioners, before he turns to waiting patients. *Ācāṉ*s, it is held, should act only after contemplating their teacher (*kuruvukku niṉai-ttal*). Before diagnosing or treating a patient, physicians repeat this, in order to accord their respect (*mariyātai*) and reverence (*vantaṉam*) toward their teachers and lineage. Likewise, students may start their day by venerating their present *guru*, often by bowing down to touch the *ācāṉ*'s feet and showing their devotion toward him or her. This structure of practice is replicated in martial arts training ground.

Inside the Vital Spot Training Ground

As pointed out in chapter 1, the earliest references to vital spots in India are not found in a medical setting, but in contexts of war and battle. Some martial art forms in contemporary South India—*varma aṭi* in Tamil Nadu and *kaḷarippayaṭṭu* in Kerala, to be precise—are still intimately connected to body loci. *Varma aṭi* translates as "striking the vital spots," a description which hints at this practice's focus on spots for defensive and offensive techniques.[1] Only advanced students, that is, usually only those who

---

1. Zarrilli (1998, 27) has mentioned different names for *varma aṭi*, such as *aṭi taṭa* (strike and defend), *aṭi muṟai* (way of fighting), and *kuttuvaricai* (punching series) (see also Balakrishnan 1995). I found such terms used all over Tamil Nadu to describe martial art practices with regional variations. *Kuttuvaricai*, for instance, is popular around Thanjavur. Not always, though, do such martial practices incorporate all constitutive elements of *varmakkalai* or utilize vital spots.

have received instruction in medical techniques for years as well, receive detailed instruction on the locations of vital spots, as well as on how to attack them in an adversary and defend their own. This is primarily done using the hands and legs, but also with different instruments, such as the wooden longstaff called *cilampam*—a weapon which is prominent among martial practitioners in most of Tamil Nadu (Raj 1975; 1977).

The place where vital spot martial training occurs is called *kaḷari*. This means "training ground," and is in some ways similar to the *ākhāḍā* gymnasium of *pahalwān* wrestlers in North India (Alter 1992a, 319). *Kaḷari*, a term of Dravidian origin, has an ancient history, and is encountered in early Tamil *Caṅkam* poems dated to about the first century CE (Burrow and Emeneau 1984, 98). Here, it denotes "ground, battlefield" or the gymnasia for the training of soldiers (Zarrilli 1998, 25). Similarly, in Malayalam the term *kaḷari* is closely connected with *kaḷarippayaṭṭu*, literally meaning "practice-ground exercise," the popular martial art form of Kerala. *Kaḷaris* in Kerala are generally dug out arenas, called *kuḻikkaḷari*, "pit ground." In these, the actual training floor is situated about one meter beneath the ground level. *Varma aṭi kaḷaris* in Kanyakumari, on the other hand, can be of various appearances, though normally this does not include dug-out pits. Rather, a *varma aṭi* training ground might be a small, thatched shed, or an open space, in the shade of coconut palms. Some *kaḷaris* are located on the rooftop of a house, or in the premises behind or inside a temple. Of importance in this regard is the fact that in *varma aṭi* it is not only the place of training that is designated as *kaḷari*, but also the training itself and the persons training together—the combination of martial master and students. Virtually any place can, at any time, be utilized ad hoc for exercises and thus be a *kaḷari* training ground.

A few requirements, however, should be met. Often, the ground of a *kaḷari*, like that in *kaḷarippayaṭṭu* (Zarrilli 1998, 66) or the *ākhāḍā* in *pahalwāni* wrestling (Alter 1989, 90), is made up of special mixtures of soil or sand, to assure softness of the ground. This allows for throws, jumps, and falls to be conducted without injuries. Further, and of greater importance, although most *kaḷaris* are found outdoors, visibility or easy accessibility are not implied, and the training areas are in fact most often found screened from curious eyes by thick vegetation. Thus is preserved the seclusive character of the vital spot dispensary, to which many training grounds are attached. Martial exercises may also be conducted behind a dispensary or on its rooftop. The *kaḷari* of Velayudhan, for instance, is a compound *within* a compound. In the rearmost part of the garden surrounding the practitioner's house, which also accommodates his dispensary, a compound wall separates an area of about 20 square meters from the rest of the garden. This is the *kaḷari*, and can be accessed only through a small gate, which is closed when training is going on. A head-high wall running within the *ācāṉ*'s garden prevents patients and passersby from observing the training. The choice of timing for the exercises also helps in this regard: they begin only after the dispensary has dealt with its last patient for the day, rarely before 9 p.m., by which time the training ground is enveloped in darkness.

Ritual inside the Training Ground

Martial practices around the world have been universally described as concentrating on a kind of internal power, or seeking an external force which can be internalized for greater prowess (Jones 2002, xii). For instance, Zarrilli (2005, 30) emphasizes the ritual life of *kaḷarippayaṭṭu*, about which he writes that "from the very first day of practice in a traditional Hindu *kalari*, students must participate in the devotional life of the *kalari* from the point of ritual entry into the sacred space through the practice of personal devotion to the *kalari* deities and to the master." When entering the place of training, students of *kaḷarippayaṭṭu* start by honoring the deities installed inside the training ground (1998, 65). Students perform different movements from the martial repertoire in front of these deities and in front of their teacher, in order to express their devotion. The concerned movements and performances enact in a prescribed manner the hierarchical learning relationship of students and masters, on the one hand, and are thought to provide access to divine powers, on the other. Ritual thus is a major factor in the process of students' *kaḷarippayaṭṭu* instruction and practice, as it combines and helps to internalize exercises and devotion toward gods and preceptors. A somewhat similar practice is found in *varmakkalai* martial training as well. However, although I saw training grounds in which an idol or picture of a god was installed and worshipped before commencing training, this is the exception rather than the rule. Students largely focus their attention on the *guru*, or *ācāṉ*, and on the ground itself.

Vital spot martial training therefore routinely starts with greeting the gods in the form of the soil, and then one's *guru*. This is called "saluting method," *vaṇaṅkum muṟai* (Raj 1977, 96; Jeyrāj 2000, 9). When entering the place designated for martial practice, a student makes sure to place the right foot inside first (the right side of the body being considered more pure and auspicious); this mirrors the behavior of Hindu devotees when entering a temple. A student then bows down to touch the ground, the forehead, and throat or chest with the right hand, this way revering the earth like one does a deity. Velayudhan explained that when entering a *kaḷari*, a practitioner asks Pūtēvi, the "earth goddess," for permission to use the ground for exercises. When leaving after concluding training, the same action is repeated, this time to apologize for having used the ground, according to the *ācāṉ*. By revering the earth (*maṇ*) thus, all gods (*teyvam*) are said to be venerated as well, and their blessing is sought in this way.[2] The actual performance of such "saluting methods" varies from practitioner to practitioner and may include silent uttering of *mantras* or inward prayers in order to honor different gods (see Jeyrāj 2000, 11).

Movements called "saluting the *guru*," *guru vaṇakkam*, are invariably performed next by students, who individually approach the *ācāṉ* and bow down, sometimes kneeling or prostrating flat on the ground in front of their teacher. Students touch their *guru*'s feet, a meaningful performance in South Asia and the core part of "saluting the *guru*" (Jeyrāj 2000, 9). This is called "to greet by touching [someone's] feet," *kāl toṭṭu vaṇaṅku-tal*, an act which conveys the highest respect of the person greeting toward the person or deity being thus revered (Alex 2008, 537).[3] Jeyrāj (2000, 14) adds that, while bending down before the *guru*, a student should never look into the *ācāṉ*'s eyes, thus demonstrating all-embracing trust and obedience. After being thus revered, the *ācāṉ* responds by touching the student's head. This is called "touching the head," *talai toṭu-tal*, a gesture which conveys acceptance and blessing.[4] If the *guru* is absent, the most advanced student directs the training and may adopt the *ācāṉ*'s position, toward whom the saluting is then performed. Yet, as I was told frequently, a kind of inner reverence of one's actual master is still to be performed

2. Such veneration of gods in the form of the soil is reminiscent of the ancient Dravidian concept of *aṇaṅku*. Several scholars have described *aṇaṅku* as a kind of impersonal power or force, mostly connected with mother deities or female power, which can be resorted to, internalized, and possessed (Hart 1973; Rajam 1986; Pechilis 2006).

3. Both human beings and deities can be accorded devotion or reverence in this way in India (Alex 2008, 537).

4. I will come back to and describe this somatic performance of the teacher-student relationship in greater detail in chapter 6, with regard to its meaning for initiation and the instruction of *varmakkalai*.

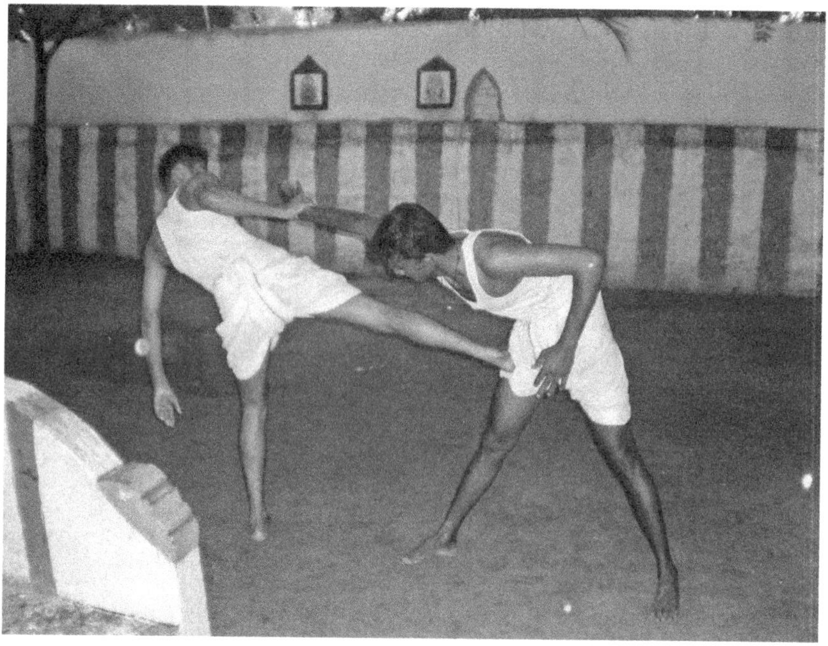

FIGURE 3.2 Early morning practice in a training ground

in the minds of students, regardless of the *guru*'s presence, and even full-fledged practitioners honor their (often long deceased) former *ācāṉ*s (compare Jeyrāj 2000, 14).

Varying patterns of "saluting of the *guru*" are exhibited in *kaḷaris*, while touching of the teacher's feet on the part of the student, and touching of the student's head in return, constitute its ubiquitous core. However, miscellaneous preliminary body moves, punches, and kicks in different directions or rapid clapping on different limbs or parts of the body are frequently performed as well, depending on the style of the martial training (figure 3.2). For all these movements there usually is a set of commands, which an *ācāṉ* calls out as explanation for new, inexperienced students, but which otherwise may remain mute. As in *kaḷarippayaṭṭu* (Zarrilli 1998, 112), these are called *vāyttāri*, "oral commands." For "saluting the *guru*," a *vāyttāri* might sound like the following:

> [Place the] right leg in front; assume a standing position! Swing both hands from the left to the right side and place your right leg behind! The left leg [being] in front, hit with your left hand straight up, then kick with your right foot and touch the [left] hand [high in

> the air], then hit with your right hand straight up, kick with your left foot and touch the hand [with your foot high in the air]! Pull back your right hand, turn to the left side and repeat . . . ; turn to the right side and repeat. ... Look in front and salute the *guru* [by bowing down, touching the *guru*'s feet]!

In contrast to what has been described for *kaḷarippayaṭṭu*, in which the ritual life is centered on one or several deities within the *kaḷari*, or for wrestling *ākhāḍās* in North India (which are often devoted to the god *Hanumān*; see Alter 1992a, 319), the martial aspects of *varmakkalai* do not normally involve idols of deities. Apart from this, the devotional life of training grounds is centered on the person of the *guru*, the *ācāṉ*, thus paralleling the focal point of the vital spot dispensary. The close relation between both spheres, and even more so, between therapeutic and combat applications of vital spots, becomes all the more apparent when analyzing the process of instruction of students, who have to progress gradually in different learning procedures that blur the delineations between medicine and martial arts.

Learning the Vital Spots

Students of vital spot practices are required to undergo a process of learning for which both physical and mental progression are central. *Ācāṉs* describe this as the development of "body power," *uṭalcakti*, and "mind power," *maṉacakti*. Stamina is needed for performing long, deep, and strenuous massages, for body manipulations in the dispensary, and for exercises in the training ground. Physical endurance is also developed by both receiving and administering therapeutic techniques, on the one hand, and by gaining proficiency in martial practices, on the other. Students are furthermore expected to be mentally strong, exhibiting determined will-power, self-confidence, and restraint. This is thought to allow for the development of both flawless mastery of combat techniques and therapeutic intuition for diagnosing diseases and treating patients. The means to achieve these strengths are the martial and therapeutic techniques and exercise of yoga, breath control, and meditation. All these resources merge the mental and physical progression of students, help them to advance in the training ground as well as in the dispensary, and serve to develop their therapeutic and combat intuition.

Progressing Physically in the Study of the Vital Spots

Massage methods (*taṭavumuṟai*) are not only an integral part of most vital spot therapies, but are also important with regard to its martial training. Practitioners of *kaḷarippayaṭṭu* receive as part of their training routine regular massages, before or after training sessions, especially during the rainy season. For this, medicated oil is massaged into practitioners' bodies, using intense, deep strokes, often administered with the feet of the master, who balances while holding on to ropes tied to the ceiling, thus utilizing his or her whole body weight. Such massages are supposed to render the body of a student supple and flexible, and to support martial practice (Zarrilli 1998, 88; 1995). Students of *varma aṭi* in general do not receive regular massages before or after training. Still, massage with medicated oils is frequently administered to students in order to address specific ailments. Such treatments mostly counter the injuries and unpleasant effects resulting from martial training. Massage, or *taṭavu*, is administered if a student, or *ācāṉ*, feels that his or her body is tense, or that a particular body part aches, or in order to treat sprains, bruises, or other injuries which frequently occur in the course of martial training. For this, medicated oils (*eṇṇey*) are deployed, which generally are produced by the *ācāṉ* and students themselves. The same oils are utilized in the therapeutic practices of the dispensary to address vital spot ailments. Such oils effectively render the body supple, soft, and flexible, straightening the nerves (*narampu nērākum*) and activating the flow of *pirāṇam* life force, which are the main objectives of vital spot massage methods.

Unless there is an immediate problem such as a fracture in the area which is massaged, strong pressure is applied, utilizing deep, intense strokes, on students as well as patients. Persons being thus massaged often groan under the immense force of strokes, which are delivered by various body parts of practitioners; from hands to feet, or by (mostly wooden) instruments such as sticks and clubs, depending on the desired intensity or body part to be massaged. The first time Velayudhan entrusted me with massaging a patient, he guided my hands with his, this way directing me how to proceed. The massage included several different techniques, and was mostly centered on the patient's spinal column, an area which houses many important spots. Initially guiding my hands in each new stroke technique by placing his on top of mine, the *ācāṉ* finally had me continue on my own. This kind of massage takes barely ten minutes, but is full of deep, intense strokes. Velayudhan repeatedly told me to press harder, and took my hands to demonstrate how much pressure to administer. I was struck by the force I was to use, under which the patient groaned as if in pain. I myself had experienced this massage being administered to me before, and had found it hard to relax my muscles. Velayudhan however insisted on my using a lot of pressure:

VELAYUDHAN: Strong! Strong! You must use pressure, otherwise there is no effect [*vacam illai*]. (*Toward the patient*) Is he massaging like a woman?
PATIENT: (*laughingly*) No, it's okay.
VELAYUDHAN: Always massage strongly. If it hurts, the patient will tell you, if there is any other problem, then you will feel it in your hands.

For the persons administering massage thus, that is, generally an *ācāṉ*'s student(s), this can be a tiring and strenuous activity as well. Since I was not used to giving massages, I found this to be an especially exhausting act at first. During the times when patients thronged Velayudhan's dispensary, which happened especially before and around noon-time, the *ācāṉ* himself would be occupied with diagnosing patients and the more delicate techniques of stimulating vital spots. Meanwhile, one of his two students would constantly bottle and hand out medicines to patients, while the other one had to remain at the massage table, barely able to wash the oil off the hands in between attending to patients.[5] I estimate that during such onrushes about twenty-five patients were tended to per hour. Oddly, some days I was thankful for every fracture case we had to attend to, as it meant a welcome change from the demanding massage routine. Thus, administering vital spot massage can itself cause strain and tightness, which the *ācāṉ* or a costudent deals with by administering massage.

After finishing a massage, struggling in vain to fully wash off the oil, Velayudhan one day asked me to feel his hands. They seemed exceptionally rough. He explained: "An *ācāṉ*'s hands must become rough and strong! Do you agree now that this is hard work?" I agreed without any hesitation! Strong hands, Velayudhan added, were necessary for strong massage strokes, but would also come in handy when fighting. And the

5. When I first visited his dispensary, Velayudhan already had two students who, though friendly, were understandably suspicious as to my aims in the beginning. They were glad, though, and I earned their respect and friendship, when I began assisting in the dispensary and after some months even took over the massaging of patients.

practice of powerful blows, in turn, helped to intensify massage strokes. Indeed, to improve strength in their hands and fingers, many *ācāṉ*s have their students hit plantain and bamboo stems.[6] These plants are thought to be similar in structure to a human body, and thus students practice to penetrate vital spots by hitting banana stems, but also to train their hands' strength. Velayudhan advised me how to do this correctly, by keeping the thrusting finger erect and firm, in order to prevent an injury. The hereditarily trained practitioner Caṇmukam recounts that his *guru*, while teaching him *varma aṭi*, ordered him to perform numerous arduous exercises, which he did not understand back then, but the use of which he comprehends today. As a student, he was ordered to collect the small fruit of the *neem* tree (*vēppappaḻam*) and to press it between his fingers, squeezing out the interior kernel, which is easy. Then, his *ācāṉ* would ask him to try and squeeze the kernels as well, until it gave in and cracked open, which is difficult, considering its sturdiness and density. After having struggled to do so for some time, holding the *neem* kernel between his thumb and index finger, his *guru* had him try different finger combinations; pressing the kernel between thumb and middle finger, between thumb and ring finger and so on. Caṇmukam thus slowly built superior strength in his individual fingers (Caṇmukam 2010, 29).

The day after I had delivered my first massage, the muscles of my arms felt sore, as I had had to massage the next two patients as well. Velayudhan noticed this and said, "Your arms are hurting already? That's good. Let's see how fast you will be able to spin the *cilampam* staff after some days!" Indeed, sometimes I did not know whether the sore muscles in my body were caused by the massage or by martial training, as both were physically challenging. Martial training is arduous and may sometimes also require massages to overcome stiffness of muscles and nerves, or injuries. However, there are still more connecting points between therapy and fighting in *varmakkalai*.

Velayudhan divided his martial training course into eighteen steps or "forms," *muṟai* (compare Aleksāṇṭar Ācāṉ 1998, 5), in all of which a practitioner had to excel before being considered a full-fledged *ācāṉ*. These eighteen forms include *cilampam* or *neṭuṅkampu*, which is a long staff used in individual training or sparring exercises; *ciramam*, or

6. See also Jeyrāj (2000, 234–238), who mentions hitting the stems of coconut trees among methods for improving finger strength.

medium staff, about one meter in length; and *kaṭṭaikampu*, which is a short stick, about the length of a hand. Further forms include *aṭi taṭa*, literally "hit and defend," a bare-handed fighting method consisting of blocking, punches, and kicks; *piṭitteṟittal*, grappling; *pūṭṭu*, interlocking techniques; and *tūkkiyeṟittal*, throws, all of which are normally practiced by two sparring practitioners. A few nonwooden weapons are also included in the eighteen forms: *māṉkompu*, or *māṭukompu*, a weapon made of the "horns of a bull or a deer"; *veṭṭukatti*, machete; *kōṭāri*, axe; *veṭṭuvāḷ*, short sword; *vīccuvāḷ*, long sword; *vāl kēṭakam*, sword and shield; and *vēlkampu*, lance, a staff with a sharp, metallic point at one end. All of these weapons are also generally practiced with a sparring partner. The eighteenth form is *varma aṭi*, the direct attack upon and defense of vital spots.[7] A student has to progress sequentially through these forms, being allowed to pass on to the next *muṟai* only after having successfully mastered all the previous ones. Learning how to utilize the vital spots in a combat situation, or *varma aṭi*, is thus ideally revealed to only the most advanced among students at the final stage of their instruction.[8] Often, though, even beginners may be taught a number of vital spots alongside simple, less dangerous techniques, with the aim of providing the student with one or two effective but nonlethal self-defense methods.

To instruct and practice these forms, some *ācāṉ*s make use of *taṟaippaṭam*, literally "floor pictures." These are pictures, drawn with white rice flour on the training ground. *Taṟaippaṭam* pictures are similar in appearance to the ornamental drawings called *kōlam*, which consist of complex geometrical patterns (sometimes colored) drawn in front of the thresholds of houses in South India (the North Indian counterpart being *rangoli*).[9] *Kōlam* floor ornaments abound during festival times, but are laid out in most areas of Tamil Nadu in the early morning as a daily routine

7. This list contains only fifteen *muṟai*s. However, training for the first three—*cilampam*, *ciramam*, and *kaṭṭaikampu*—begins alone, and only later includes a sparring partner, and since both stages are counted as separate forms, we get a total of eighteen *muṟai*s.

8. Similarly, Zarrilli (1998, 97) describes the progression of *kaḷarippayaṭṭu* students as starting from body poses (*vaṭivu*), bare-handed combat, weapons practice, learning, and application of *kaḷari* massage, and finally culminating in vital spot applications.

9. Zarrilli (1998, 106) and Pati (2010, 185) mention *kaḷam* drawings as being used in both *varma aṭi* and central-style *kaḷarippayaṭṭu*. Zarrilli also mentions that these drawings are considered *yantras*, sacred diagrams used in tantric rituals, and that "esoteric interpretations abound."

by the women of the household. *Kōlams* are supposed to ward off evil spirits, and it is also said that their often highly complicated geometric patterns boost the concentration of the person who draws them in a kind of meditation (Cārōjā 1995; Nagarajan 1998). In *varmakkalai*, such "floor pictures" are not complicated ornaments, but simple drawings, consisting of only three to seven dots or marks, spread over an area of about one and a half meters. The dots, often one in each corner of a square and one in the middle, can be connected by lines, going in zigzag or triangles. Standing on a floor picture, as Zarrilli (1998, 106) has noted, "the central spot is the one to and from which steps are made as the practitioner steps between and among these . . . steps, moving in triangle or zigzag patterns." Using the pattern of a floor picture, students are taught every possible stance and movement by going through all spots on the ground. This is done by first concentrating on the "step sequences," *cuvaṭu*. The same steps, once understood and incorporated by the student, can be applied in any combat sequence and in combinations with each weapon or combat form, that is, irrespective of whether the practitioner bears a staff or fights bare-handed. One basic exercise practiced within a floor picture is the "single-step exercise," *oṭṭaccuvaṭu* (figure 3.3). For this, one leg remains stationary, usually on the central spot of the floor drawing, while the other leg rapidly moves from one spot to the next. Accompanying these leg movements, any set of attack or defense forms can be executed. Here is an example of Velayudhan's oral command of for a single-step exercise, as reconstructed from my field notes:

> [Place the] left leg in front, speed up the left arm, strike the left thigh and swiftly swing the left arm and turn back! Repeat this towards the right-hand side, without moving the right leg, keeping it firmly in position! Repeat this in all the four directions, keeping the right leg on the same position! This is the single-step exercise.

As Zarrilli (1998, 106) states, the aim of using these floor pictures is to develop "the instinctive ability to step in any direction." Especially in *cilampam* staff fighting, Robert Crego (2003, 33) remarks, "fast foot movement either to create a large sphere of control or to establish a defensive posture is crucial." Such motion sequences have to be practiced over and over again, until the movements become second nature and can be performed automatically and rapidly. One obvious result of training is that students learn to execute hits or blows in every direction,

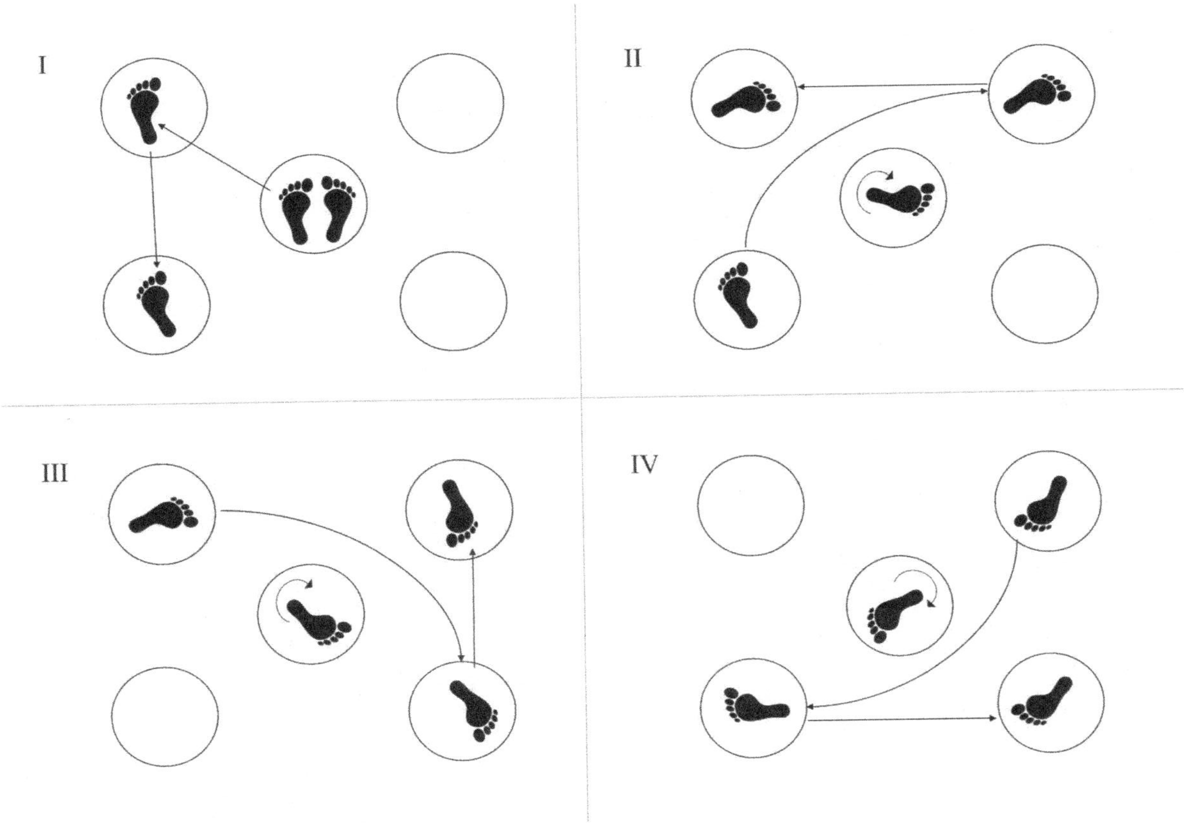

FIGURE 3.3 A “floor picture” with a schematic depiction of a “single-step exercise”

as they practice successive directions with the help of the floor pictures.[10] These drawings can therefore be seen as graphic tools assisting kinesthetic learning. In fact, one practitioner insisted on the correct spelling being *taṟaippāṭam* (with a long *ā* in *pāṭam* instead of *paṭam*), which literally translates as "floor lesson."[11]

Importantly, however, the purpose of such lessons or drawings is training, and to prepare students for eventually abandoning them. In vital spot practice, endless repetition of the steps and movements results in embodied kinesthetic learning. After an initial phase of learning steps and movements within the matrix of the drawings, students can, having internalized its pattern, do without it. By this time, ideally, practitioners have repeated the step exercises countless times and will not require the drawings to guide their movements any more. This is reminiscent of hereditary Chinese *qigong* practitioners, who instruct novices into their practices incorporating martial and medical techniques through repetitious body movements. Elisabeth Hsu (1999, 49) notes that such training was "directed at mindful being in the body," which produces "sensations, feelings, emotions and visions," important in the learning process of hereditary Chinese medical and martial practitioners and their students. Students of *varmakkalai* also learn to abandon the floor drawings after endless repetitions, having not only deeply incorporated the patterns, but having also developed a certain intuitive feeling for the movements and techniques. As Zarrilli (2005, 30) has remarked in the case of *kaḷarippayaṭṭu* martial training, endless repetitions of body exercises help to foster a kind of outer control, and observance of rules and rituals fosters an "inner connection to practice." This inner connection to practice is described as a state of being "all eyes" (Zarrilli 1998), a state which students may eventually attain through the physical exercises, but which also positively influences their martial performances.

Similarly, *varmakkalai gurus* emphasize the meditative qualities of certain drills, especially those deploying the long staff, *cilampam*. These staffs

10. This must be noted as different from *kaḷarippayaṭṭu* martial training, where many body exercises are executed in one direction, after which a 180° turn is taken and the same movement is practiced again in the opposite direction. Notably, moreover, every movement exercise in *varmakkalai* training appears to have a direct combat application, whereas many body poses and moves in *kaḷarippayaṭṭu* appear as primarily designed to cultivate and support flexibility and balance (Zarrilli 1998, 108).

11. Similarly, Makovicky (2010) shows how schematic drawings function as a kind of bridge in teaching for Central Slovakian lace makers, who transmit their knowledge in apprentice-style methods, and for whom it is difficult to articulate their skills verbally.

are similar in appearance to English quarterstaffs, yet generally made of bamboo,[12] and should be slightly shorter than the practitioner's height. *Cilampams* are used for fast twirling around a practitioner's perpendicular and horizontal axes for attack and defense, and for controlled, direct offensive blows or defensive blocking moves. For twirling, a staff is normally held in one hand, in the middle, while the weapon is rotated horizontally and vertically around its axes in various patterns. Skilled practitioners spin two staffs at a time, one in each hand, often achieving high circulation speed. These techniques are popular in public shows, as is the use of fire-lit *cilampams*. However, staff twirling does not have merely aesthetic value, and it is held that if twirled fast enough, even arrows and projectiles can be fended off. Grasped with both hands, a staff can be used in direct combat as well, and usually this is practiced with a sparring partner, who delivers strikes and blows that the opponent has to parry. Once practitioners have achieved a certain degree of skill in handling this weapon, then, in the words of the practitioner Palanisami *ācāṉ*, when exercising a particular form, "the staff moves by itself; you don't have to think but start to meditate." To achieve this, one has to control knowledge and mind (*aṟivum maṉamum*), which is a crucial part of the mental progression of students and practitioners.

Progressing Mentally in the Study of the Vital Spots

Many *ācāṉ*s emphasize that except for self-protection, the knowledge of the vital spots ideally should not be put into practice. Practitioners and manuscripts explain this as being due to the dangerous and potentially lethal nature of some combat techniques that involve vital spots. Therefore, students are incessantly advised to practice self-control, *oṭukkam*. The *Varmakkaṇṇāṭi* (4; Mariyajōcap n.d., 2) advises practitioners to desist from fighting even under provocation, and to peacefully withdraw instead of fighting back, noting, "On earth, whoever may oppose you, be cool-headed and recede just like an honorable person [would]. Talk friendly with [the aggressor] and withdraw." Knowledge of the vital spots can become a deadly weapon in the hands of a wrong kind of person, with terrible consequences, and practitioners are cautioned about such a possibility. As the *Varmakkaṇṇāṭi* (4; Mariyajōcap n.d., 2) states, an opponent attacked at a vital spot will "obey and perish."

12. Sometimes, *cilampam* staffs are cut from cane as well, especially for training purposes, as this material is lighter than bamboo, and hence unintended hits, particularly to the performer's own body during practice, do not hurt as much as might the heavier bamboo staffs.

The reticent behavior required for not misusing or even not using vital spots at all is possible only in the absence of intense desire such as avarice, Velayudhan explained. Moreover, according to him, a suitable mental state is of vital importance for the efficacy of and success in both martial arts and medical therapies. In case of any agitation or dangerous situation, the practitioner has to remain mentally detached. If one has desires, so the *ācāṉ* told his students, one is prone to become a slave to these desires. At the time of the infamous attacks on several public places in Mumbai in November 2008 by alleged Pakistani terrorists, Velayudhan, after having studied the local Tamil newspaper, explained that the aggressors had "desires," *ācai*. Even more,

> terrorists or anyone killing someone else has intense desire [*pērācai*]. This is bad; one should live without intense desire, otherwise one will never be content. One must also practice medicine without desire. Of course, desires will always be there, but intense desire mustn't. If you strive to achieve something too much, it will become an obstacle—even if one wants to help people. Especially for *varma aṭi*, one has to be completely free from desires.

Controlling one's emotions for Velayudhan not only prevents a practitioner from misusing the potentially deadly *varma aṭi* techniques, but also enhances therapeutic efficacy.

The potentially dangerous knowledge of the vital spots and their penetration should remain concealed except in the case of self-defense. Still, practitioners teach various defensive techniques, such as locking techniques, throws, and grapples, which render the actual deployment of vital spots or injurious stimulations redundant. *Ācāṉ*s and manuscripts clearly proscribe actually striking the vulnerable loci in combat situations, as is illustrated, for example, by the *taṭṭuvarmam*, "tapping spots." According to most accounts, the eight *taṭṭuvarmam* are amongst the *paṭuvarmam* "lethal spots." A physical impact, depending on the specific force applied, causes instant death, and hence the tapping spots are called "*ācāṉ*'s spots" (*ācāṉ varmam*) by many practitioners. They are reserved for the accomplished practitioner to know due to their dangerous or lethal nature. While many know the locations of these spots, the actual and very specific way of penetrating a tapping spot, the particular hand movement to strike a spot, remains concealed and a prerogative of *ācāṉ*s. I will come back to notions of morality and ethical behavior in chapter 6, and especially to their relation with secrecy and therapeutic and martial efficacy, in a discussion that is intended to demonstrate that secrecy and morality are pivotal for efficacy and practice in *varmakkalai*.

To resist making use of the potentially dangerous vital spot knowledge is difficult and requires, amongst other things, attaining a kind of inner peace or, in the words of several *ācāṉ* informants, "mind power," *maṉacakti*—strength of mind. According to Velayudhan, such mental strength is not only crucial in ensuring success against an adversary, but in ensuring that practitioners do not deploy their knowledge of vital spots in an adversary. Moreover, mental strength can help to avoid conflicts in the first place in most cases. Different *gurus* stress various mental and physico-mental issues as paramount for attaining such a state. Some advise their students to practice yogic exercises and meditation, or combinations of both, such as *pirāṇāyāmam* breath control (Jeyrāj 2000, 19).

As Zarrilli (1998, 35) points out, we find the connection of meditative concentration with military and combat training in relatively early texts. For instance, in the *Dhanur Veda*,[13] the "science of archery," a Sanskrit text setting out rules for fighting techniques and weaponry,

> [p]ractice and training were circumscribed by ritual, and the martial practitioner was expected to achieve a state of ideal accomplishment allowing him to face death. He did so by combining technical training with practice of yoga/meditation and *mantra* thereby achieving superior self-control, mental calm, single-point concentration and access to powers in the use of combat weapons.

Similarly, Velayudhan advises his students to practice sets of yoga body postures (*yōkācaṉam*; Skt. *yogāsana*). These include *patmācaṉam*, or "lotus pose," sitting in cross-legged position on the ground; *pujaṅkācaṉam*, or "cobra pose," which consists of stemming the upper body off the ground while lying flat on the stomach; *cakrācaṉam*, or "wheel pose," a backbend in a standing position; *pātacakrācaṉam*, or "semicircle pose," a variation of *cakrācaṉam*, which includes lifting one leg in a straight line while in a backbend; *paccimācaṉam*, or "bird pose," a sitting position with both legs being stretched out on the floor while simultaneously bending one's

---

13. There is considerable disagreement regarding the dating of the *Dhanur Veda* texts (Zarrilli 1998, 35).

uppers torso to grab one's soles with the hands; *vīrācaṉam*, or "hero pose," a position of squatting on one's knees; *carvāṅkācaṉam*, the "entire body pose" or shoulder stand; and *cavācaṉam*, or "corpse pose," consisting of lying calmly on the back.[14] Some of these exercises are meditational, recreational, or calming, others are physically challenging, and many include both these aspects at the same time.

According to Mircea Eliade (1970, 54), the purpose of such yoga poses is the realization of "a certain neutrality of the senses [when] consciousness is no longer troubled by the presence of the body." In other words, practitioners attempt to achieve a state in which sense perceptions but also bodily and mental desires are shut down and controlled. Yoga is therefore equally stressed for its value in training the senses and one's perception, in making the body fit and flexible, and in calming the mind through its meditative aspects.

However, even on a physical level, its effects go deeper than merely causing relaxation of muscles, and a protective function is ascribed to different yoga poses. According to one informant, Thangaraj *ācāṉ*, all vital spots can be "locked," by assuming the "pose of the wild boar," *varakācaṉam*. Assuming this deep squatting position provides protection to the lowermost *cakra* in the coccyx region, *mūlātāram*. This, in turn, protects all other vital spots in the body, according to Thangaraj. Dharmalingam (Balasubramaniam and Dharmalingam 1991, 24), a practitioner from Chennai, who notes in a published interview that vital spots can be stimulated when practicing yoga, by strengthening *pirāṇam* and its circulation, supports this view. Velayudhan, too, stated that yogic practices convey the ability to protect vital spots from attacks, and related this to the circulation of life force. Protecting vital loci is not achieved only by particular body stances but even more so by breathing exercises. Again, Dharmalingam (Balasubramaniam and Dharmalingam 1991, 26) notes that "a person 'holding' the breath does not get affected by any force applied on the varma points [which] get 'bound' when we hold the breath. This . . . paralyses the points." Describing his body as "airtight," one of Zarrilli's

---

14. Other *yōkācaṉams* that I have seen utilized by practitioners include: *cittācaṉam*, or "pose of realization," a variation of *patmācaṉam; kukkuṭācaṉam*, or "rooster pose," standing on the hands in a cross-legged position; *muktācaṉam*, or "liberation pose," lying on the back, tucking up one's legs, reaching around with one's arms; *muttirācaṉam*, or "mudra pose," sitting cross-legged, reaching with the arms behind one's own back and touching one's toes; *varakācaṉam*, or "pose of the wild boar," a deep squatting position; and *ciracācaṉam*, or "head [stand] pose."

kaḷarippayaṭṭu informants similarly claimed to be able to stop and hold *pirāṇam* in any desired body part. Controlling this life force and concentrating it in particular places and thus "locking up" vital spots, is indeed the objective of *pirāṇāyāmam*, or "the control of *pirāṇam*" as exercised by many vital spot practitioners. Velayudhan attached much importance to being able to control *pirāṇam*, an exercise which he also called *nāṭicutti*, "cleansing of the *nāṭi* [channels]." The *nāṭis*, as discussed in chapter 2, are the routes of transport of *pirāṇam*, which is of utmost importance to a person's life and to the functioning of the vital spots. Controlling the flow of life force through the body is thus not only a tool for meditative purposes, calming the mind and cleansing the transphysical body—the functioning generally emphasized in literature on yoga (Eliade 1970, 56)—but can also be deployed to "control the circulation of *pirāṇam* and 'lock' the *varmam*," and hence to directly influence one's own vital spots. This is crucial for both martial and therapeutic applications in *varmakkalai*.

Breath control consists of the manipulation of breathing through controlled inhalation (*pūrakam*), retention (*kumpakam*), and exhalation (*irēcakam*). All three are conducted according to stipulated amounts of time, in attempts to deepen and slow down respiration. The semimythical founding fathers of siddha medicine, the Siddhars, had observed a curious fact, which they report in numerous of their writings: In breathing, exhalation normally involves a larger quantity of breath (that is, eight *aṅkulam* or fingerbreadths) than inhalation (four *aṅkulam*). The Siddhars thought to have recognized the main reason for the finitude of life in this way, as they understood every life as characterized by a stipulated amount of breathing cycles, upon termination of which life expires. Thus, with every respiration sequence, vital breath is lost and a person approaches expiration of life according to siddha medical theory. The aim of breath control therefore is to counter this loss of breath both by synchronizing inhalation and exhalation and slowing down the respiration cycles considerably. Ideally, the continual practice of breath control thus enables a prolongation of life or even immortality, the ultimate goal of the ancient Siddhars, as the *Tirumantiram* of Tirumūlar, for instance, shows (Tirumūlar 1991, 89).

The same method of breath control is pursued by vital spot *ācāṉs*, albeit not necessarily with the intention of attaining immortality. As Velayudhan elucidated, forging the respiration in the way described, during retention of breath, *pirāṇam* becomes "locked" inside vital spots. As we have already seen, *varmam* loci are vulnerable precisely due to their housing of *pirāṇam*, and disease or death can result when this life force is exhaled from them. Vital spots can therefore be guarded from attacks and disease by consciously controlling one's respiration, since *pirāṇam* is forcibly retained and locked within the vital spots, not allowing any impact to extract or disturb this life force. *Pirāṇāyāmam* hence attains particular importance for the martial art practitioner, since skilled breath control facilitates the protection of one's vital spots, among other things. Moreover, *pirāṇam* and its regulation are effective tools for an outstanding combat performance, in *varmakkalai* as well as in *kaḷarippayaṭṭu*. As Zarrilli (1989, 1302) has noted, "in martial practice, control of the wind [*pirāṇam*] eventually leads the practitioner to power (Śakti). ... [*Pirāṇam*] courses through the body-in-movement, and power becomes manifest in the accomplished performance of exercises, in potentially deadly combat blows." If a practitioner has attained skill in controlling *pirāṇam*, this becomes manifest in martial exercises: blows delivered can be observed or felt as particularly "heavy," and of a deadly power (1302).

According to Velayudhan, control of *pirāṇam* attains a therapeutic value. This is true for a practitioner's own condition and health. Moreover, and more importantly, being sensitive to this subtle life force and being able to control it enhances a practitioner's therapeutic efficacy for curing patients. The life force can therefore be utilized not only for fighting purposes: "[a] master's hands, feet, forearms, and elbows control [*pirāṇam*] vital energy also to heal" (Zarrilli 1989, 1302). Practitioners ideally direct *pirāṇam* through their limbs while administering manual therapies such as massages, in which they carefully transmit life force through each massage stroke, conveying strong but steady force. Breath control, Velayudhan elucidated, was a way of training students to direct this energy through their own bodies, and how to utilize this in martial and medical applications. Administration of massages and the manual stimulations of loci in particular require *ācāṉs* to be experienced in controlling and directing *pirāṇam*. Only the hands that deploy this life force will deliver strong and therapeutically effective massage strokes. Moreover, since vital spots are the places where life force exists in a condensed form, practitioners who have become sensitive to this vital force—both to their own and the *pirāṇam* in patients' bodies—unerringly detect a vital spot, by sensing the life force inside of it.[15]

15. Again, it may be interesting to note that anthropologist Elisabeth Hsu (1999, 22) has observed how Chinese martial and healing practitioners alike use *qigong* meditative practices. Like *pirāṇāyāmam*, controlling of one's *qi* energy within the body is said to confer abilities with regard to both therapeutic and combative effects. In fact, *qigong* techniques also draw on various breath exercises, amongst others.

Most of my informants in Kanyakumari stressed the need to practice yoga and breath control to achieve specific abilities, a state of inner peace and strength to perform both martial exercises and therapeutic techniques, the two disciplines that must be regarded as essential parts of *varmakkalai*. Zarrilli (2005, 20) has defined *kaḷarippayaṭṭu* "as an active, energetic means of disciplining and harnessing (*yuj* the root of yoga) both one's body and one's mind as a form of moving meditation." One practitioner similarly described *varmakkalai* as a "way of meditation," *tiyāṉamārkkam*, noting that unless meditation was practiced daily, one would not attain proficiency in *varmakkalai*. As such, meditative aspects are at the same time a prerequisite and an inherent characteristic of vital spot practice; only through austere practice of yoga and breath control, it was often explained to me, was it possible to fully learn and to successfully practice martial and therapeutic aspects of the vital spots. If correctly incorporated into one's regimen, Rājēntiraṉ (2008, 40) maintains, the combination of meditation and physical training would convey superhuman powers. *Nōkkuvarmam*, "gaze spot," or the esoteric ability to affect vital spots by the power of sight alone is often cited as an example of such "superhuman powers," which some *ācāṉ*s attain.

Attaining a particular mental and physico-mental state is important in *varmakkalai* with regard to a practitioner's performance in both martial and medical arenas. This physico-mental state allows for self-confident behavior, assists in combat situations and in therapies, and fosters a kind of intuition for diagnosis and treatment on the one hand, and for fighting efficiency on the other. Time and again, Velayudhan advised me to "foster my mind power" (*maṉacakti vaḷaraṇum*). He claimed to have detected a kind of reluctance in me, exhibited, for instance, when I was massaging patients. In fact, I somehow expected patients to feel uncomfortable being massaged by me, obviously an outsider, at best a student of the *ācāṉ*, but ultimately only a student and not a "professional," full-fledged practitioner. I was upset for this same reason when one day Velayudhan announced that the local association of siddha medical practitioners, the Siddha Vaidya Sangam in Nagercoil, would conduct a "free medical treatment day,"[16] at which he would offer his services and I was to assist him!

16. All over Tamil Nadu, such siddha free treatments and camps (*mukām*) are becoming popular with practitioner associations and are regularly organized with the aim of providing free treatment and promoting siddha medicine. Often, apart from giving free treatment and handing over samples of medicine to patients, producers of siddha pharmaceuticals are present and exhibit their products.

I immediately expressed my reluctance to massage in public, and especially to assist him under the gaze of other medical professionals, since I was, after all, neither a *vaittiyar* nor a doctor. But Velayudhan would hear none of it, and encouragingly responded,

> You should never think like that! You have to be brave; only if we become lions [*ciṅkamāṉā*], we will have success in life. Don't you understand? Aren't you yourself a Siddhar now? Isn't even someone who is studying siddha a Siddhar? But in siddha it is necessary to be brave, otherwise you will not be able to diagnose a disease or trace the right spot! So wherever you go from now, you will go there as a *vaittiyar*! Treatment will only work like this. And of course, this is important for fighting as well!

After some convincing from Velayudhan, I finally accepted and assisted him at the event, although I did not feel very confident at first. Subsequently, the *ācāṉ* repeatedly advised me to develop my "mental strength," *maṉacakti*.

I had plenty of opportunities to observe Velayudhan's and his students' mental strength. One late evening, a young man, who obviously had met an accident, was brought into the dispensary, accompanied by a group of six other young men. It did not take long to realize that they had been drinking, judging from the smell and the commotion they created. While Velayudhan diagnosed the patient's hand as dislocated at the wrist joint, the mob was busy squabbling. Feeling disturbed in his examining the patient, the *ācāṉ* scolded the youths, telling them to be decent and quiet, so he could treat their friend. The group however was agitated enough to talk back to Velayudhan, not lowering their voices. Calmly, yet authoritatively, the *ācāṉ* explained to them that they had no right whatsoever to raise their voices inside his dispensary, but had to obey his orders. Enraged by this, and far from being pacified, the group got even more agitated. Velayudhan remained calm and simply gazed at the youths, his two students, Murugan and Manikandhan, at his side. The room went silent for some moments; the atmosphere was tense. Perhaps the drunken youths had initially considered taking a chance and testing these practitioners' actual fighting skills; but in any case they now had no such thoughts. After a few moments Velayudhan asked them politely to leave the room and wait outside, to which they immediately and silently complied. Although the young men kept quiet, the *ācāṉ* sent Manikandhan, the elder of his students, outside to keep an eye on the group, and proceeded to calmly treat the patient.

Directly after this incident, Velayudhan summoned his students, again advising us to abstain from fights, except for the purpose of self-defense. Only after warning an opponent three times by expressing our wish not to fight were we free to counteract aggression. Most dangerous situations thus would be avoided, precisely by proving one's mental strength. According to the *ācāṉ*, this was of the nature of a lion's strength. To explain this, he asked us a question:

VELAYUDHAN: What characterizes a lion?
MANIKANDHAN: A lion is ferocious.
VELAYUDHAN: Correct, but a lion is also proud and brave. If you walk outside late at night, you have to be proud and brave, your head held high. If anyone talks unfriendly to you, if there is any trouble, then tell them you are my student. Saying that should suffice. If then there is still trouble, then you must warn three times, saying "I don't want to fight." If still you are confronted, then bravely, without fear, hit here (*pointing out a specific point*); like that; you know the place. He will tumble and fall down, unconscious.

As it is important to not make use of the knowledge of the vital spots without being forced to, Velayudhan repeatedly stated that only a Śiva *yogin* should be selected to become a student. This is found in several manuscript sources on vital spots as well (*Varma Cūttiram*, 3; Subramaniam 1994, 14; Zarrilli 1998, 45–46). This means, amongst other things, that for the student it is of the utmost importance to practice self-control, both physically and mentally.

Modalities to achieve this special state include yoga, meditative exercises, and breath control, which merge physical and mental training in order to produce such a desired body-mind. This is parallel to what Zarrilli (1998, 46) has described in the case of *kaḷarippayaṭṭu*, where students ideally develop "one-point focus," or *ekāgratā*, achieved by repetitious practice of correct body movements, and cultivation of ritual habits inside the training ground. In *varmakkalai* as well, students strive to attain a physical and mental balance that will assist them in their practice. *Ācāṉ*s in this regard stress the need for simultaneous development of "physical strength," *uṭalcakti*, and "mental strength," *maṉacakti*. When fostered in a parallel way through the practice of martial exercises, therapeutic manipulations, and yogic techniques, this triggers an effective *maṉa utti*. This term is composed of *maṉam*, "mind," and *utti*, which is defined as "intuitive perception . . . tact," by the Madras *Tamil Lexicon*. In combination, *maṉa utti* may be translated as "intuition" (Sujatha, Aruna, and Balasubramanian 1991, 74). This kind of intuition, which vital spot practitioners ideally develop, is deeply connected to the efficacy of all practices of both training ground and dispensary. Intuitively, a practitioner must develop a sense of confidence in his or her practices beyond any doubts, a doubtless mentality (Zarrilli 1998, 198), which is intrinsically related to both the healing and fighting practices.

Medicine and Martial Arts Intertwined

I was sitting together with Velayudhan in the backyard of his house one afternoon, enjoying a short break from the rush of patients. The *ācāṉ* picked up two *cilampam* staffs which had been leaning against a coconut tree, and after throwing one over to me, started to playfully exchange a few strikes and blocks, a common pastime during such breaks or in the evening hours. In between delivering blows or parrying mine, he explained that by handling a *cilampam*, one became more aware of the vital spot locations, but a knowledge of them should also be considered a prerequisite for such martial training. Injury to prominent places is a common occurrence when staff fighting, and *ācāṉ*s therefore have to be prepared to deal with any related traumata. Though normally nothing serious happens, sometimes staff training results in severe injury, and this is also true of other weapons and bare-handed fighting forms. Velayudhan said, "A practitioner of *varma aṭi* [vital spot martial arts] must be skilled in *vaittiyam* [medicine] as well; otherwise injuries happen and cause chronic ailments or even death." This is, according to most practitioners, exactly the reason why staff training, "hitting the vital spots," and similar martial exercises and vital spot treatments are practiced in combination (*Varmakkaṇṇāṭi*, 319; Mariyajōcap n.d., 164; Jeyrāj 1999, 12). Each and every martial application of a vital spot must be completed by therapeutic techniques, and every possible effect to a *varmam* must be treatable by corresponding measures. Also, numerous shared concepts characterize both combat applications and therapies of vulnerable loci; these include stimulation and penetration techniques as well as underlying concepts of timing, force, and effects.

The Vital Spots in Therapy and Martial Training

A spot called *tiṭavarmam*, "sturdy vital spot," is located on the upper side of the foot, about one inch above the big toe, and due to this prominent position it is frequently hit with staffs during training. If injured, even by only slight impacts, the toe and consequently the entire foot swells up, a blood-clot forms, and pain, which can be severe enough to cause unconsciousness, sets in (Jeyrāj 2000, 39). To assuage these symptoms and to prevent or reverse fainting, one stimulates a particular *aṭaṅkal* "relief spot." This must be followed up by massaging the foot with medicated oil. A similar case in point is the spot called *aṭappakkālam*. When Velayudhan and I were outside exchanging *cilampam* blows, the *ācāṉ* would repeatedly deliver a speeding blow in the direction of a specific part of my body, but stop short of actually touching the particular point with the tip of his staff at the last moment. To me, it was each time obvious that such locations were significant loci, and in the case of a real fight, each blow would have had serious effects. One of those spots is situated on each side of the ribcage. This is a delicate offensive move, as these spots, *aṭappakkālam*, are by most accounts considered lethal spots. As soon as the *ācāṉ* had delivered a mock strike in the direction of this spot, he listed the symptoms of an affected *aṭappakkālam*, apparently reciting from a manuscript: "If *aṭappam* is hit, blood oozes from mouth and nose; [he] will not be able to breathe, unconsciousness will set in and he will faint." Immediately, Velayudhan pointed out *kūmpuvarmam* as relief spot in the case of *aṭappakkālam* being affected and how to stimulate it, thus countering the ill-effects. In this manner, no attacking blow to a vital spot would be imaginable without knowing the relevant countermeasures required to counteract the effects of an affliction for saving a victim or opponent from an impact. Practitioners frequently cautioned that there was no "combat method" (*aṭi muṟai*) without "treatment method" (*iḷakku muṟai*), since it is every *ācāṉ*'s duty to retrieve and treat an opponent he has struck on a vital spot (provided the ailment is curable).

In *kaḷarippayaṭṭu*, *oṭṭa kol*, or simply *oṭṭa*, is a curved, wooden, dagger-like instrument. Balakrishnan (1995, 105–106) explains this to be amongst the most important weapons for *kaḷarippayaṭṭu* training, although he is puzzled why this is so, as *oṭṭa* never seems to have been used in duels or actual fights; it is pointed, yet blunt at its tip. As Zarrilli (1998, 304) shows, *oṭṭa* is introduced to students rather late in their training and is regarded as an important weapon precisely because it is understood to be ideal for penetrating the vulnerable *marmmam* loci. In *varmakkalai,* a rough approximate to this weapon is the *kaṭṭaikkampu,* "short stick," which can be used to penetrate vital spots. Unlike *oṭṭa* of *kaḷarippayaṭṭu,* these short, wooden sticks are not normally finished in an artful, dagger-like style. Most "short sticks" have a plain, cylindrical shape, are on average about one-half to one inch in diameter, and correspond more or less to the width of a hand in length. It can therefore be easily concealed in its bearer's closed fist, and hence makes for a weapon, which should not be underestimated.[17] However, the *kaṭṭaikkampu* is not merely a weapon. Intriguingly, the same device may be utilized not only in martial practice, but also for therapeutically stimulating vital spots. The same short sticks are often used to penetrate spots which are difficult to reach with the bare hand, or which require greater amounts of pressure. Yet, despite the occasional use of instruments to address vital spots in general, the tool perceived as best suited to achieve this are the hands of an *ācāṉ.*

Whereas the *Dhanur Veda,* the ancient Sanskrit treatise on war and military training, describes bare-handed combat as the least valuable fighting form (Balakrishnan 1995, 17), in the case of *varmakkalai* it has been correctly recognized that "very quick movements of the feet and dexterity of hands with lightning speed both for attacks and defense are the basic skills practiced" (105–106). In contrast to *kaḷarippayaṭṭu* and many other martial arts, vital spot *ācāṉ*s do not consider bare-hand combat a primitive or rudimentary form of type of practice. To the contrary, bare-hand skills and particularly the use of "hand postures," *mudrā,* are esteemed as the most advanced levels of practice, and the device through which vital spots are best accessed. Vital spot martial training does not exclude the use of weapons, a supposition on the basis of which *varma aṭi* has been differentiated from *kaḷarippayaṭṭu* by Zarrilli (2005, 32). The importance given in *varma aṭi* to the staff training disproves that belief. However, it must be said at the same time that, at its core, *varma aṭi* is about penetrating the vital spots, a task best accomplished by the practitioner's hands. Again, the manual techniques to achieve this highlight the double characteristics of healing and harming.

---

17. See also Zarrilli (1998, 180), who mentions "cottacan," small sticks designed to be easily concealed in the hands for the penetration of vital spots.

The Healing and the Harming Touch

Many practitioners utilize a set of hand gestures designed for penetrating the vital spots. *Mudrās*, translated by the Monier-Williams *Sanskrit-English Dictionary* as "particular positions or intertwinings of the fingers ... commonly practised in religious worship, and supposed to possess an occult meaning and magical efficacy," are found in many forms in South Asia. Such gestures or hand postures are, for instance, utilized in day-to-day practices, such as forms of greeting, and also enjoy a special meaning in worship in Hindu temples. In theatrical performances, such as Bhāratanāṭyam dance, a specific set of *mudrās* contributes to the dramatic action, which literally "draws [the audience] towards" (*abhinaya*) the narrative or moods of a play or performance. Vital spot practitioners draw on yet another set of *mudrās*, for both combat and healing needs.

Penetration of a vital spot, no matter which of the two purposes it is intended to serve, has to be done in a very particular way: by "opening" (*tiṟa-ttal*) a specific spot. The form of manipulation employed, whether a rotating movement, a quick jerk, a twisting movement, or a plucking movement, is determined by the type of spot that needs to be stimulated. Only if the right technique is deployed will a particular spot be opened, which otherwise would remain undeterred (Rājēntiraṉ 2008, 53). Every spot thus is associated with a specific technique, and it is the *mudrās* which facilitate such openings. Practitioners frequently refer to such hand postures as keys (*cāvi*), which they use to unlock or open a vital spot. Only the right key will open a *varmam*.

Most vital spots can be opened by the means of a practitioner's hands and, to a lesser degree, feet. The heels, soles, instep, toes, and balls of the feet can all be utilized to massage and to stimulate spots and themselves count as *mudrās*. Though there is considerable variation in the usage, forms, and names, some common hand postures include: "elephant-face *mudrā*" (*yāṉaimukamuttirai*), "horse-face *mudrā*" (*kutiraimukamuttirai*), "power *mudrā*" (*caktimuttirai*), "wheel *mudrā*" (*cakkaramuttirai*), "conch *mudrā*" (*caṅkumuttirai*), "heel or instep *mudrā*" (*puṟaṅkālmuttirai*), *Viṣṇumudrā* (*viṣṇumuttirai*) "*Vēl* (Murukaṉ's spear) *mudrā*" (*vēlmuttirai*), "Śiva's spear (*triśūla*) *mudrā*" (*tiricūlamuttirai*), "snake-(head) *mudrā*" (*carppa(muka) muttirai*), and "five-(finger) *mudrā*" (*pañcamuttirai*) (figure 3.4).[18] Some of

18. This list has been taken from Velayudhan's repertoire of *mudrās*. Other practitioners may incorporate different *mudrās* or terms (compare Kaṇṇāṉ Rājārām 2007b, 310–314;

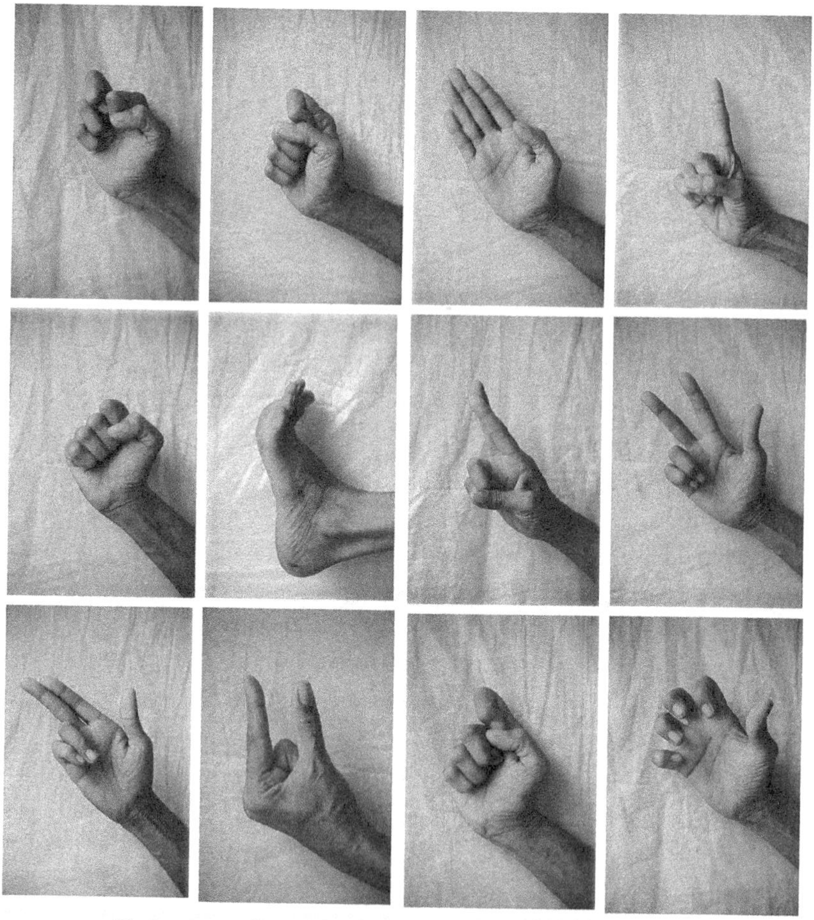

FIGURE 3.4 Vital spot *mudrās*. From left to right and top to bottom: "elephant-face *mudrā*," "horse-face *mudrā*," "power *mudrā*," "wheel *mudrā*," "conch *mudrā*," "heel or instep *mudrā*," *Viṣṇumudrā*, "*Vēl* (Murukaṉ's spear) *mudrā*," a variation of *Vēl mudrā*, "Śiva's spear *mudrā*," "snake-(head) *mudrā*," and "five-(finger) *mudrā*"

these gesture-like intertwinings of fingers can be found in artistic expressions, such as dance, while others are apparently unique to *varmakkalai*.

Practitioners are required to perform these positions quickly, and in the correct form. Thus, students practice making one *mudrā* after the other in rapid succession, so as to internalize all postures. Practitioners

---

Aleksāṇṭar Ācāṉ 1998, 335–339; Kaṇapati n.d., 8–9; Rācā [1997] 2002, 53–54). Refuting the use of *mudrā* altogether, Dharmalingam declares: "There is no specific recommendation for the use of a particular finger—it depends upon the talent of the *aasaan*" (Balasubramaniam and Dharmalingam 1991, 21).

further may train using these finger positions on surfaces that closely resemble the structure of a human body or different body parts and limbs. These include: banana stems, being somewhat similar to a body's trunk; pumpkins, resembling a head in shape and stability; or gourd varieties, which correspond to the limbs. Hitting such objects is believed to strengthen one's blows, and to help one become accustomed to a particular hand gesture.

Every hand posture can be assigned to one or more vital spots, the opening of which is affected through it. For example, *tilartakkālam*, situated on the forehead, in between and slightly above the eyebrows, has to be penetrated utilizing the power *mudrā* (Rājēntiraṉ 2008, 53–57). It is indispensable to intimately know which finger positions to utilize for stimulating a particular vital spot. This applies equally to the opening of vital spots in combat techniques and in therapeutic methods.

Force and Timing

Closely related to the hand postures and to the knowledge about penetrability of, and effect on, vital spots is the taxonomy of force and timing called *māttirai*. According to the Madras *Tamil Lexicon*, *māttirai* means, among other things, "moment, measure of time ... of winking one's eyes or of snapping one's fingers; ... limit, as of time." The implications in vital spot theory go beyond these meanings. As several informants told me, it denotes the measure of time, and the measure of impact or force of a vital spot penetration. It thus relates both to combat applications and to therapeutic techniques. One informant, Samuel *ācāṉ*, who practices about 20 km southwest of Thackalai, explained this to me while simultaneously treating a young boy by stimulating several relief spots:

> If I stimulate this spot, by using half *māttirai*, [the disease] will be cured. *Māttirai* can mean different things: It is the pressure which is applied for treating; the indentation of massage. In case of an injury to a vital spot, *māttirai* describes the degree of the trauma and therefore the severity of an ailment. Even the time of day [*camayam*], including how and when an injury happened, belongs to *māttirai*.

Māttirai thus describes the time, timing, and force of injury or attack, all of which together determine the extent of impact and the virulence of a resulting disease. *Māttirai* further is a measure for describing the force and timing used in treatment measures, laying down the force of indentation and penetration of a vital spot by the practitioner. Thus, diagnosis of an ailment and correct treatment are intimately connected to, and determined by, *māttirai*.

Generally, as a force of striking or therapeutic indentation, *māttirai* is described as less than one-quarter, one-quarter, one-half, three-quarters, one, or as more than one *māttirai*. There are several notions regarding how to assess such degrees, a knack which can be learned only through experience. Hence, exactly how much force *māttirai* involves is difficult to specify, and different *ācāṉ*s describe this in varying terms. It has been noted that one full *māttirai* equals the force needed to penetrate the stem of a banana tree (perceived as similar to the structure of a human torso) up to the first metacarpal of the index finger (Balasubramaniam and Dharmalingam 1991, 32; Maṇiyaṉ 2012, 215).[19] Velayudhan instructs his students on *māttirai*, by pointing out that "if the finger penetrates the [human] body until the first line, or wrinkle, of the finger, then it is one full *māttirai*. [If the finger penetrates the skin] from the tip of the finger three-quarters to its first crease, it is three-quarter *māttirai*. Half and one-quarter *māttirai* mean penetration of the finger half or one-quarter to that line, respectively" (compare Jeyrāj 1999, 66). Another *ācāṉ* described one *māttirai* as the power required to lift a weight of 100 kg above one's head. Similarly, Rājēntiraṉ (2008, 36) notes that lifting weights of 75, 50, and 25 kg equaled the energy required to produce three-quarters, one-half, and one-quarter of *māttirai*, respectively.

Rājēntiraṉ (2008, 38) also notes that whereas, in earlier times, Siddhars were more physically powerful and muscular because of their hard work and were therefore fit to apply one *māttirai*, nowadays people were generally too weak for this, unable to realize the force of one full *māttirai*. For attaining the power of delivering blows as powerful as one *māttirai*, a lot of training had to be undergone. Proponents achieved this by lifting weights or trading punches while carrying weights. In this way, their blows would become heavy like the weights itself, the author states (38). Nevertheless, if the intricacies of right timing and force are intimately understood and

---

19. Contrary to what Dharmalingam (Balasubramaniam and Dharmalingam 1991, 42) states, I have not observed practitioners experiment on animal or human bodies to learn *māttirai* force, or to practice stimulating vital spots.

combined, astonishing effects can, according to Velayudhan, be obtained without requiring a lot of pressure:

> For boxing a lot of energy is required, and after some time you will feel tired and weak. But in *varmakkalai*, not much power is required; it can be practiced easily [*eḷimaiyāka*]. Come; strike my face hard, as hard as you can. (*I try to hit him, reluctantly at first, but he blocks me, with great ease*) You see, you become strained, but I need no energy at all. It is all about *māttirai* and *mudrā*. "Hitting the vital spots," my son, is all about timing/force and hand positions; that is the way of the *ācāṉ* [*ācāṉ vaḻi*].

However, *māttirai* cannot be reduced to either combat or therapeutic relevance alone. For instance, *naṭcattirakkālam*, "star vital spot," a lethal spot, which is located one fingerbreadth from the exterior corner of both eyes, was demonstrated to me as best attacked using the snake *mudrā*. But only one fourth of a *māttirai* pressure should ever be applied to this spot as both the forces which accord to half and full *māttirai* might lead to immediate death, due to this spot's extreme sensitivity. If a "star vital spot" is affected, the victim starts sweating profusely, the eyes turn yellow, and the ability to see and hear diminishes. If these signs are noticed, treatment has to be given quickly, otherwise death is certain, as Velayudhan cautioned. To counter these ill-effects, the practitioner presses on the sides of the patient's forehead by again using the same amount of one-fourth of *māttirai*. Another example is *kūmpuvarmam*, or "bud vital spot," located on the breast, which becomes a therapeutic spot in the event of *naṭcattirakkālam* being injured, and hence must be stimulated using the thumb, also applying one-fourth of *māttirai* (Jeyrāj 1999, 51–53).

Another vital spot, *aṭappakālam*, located on both sides of the rib-cage, can be penetrated by way of an offensive method, which utilizes either the foot or the snake *mudrā*. If attacked with one-half *māttirai*, an opponent is said to fall unconscious or roll on the ground in pain. Full *māttirai* is understood to kill, and hence has to be avoided at all costs. For treatment, as above, *kūmpuvarmam* on the patient's breast must be stimulated with a thumb indentation using a half-*māttirai* pressure. After stimulating *maṉipantavarmam*, the "wrist vital spot," and massaging the patient's back with the feet, the patient regains consciousness (compare Jeyrāj 1999, 147–150). This shows that the interrelations and influences of *māttirai* (force and timing) and *mudrā* (hand positions) characterize both combat and treatment of vital spots.

Time Limits

If a vital spot is physically impacted, the injury must be addressed by therapeutic countermeasures within a stipulated period of time, provided the impact has not exceeded a lethal degree. Each vital spot, if afflicted, has a particular time limit, within which treatment is still feasible. Exceeding a specific period, the symptoms cannot be reversed, and in many cases, incurability (*acāttiyam*, Skt. *asādhya*) of an ailment, sometimes even death of the patient, is certain. To ensure survival, treatment has to be administered within a stipulated period of time, as described by manuscripts. This time frame, *kālam*, translating simply as "time" (Skt. *kāla*, time), is defined by the force of impact. The more forceful the impact, the less time will be available for treatment. Manuscripts and practitioners measure the duration during which treatment is possible in *nāḻikai*, a time category that roughly corresponds to twenty-four minutes; one hour therefore consists of two and a half *nāḻikai*. For every vital spot, the period from an impact to the onset of certain symptoms and to the manifestation of incurable situations differs. If the stipulated time frame is exceeded, complete cure cannot be guaranteed. Rather, the manuscripts caution that an ailment is likely to have turned *acāttiyam*, "incurable," by that time, and that an *ācāṉ* should abstain from administering treatment (*Varmapīraṅki Tiṟavukōl*, 3; Nicivilcaṉ 2003, 52). For instance, if *tilarttakkālam* on the forehead is affected, treatment must be administered within one and a half hours (three and three-quarters *nāḻikai*) to ensure recovery of a patient, according to the *Varmakkaṇṇāṭi* (183; Mariyajōcap n.d., 95).[20]

There is an interconnection between *māttirai* and *kālam*, the severity of impact, time, and harm. Velayudhan tried to explain this, deploying the metaphor of archery:

> If you want to shoot an arrow using a bow, you need to know exactly how to aim for your target. Carefully holding the bow's string you

20. This is not to say that all manuscripts or *ācāṉ*s agree on these time limits. In fact, they vary considerably. Irājēntiraṉ (2006, 167), for instance, notes that in the case of *katirvarmam*, the manuscripts *Varma Cūttiram* and *Varma Kurunūl* give conflicting time periods of nine and fifty *nāḻikai*, respectively. Probably this huge difference (of about four as against twenty hours) is to be explained by a mistake in copying manuscripts, as Tamil "nine," *oṉpatu*, and "fifty," *aimpatu*, are lexically and phonetically very close. Yet there are more instances of considerable deviations, such as between the manuscripts *Varma Tiṟavukōl* and *Varma Cūttiram*, which state the *nāḻikai* of *aṭappavarmam* to amount to eighteen and twenty-eight, respectively (218).

> must decide how to release the arrow, how to speed it up and how much speed is needed. This is *māttirai*. Depending on how much speed and power you apply, the arrow will reach the aim more or less quickly; penetrating more or less deeply. As in the case of the arrow, an effect [*pinpōkku*] on the body is seen after a spot is struck. Some are affected fast, within one or two *nāḻikai*, others take longer. If you strike a vital spot very powerfully, then *nāḻikai* is reduced, like the powerful arrow, which reaches its target very fast.

Velayudhan's statement elucidates that *māttirai* and *nāḻikai* are closely interrelated and several factors relate to both. First, as in archery, the distance from which a shot is being delivered determines the force of impact, as does the speed of an arrow. Released from a short distance and at high acceleration, the impact is more powerful and deep. Second, the time limit given for treating a vital spot affliction invariably depends on the force of impact. In many cases, an impact of one full *māttirai* forecloses any therapy, because such a powerful injury causes an incurable trauma or considerably minimizes the time frame for treatment.

Thus, all concepts described here not only define vital spot practice and determine related practices. All share the dual importance for aspects relating to both dispensary and training ground, or which, in other words, epitomize the close interrelation of therapy and combat, the intertwining of healing arts and martial arts.

Conclusion

It may be interesting to note that, in the Indian context, the double character of harming and healing or, in other words, of destroying and (re) creating, is reminiscent of god Śiva, who is generally perceived as incorporating both devastating character traits and the power to create anew. According to Wendy Doniger (1973), it is precisely the joining and mastering of such apparent opposites—of creating and destroying, but also of asceticism and eroticism—from which Śiva derives his ultimate power.[21] In the case of vital spot practice, it is the very combination of fighting and healing by which this practice functions and derives its meaning, and

21. Historically, the combination of apparently antithetical character traits is also an expression of the circumstance that several religious traditions and ideas became joined within the god Śiva (Michaels 1998, 240).

through which *ācāṉ*s understand what they do. However, most publications on *varmakkalai*, though being few and mostly in Tamil, stress either its medical or its martial aspects, or hold that one aspect has developed first, and has facilitated the evolution of the other (Caravaṇakaṇēṣ 2009, 7; Aleksāṇṭar Ācāṉ 1998, 7). On the other hand, most of the *ācāṉ*s I met in Kanyakumari were outspoken about the inseparability of vital spot treatment and martial arts. Velayudhan, for instance, related the origin of *varmakkalai* as follows:

> The Siddhars have created *varmakkalai*. Agasthiyar analyzed the body and found the vital spots. The meaning of *varmakkalai* is preservation. Learning the vital spots includes protection and self-protection. One part alone will not suffice; they have to be combined. It is not me who is saying this, Agasthiyar himself has stated so. If one knows only one part, lives will perish. *Varmakkalai* is a method for taking life, but it is a method of conferring life as well.

Similarly, although *kaḷarippayaṭṭu* is popularly understood as an exclusively martial art, Zarrilli shows in his study that a student's progress toward psychophysical accomplishment in martial practice is inseparable from abilities as a potential healer. In the same way, *varmakkalai* highlights how closely aspects of martial art and therapeutic treatment can be interrelated. Here they are not opposed, but mutually supportive. Hence, combat training is complemented by manual therapies and massages, often administered to students to ensure flexibility and softness of muscles and tendons, strained by exercises. Practitioners of *varma aṭi*, "hitting the vital spots," are often accomplished medical practitioners who offer their services to patients. Analyzing the process of learning *varmakkalai*, this becomes all the more apparent, as, while a student learns about broken bones, strains, and so on, during martial exercises in the training ground, the same skills are required when dealing with patients in the dispensary, and vice versa. Experiential learning about the body and anatomical concepts takes place both in a medical setting and in physical combat training. Encounters in the dispensary give a highly developed and precise sense of the anatomy of the body, which is used for combat training as well. As Velayudhan once put it, "you learn which bones break if you apply a certain amount of force and which fractures really hurt a lot." This is crucial knowledge for any fight; and for any treatment for that matter.

However, when one takes a closer look at attempts to institutionalize, promote, and spread the lore of the vital spots in contemporary Tamil Nadu (as I will do briefly in chapter 6 and in the epilogue), we find that the amalgamation of martial and medical practices is a delicate issue. Institutions of comparatively recent origin, like siddha medical colleges, NGOs, and private education facilities, tend to divide and fragment this combined practice. For instance, it appears that within the setting of siddha medical colleges, where textbooks and the medical curriculum dictate the form of education, it is precisely martial arts components that are being omitted. Is it justifiable to speculate that within academic frameworks, martial arts, yoga, astrology, and so on, suffer from their alleged "unscientificity," which inhibits them from being paired with therapeutic practices?[22] Whereas dispensary and training ground are closely interrelated institutions in the practices of hereditary *ācāṉ*s in Kanyakumari, they pertain to clearly demarcated concepts in modern educational imaginings. This is a demarcation of practices and objects, which has affected the framework of modern education institutions as well, classifying some of its objects as science and others as arts, but never as coinciding or as applying to both (Scheper-Hughes and Lock 1987).[23] One practitioner in Chennai has characterized *varmakkalai* as "an art as well as a science" (Citamparatāṇuppiḷḷai 1991, 39). As an art, it was employed to attack a person, and as a science, it helped patients to recover from physical impacts.

I suggest that an academic dichotomy between (healing) science and (martial) arts, together with its corresponding taxonomies, has ensured distortions in the study of medical and martial arts in South Asia. Often, both in martial arts literature and in public discourse, it is alleged that India has been the cradle of martial arts that diffused to other parts of the world, to China and Japan in particular (Payne 1981, 5; Varghese 2003). However, contemporary India is not as closely associated with combat sports as are East and Southeast Asia. With the exception of *kaḷarippayaṭṭu*, martial arts and India are not intimately connected in the popular mind. Of course, this does not mean that there is not a rich and varied tradition of martial practices in South Asia. Different regions display varying martial practices and have been

22. Alter (2004) has described projects to put yoga on a scientific footing. Similar attempts and arguments have been made for siddha medicine as well. Nevertheless, such attempts at conferring a scientific gown to yoga, siddha, or other Indian practices in fact accentuate the asymmetries that remain between officially accepted subjects of study and practice, as per a Western model, and the nondisciplined ones.

23. As Scheper-Hughes and Lock (1987) have tentatively argued, the academic division of the sciences and the arts and humanities may go back to the Cartesian mind-body dichotomy.

subject of scholarly research. Notable amongst these are *thang-ta* of Manipur (Dutta 2006), *pahalwān* wrestling of North India (Alter 1989; 1992b), and *gatka* of the Panjab. Zarrilli is, however, right in noting that Indian martial arts are "founded on a set of fundamental cultural assumptions about the body-mind relationship and health and well-being that are similar to the assumptions underlying yoga and Ayurveda" (Zarrilli 2005, 20). Therefore, he calls *kaḷarippayaṭṭu* a "martial/medical/meditation discipline" (Zarrilli 2005; see also Pati 2009; 2010). It might indeed be argued that, in South Asia, martial practices have seldom been practiced as martial arts alone. Yet on those rare occasions when they have been addressed by the scholarly literature, this has been done by considering their combative, performative, or ritualistic aspects (Jones 2002, xiii), but not their therapeutic dimension, for instance. This might well be a reason why the idea of martial arts in general imagination is not connected to India.

Equally distorted would then be the analysis of Indian healing modalities, which has hitherto tended to overlook performative aspects and physical exercises, such as those described in this chapter, possibly because these correspond to "arts," as defined by modern taxonomies and curricula, and therefore do not square easily with healing "sciences." The striking involvement of many manual medical practitioners, such as "bonesetters," with martial traditions in India (Alter 1989; Lambert 1995), and the apparently close connection of ayurvedic practice with dance and theater performances in Kerala, for instance,[24] should, however, sound a note of caution in regard to a temptation to apply rigid dichotomies to Indian traditions. In South Asian culture, I would argue, distinctions between arts and science have only a recent footing. This is highlighted by *varmakkalai*, which is as much an art as it is a science: a healing art or science and a fighting art or science.

24. For instance, P. S. Varier, founder of the Kottakal Arya Vaidyasala, started a dance and theater group, run by employees of his enterprise at the beginning of the twentieth century, which still functions today (Varier 2002, 52). With this, Varier seems to have continued a long tradition of medicine and performing arts. Moreover, many indigenous healers in South India appear to have a strong connection with different performing art forms. This is exhibited at Pūṅkuthil Maṉa, a famous place for the treatment of mental disorders in Kerala, which has a tradition of housing *kathakaḷi* dance performances in its premises (personal communication with Narayanan Nambudiri of Pūṅkuthil Maṉa).

4

Healing the Hidden

SOMATIC MODES OF ATTENDING TO BODIES

THIS CHAPTER CONTAINS an analysis of "vital spot medicine," *varma maruttuvam*, as practiced in Kanyakumari. Here, *varmakkalai* is found in a high concentration, and the numerous vital spot dispensaries that one finds here evidence this. Practitioners, have, to a large degree, enjoyed a noninstitutionalized but hereditary type of education and are therefore frequently not registered or licensed to practice medicine. However, they offer treatments for ailments of the vulnerable loci of the body, including stimulations of particular spots to retrieve patients from unconscious states, but also long-term treatments for chronic ailments, or setting of fractures and massage therapies. While *ācāṉ*s may use a rich stock of medicinal substances for the production of drugs, they mainly conduct manual therapies. Vital spot medicine follows concepts of health and disease common to both ayurveda and siddha medicine, and in particular addresses and manipulates *pirāṇam*, life force or "vital energy," a trans-physiological category present in all vital spots. The analysis of *pirāṇam* and *varmam*, and how *ācāṉ*s utilize these in their manual diagnostics and therapies, allows for an insight into the healing relationship between *ācāṉ*s and their patients and into the intricacies of manual medical procedures in general. This helps to reconsider the patient-physician interaction, and thus provides a critique of hitherto argued theories and clichés prevalent in this regard.

Aspects of agency, decision-making processes, and scope of action of both sufferers and physicians have been of central importance for the socio-cultural analysis of medicine for decades. A long list of scholars—including Parsons (1951), Freidson (1970), and Kleinman (1980)—have placed the doctor-patient relationship at the center of understanding medicine, and have described issues of autonomy and dependency as crucial aspects of doctor-patient interactions (Pappas 1990). While these are indisputably important focal points of medical anthropology in particular, many related studies have tended to perpetuate clichés and dichotomies in this regard. For instance, both scholarly writing and popular discourse generally consider patient agency and physician agency as two distinct entities (Gafni, Charles, and Whelan 1998). Deriving from this assumption, it is too often and too stereotypically held that while patients of biomedicine are uninformed regarding diseases and treatment processes, and are therefore passive objects, patients of so-called Complementary and Alternative Medicine (CAM) and of "traditional" or indigenous healing modalities are active subjects, because they are involved in, and knowledgeable of, therapeutic processes (Barrett et al. 2003). This is the notion that medical approaches in the West and in the East are diametrically opposed. It has become almost a standard view in scholarly writing that biomedicine alienates patients from their ailments, from the system of medicine they are treated with (Naraindas 2006), from the physicians conducting the treatments (Foucault 1965, 202; Rhodes et al. 1999), and from understanding or contributing to these treatment processes (Taussig 1980; Mol 2008; Sujatha 2009). While biomedical patients have been described as bereft of autonomy (Illich 1975), alternative systems of healing, such as ayurveda or siddha medicine, have recently been claimed, on the contrary, to encourage patients' involvement in diagnosis and treatment and a better communication between healers and sufferers. For instance, Sujatha (2009) has put forth the argument that patients' experience is important in diagnostic and treatment processes of siddha medicine, and hence its patients could be accorded a role as "knowers," not alienated from diagnosis or treatment. This raises the question of whether patients of indigenous Indian medicines are more emancipated and active as compared to biomedical patients in healing encounters.

However, binary opposites of passive and active patients may be clichés of the "West" and of the "East" respectively, which reiterate the stereotype of the cold, distanced biomedical doctor, on the one hand, and the romanticized picture of the Oriental physician, on the other. These opposites, however, do not suffice to describe and understand the dynamics of healing processes. Moreover, opposing different therapeutic methods in such a way reveals a high degree of analytic vagueness, since this approach assumes biomedicine to be a homogeneous practice and it also lumps together diverse therapeutic techniques under the labels of "traditional," "alternative," or "complementary" medicine. Such analytic imprecision results in dualisms, such as that of active–passive patients or physicians, or that of illness–disease, which do not advance our understanding of the dynamics of healing. Annemarie Mol (2008), writing on the logics of choice and care in Europe, has similarly criticized generalizing notions of active and passive patients. She has noted that treatment is a dialectical process influenced by the logics of choice and of care. Rather than assuming either active or passive patients, it would be more inclusive to analyze the "logic of care" involved (Mol, Moser, and Pols 2010, 9). In other words, in order to adequately understand healing processes, we need to recognize interactions between patients and healers as more complex than simple dualisms suggest. Taking into account the various agencies which influence treatment choices and healing processes also dissolves the problem of patients as active (subject) or passive (object). For Mol (2008, 18), care is not a transaction, but an interaction; care is not a product but "a process: it does not have clear boundaries. It is open-ended." I propose to analyze the particular logic of care involved in a form of indigenous manual medicine in Tamil Nadu, South India, in order to emphasize its processual and physically reciprocal character.

Diagnosis and treatment in vital spot medicine are esoteric processes, conducted "behind drawn curtains," without the visual participation of witnesses, and the diagnostic insights of practitioners are not normally communicated verbally to patients. Rather, *ācān̲s* claim to "heal the hidden," which should not, and cannot, be disclosed. Thus we may question the postulated idea of a "knowing patient" and expose the notion as a cliché, based on a simple opposition of East and West. The negative aspects of biomedicine are mirrored by their positive "other" in siddha, contrasting with that of patients without autonomy. However, *varmakkalai* practitioners increasingly utilize biomedical concepts and nosologies in explaining and promoting their therapies. Concepts like "spondylosis," or "prolapsed disk," function to give patients apparent access to what *ācān̲s* are doing, to understand their ailments and treatment procedures, regardless of whether these terms accurately describe those ailments or the treatments.

Patients of the vital spots may not be "knowers" of ailments or treatments in a discursively conscious way. It is, however, important to note that their mode of knowing relies heavily on nondiscursive and nonverbalizable practices of touch. Through attending to their patients physically, a somatic mode of attention as described by Csordas (1990; 1993; 1994), *ācāṉs* directly address ailments without any auxiliary devices, such as radiographic images, but also without much speech. This manual, body-centered therapy caters to the specificities of vital spots, which are hidden inside the body. They are therefore not verbalized, and can be healed only by the *ācāṉ*'s embodied skills, but not easily captured in language. The practitioner's hands and feet, on the one side, and the lived body of patients, on the other, establish an intimate contact, in the course of which diagnosis and treatment are conducted. This allows for recognizing healing processes to always consist of curing and being cured—of "caring" and "being cared for." As will become apparent, curing in vital spot therapy rests on this embodied communication between patient and physician. In the case of vital spot medicine, describing this process of situational and physical reciprocity advances our understanding of curing more than the active–passive binary.

A Vital Spot Afflicted

On the first day of my visit to Velayudhan's dispensary, the *ācāṉ* proudly showed me his small "ward." The first floor of the practitioner's house consists of three small rooms for accommodating serious or long-term patients. Two patients were currently staying in this ward, one being a middle-aged man. Velayudhan explained his ailment thus:

VELAYUDHAN: He has problems using his arms and legs, but currently he is making some improvement. He fell and injured a vital spot. Therefore he suffers from *pakkavātam* [paralysis], or "stroke."

ROMAN: How is *pakkavātam* caused and how do you treat it?

VELAYUDHAN: There are many spots in the region of the neck; if any of these get injured—hit by stones, while working, by a blow, or falling from heights—nerves [*narampu*] become blocked, and inhibit the circulations of *pirāṇam* and blood. You see, like in a machine, there is this current in the body, if this is switched off, it will stop working. So we have to provide its "current" again. This is done by internal medicine and massages; relief spots have to be stimulated.

ROMAN: This "current," what do you call it in Tamil?

VELAYUDHAN: It is the power of the body and life moving inside the body, called *pirāṇam*. We can feel from the outside the *pirāṇam* inside, that is, with our hands. But it is difficult to talk about this; I cannot talk about it because it is secret.

The *ācāṉ* then took me into the next room, where a female patient of about thirty years was lying on a wooden bench, her leg fully bandaged with cotton and the bandage drenched amply in medicinal oil. Two long bamboo splints tied to the sides of the bandaged leg immobilized her. Velayudhan explained that this patient had approached him twenty-eight days ago, after having suffered a complicated fracture of her hip joint:

VELAYUDHAN: The fracture is here, close to the hip; inside the hip joint.
ROMAN: How did this happen?
PATIENT: I fell while standing on a stool.
VELAYUDHAN: How is it now, does it hurt?
PATIENT: It's a little better.
VELAYUDHAN: Her treatment consists of changing her bandage once in three days together with oil massage. She has to drink a decoction as well. This can be cured within one *maṇṭalam* [forty days]. She'll be home in two weeks.

Nearly all vital spot dispensaries ensure seclusion of therapeutic practices, mostly by means of a separate treatment room for concealing vital spots and related techniques from the inquisitive gaze of bystanders. Thus, differing from the norm observed in Indian patient encounters, where relatives and nonrelatives are generally allowed to be present in diagnosis and treatment (Halliburton 2002, 1127), vital spot medicine is not conducted publicly. Indeed, despite Velayudhan having shown me around his small ward on the first day of my visit, it would be months before I was allowed to witness the treatment of a vital spot injury rather than being sent out of the room. Several persons came rushing into the dispensary one day, carrying an unconscious person. Judged by the commotion this group caused among the patients waiting on the small veranda of the house, a serious injury had happened:

PATIENT'S COMPANION: Where is the *ācāṉ*? Quick, we have a patient here!
VELAYUDHAN: Carry him inside. Put him down on the bench. What happened? (*In a loud outburst, everyone in the room attempts to answer this question*) Hey! Not all at once. Get out now all of you (*addressing one of*

the patient's companions, while everyone is heading for the door). You stay here. Tell me what happened.

COMPANION: We're masons; while working on a roof top, he slipped and fell on his back.

VELAYUDHAN: On his back? When did it happen? (*Simultaneously, the* ācāṉ *grasps the patient's wrist, examining the pulse*)

COMPANION: It must have happened about half an hour ago. We were in Nelluvilai village and came here immediately by bus.

VELAYUDHAN: Good. Now leave the room.

COMPANION: What about him, is it serious?

VELAYUDHAN: You've heard what I said, haven't you? Wait outside.

Having everyone leave the room except Velayudhan's younger student Murugan and me, and having palpated the patient's pulse at the wrist attentively for about half a minute with closed eyes, the *ācāṉ* began to slightly press different spots on the patient's back, while advising Murugan and me how to carefully support him. Again closing his eyes briefly, as if focusing, Velayudhan now firmly pinched with his thumb and index fingers at a point near the root of the big toes on both the patient's feet. This, almost instantly, caused the man to regain consciousness. Opening his eyes, he looked about confused:

PATIENT: *Ayyō* [expression of pain or surprise], my back hurts (*tensed*); I cannot move my legs!

VELAYUDHAN: Don't worry; I'll take care of it. (*While slightly pressing a point on the patient's chest, Velayudhan asks the patient*) What do you remember? Do you know your name? What has happened? Do you know who I am?

PATIENT: (*apparently more relaxed*) My name is Mariyappan. I fell from a roof while working. You are the *ācāṉ* of Chandrakavilai [Velayudhan's village]

VELAYUDHAN: Okay. You have fallen badly and hit your back. This is a vital spot problem, but you will be alright (*pressing different parts of the patient's legs*). Now move your legs. (*Patient moans in pain, but is able to slightly lift the legs and feet*) Good. I will bandage your back and apply oil; it will heal. You will stay here for some days, about one *maṇṭalam*. (*Patient attempts to object*) You will definitely stay! You mustn't work for some time and we have to renew your bandage every three days together with massage. You were lucky, but don't take this lightly, you understand?

The patient was admitted to the ward and I was amazed at his fast recovery; after two weeks he left the dispensary walking by himself.

Somewhat later during my stay in Velayudhan's dispensary, an elderly man came in complaining of short breath and pain in his chest from which he had been suffering ever since he had been dashed against a pole on a bus. Reading the patient's pulse, the *ācāṉ* pronounced, without asking for further information:

VELAYUDHAN: This is where it hurts, exactly here, in this side (*pointing to the lower part of the ribcage on the patient's left side, while the patient affirmatively weighs his head. Then, to me, in a whisper*) this is *aṭappavarmam*! If *aṭappavarmam* gets hit, water will accumulate in the chest. It makes one unable to lift one's arms, and to breathe. If not treated properly, blood oozes from the mouth, breathing stops, and one falls unconscious; it's a very dangerous spot. I diagnosed it merely by reading the pulse. (*Toward the patient*) How many days since the accident?

PATIENT: Ten days. And it is true, I cannot raise my arm and I can barely breathe.

VELAYUDHAN: Ten days have passed? Don't worry, I will give you a medicine; take this decoction from tonight onwards twice daily and return after three days.

PATIENT: Will my breath normalize? (*Velayudhan moves closer to the patient, pressing a point on the patient's chest*) *Ayyō! Appā!* Stop, that hurts!

VELAYUDHAN: Now check if you can breathe normally. (*Patient seems more confused about the pain caused at first, but eventually admits an improvement, nodding his head hesitantly*) After three days of taking medicine and massages, it will be cured. My student will give you the medicine, take it and come back after three days. Dietary prescription: do not eat potatoes, lentils, or tomatoes.

I had observed that *aṭappavarmam*, which Velayudhan had pointed out to me as the cause of the ailment, and the spot which he had stimulated were different points:

ROMAN: The point which you first showed me as *aṭappavarmam* and the point to which you applied pressure were two different spots, right?

VELAYUDHAN: Yes. One is *aṭappavarmam*. (*leaning forward to me, whispering*) That which I pressed is different. It's a relief spot, called *kūmpuvarmam*. If we press such a relief spot, it will correct *pirāṇam*. If treated in this way, every pain will be reduced. If practiced carefully, this is a great treatment. But had the patient hit *aṭappam* harder, or come any later, then it would have been incurable, and he would have died.

Another time, a middle-aged woman patient arrived with a complaint of being unable to lift her arm without the movement causing intense pain. After examining her pulse, Velayudhan expertly pinched the skin near her armpit. The woman winced at this unheralded operation, apparently writhing in pain and jerking her upper body briefly, as if trying to squirm free from the *ācāṉ*'s grasp. Already though, and obviously capitalizing on the patient's initial confusion, Velayudhan had grasped her middle finger, and abruptly yanked it. This caused not only a series of impressive crackling sounds, emanating from the woman's hand and arm, but again obvious pain, judging from her distorted facial expression. Nonetheless, when Velayudhan asked her to test the range of mobility of her arm now, a considerable improvement was apparent, as the patient was able to almost fully raise and lower her arm. After applying medicated oil on her arm, the *ācāṉ* sent the patient home, "cured," as he affirmed.

Having portrayed a few therapies encountered in a vital spot dispensary, I will now analyze the depicted modalities in detail.

Vital Spot Trauma, Causes, and Consequences

Since vital spots are the locations of the concentrated presence of *pirāṇam*, a trauma to any of them adversely affects the quality of this life force and its circulation within the body. In that event, physical structures, such as the *tātus* (the body tissues, including blood, nerves, etc.), and physical functions, such as the *tōcams* (the "humors": *vātam*, pneumatic, gaseous functions and processes; *pittam*, acidic; and *kapam*, unctuous), undergo deterioration. For instance, an injured "joint vital spot," *mūṭṭuvarmam*, located in the joints (*mūṭṭu*) of the arms and the legs, might lead to fractures or dislocations in the limb or joint. Whether the injury is apparently so slight as to be barely noticeable—the patients themselves might be unaware of it—or more serious, it will have created malignant changes in the body's circulatory systems of blood (*irattam*), nerves (*narampu*), and *pirāṇam* (life force).

As detailed in chapter 2, vital spots are nodal points, connecting different aspects of the body. According to *ācāṉs*, one reason why vital spots are vulnerable is that these loci are points that connect the three bodies (the gross, subtle, and causal body), and injury to a *varmam* may therefore affect a person's (anatomical, physical) body and mind, and even non-physical, *karmic* aspects of their life and soul. An affliction, therefore, may cause manifold ailments, not necessarily confined to the physical anatomy, *uṭal*, as in the case of fractures, but also delirium, unconsciousness, or memory loss, ailments that pertain to *maṉam*, mind. The most severe vital spot injuries are incurable and deadly, and hence take life, *uyir*. In an inferential conclusion, *ācāṉ*s argue that *varmam* ailments are also caused by all three aspects. Thus, vital spot injuries may be induced by a fracture or other physical trauma and impairment, but also by mental shock, for instance. Health problems relating to the vital spots may even develop as a result of evil deeds committed during previous lives. Admittedly, not every ailment encountered by *ācāṉ*s is lethal; headaches and back pains are amongst those routinely dealt with. However, body (*uṭal*), mind (*maṉam*), and life (*uyir*) can all be treated by stimulating or influencing the vital spots (Caṇmukam 2006), and thus many *ācāṉ*s feel confident of their ability to heal all types of ailments.

Possible causes of afflictions can be multifaceted. One manuscript notes the following potential causes for injuries in men:

> [B]lows received from an enemy, dashing against something, heavily exercising or lifting, stumbling, running for a long time or jumping and falling; engaging in excessive sexual intercourse, riding a horse or elephant, fracturing limbs when falling from great heights, hiccups, carrying heavy loads on the head when tired and practicing *cilampam*; hitting and striking.

For women, the same manuscript lists:

> [B]ending to lift water pots to the hips, bearing the weight of a heavy person in sexual intercourse, walking or running long distances on rough and uneven terrain, overindulging in sex, excessive pushing during childbirth, which causes a turning and dislocation of the womb, yearning for a baby if childless. Through all these, vital spot diseases can develop. (*Varmakkaṇṇāṭi*, 318–321; Mariyajōcap n.d., 163–165)[1]

1. See Chidambarathanu Pillai (1995a, 90) and Balasubramaniam and Dharmalingam (1991, 30) for similar lists.

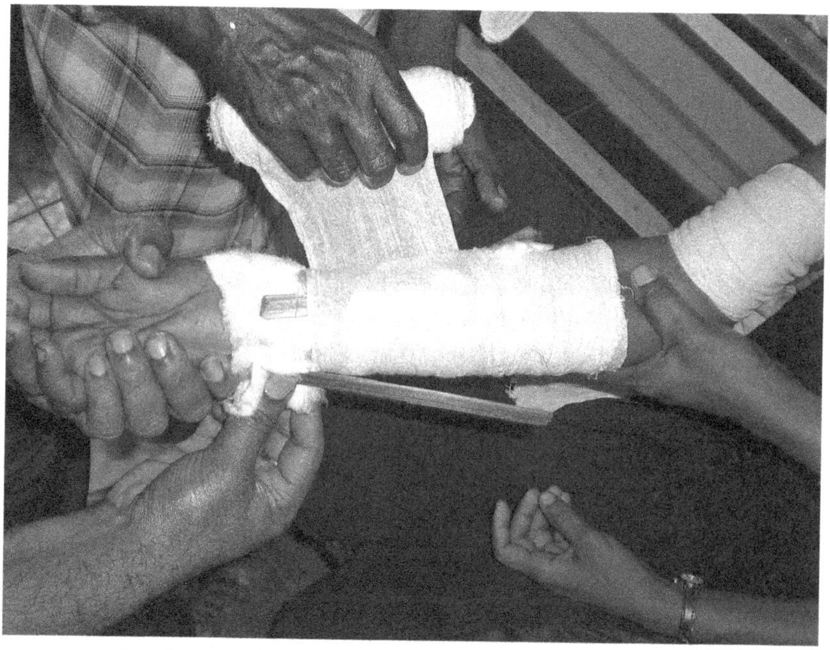

FIGURE 4.1 Bandaging a fractured forearm using bamboo splinters

Thus vital spots are particularly vulnerable to physical impacts and even a slight touch may be enough to affect such loci. As both physical *tātu* structures and the psychophysical *tōcam* functions are present in each vital spot, every injury will cause deviations among both categories. The opposite is true as well. A deviation in the equilibrium of the *tōcam* condition, that is, altered proportions of *vātam, pittam*, and *kapam*, may affect vital spots as well. Dharmalingam (Balasubramaniam and Dharmalingam 1991, 43) states that tuberculosis is caused by a derangement of the spot called *palaivarmam*, which might be affected either by an external injury or by a vitiation of the *tōcam* equilibrium.

Mending of fractured bones can be recognized as an important preoccupation of *ācāṉs* as well (figure 4.1), a fact, which in the past has brought the label "bonesetting" upon related practices (Zimmermann 1978). Yet from the view of the theoretical implications and scope of vital spot treatments, such a terminology is highly simplistic. *Ācāṉs*, mirroring this view, generally reject the term *elumpuvaittiyar*, "bone doctor," claiming their concerns embrace a much broader spectrum than is implied by that description. Thus, terms such as "manual therapy" and "manual medicine" seem to be more appropriate descriptions for vital spot medicine than "bonesetting," and are adopted here. As will become apparent, *ācāṉs*' diagnostic and therapeutic practices are conducted almost exclusively by hand—manually!

Therapeutic Practices in the Vital Spot Dispensary

Diagnosing Varmam: "Seeing" the Pulse

Upon the arrival of a patient at a dispensary, diagnosis is initially, and to a large extent, conducted by pulse examination or *nāṭi pār-ttal*, literally "seeing the pulse" (figure 4.2). In this respect, vital spot treatment does not differ from ayurveda (*nāḍī parīkṣa*) or siddha medicine (*nāṭi parīṭcai*). However, of the eight diagnostic methods, or *eṇvakai tērvu*,[2] utilized by siddha practitioners in general, only pulse examination and palpation of body parts (*toṭu-ttal, sparicam*) are deployed to

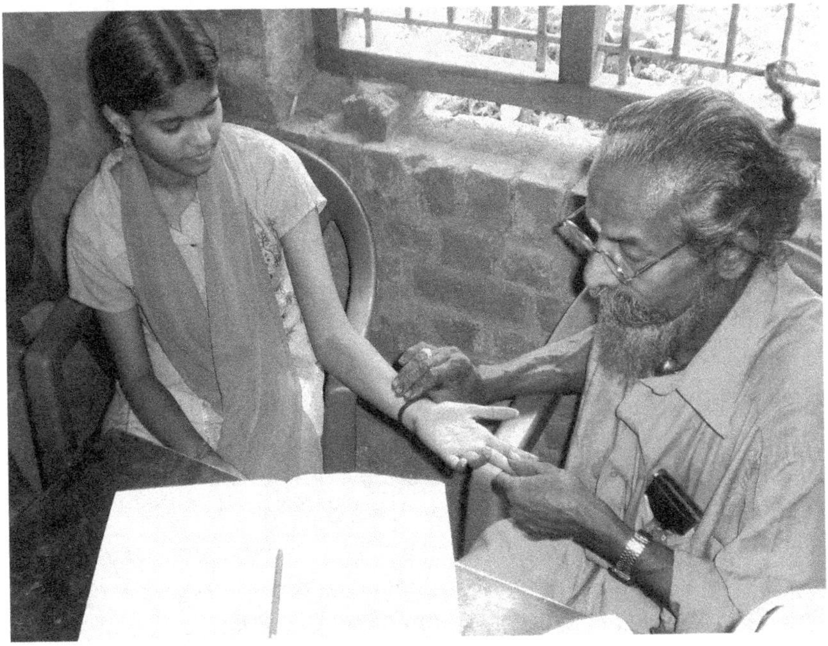

FIGURE 4.2 "Seeing the pulse": *nāṭi* pulse examination

2. *Eṇvakai tērvu*, or the "eight paths of diagnosis," consist of examination of a patient's tongue (*nā*); skin and color (*niṟam*); speech and articulation (*moḻi*); eyes (*viḻi/kaṇ*); excrement, regarding color and consistency (*malam*); urine, regarding color, consistency, and reaction to adding of oil (*mūttiram/nīr*); body by way of palpation (*sparicam*); and pulse (*nāṭiparīṭcai*).

diagnose afflictions of vital spots. Of these two, pulse examination is esteemed as the more sophisticated and of greater importance. Often practitioners claim to be able to diagnose an ailment by pulse diagnosis alone, and many do so successfully.[3] They emphasize their extraordinary skills in this, which allegedly surpass even imaging devices such as X-ray scans of biomedical doctors.

Ācāṉs hold that the vital spots are hidden, concealed parts of the body, hidden not only to the eye, but also nonexistent in the sphere of gross matter, and hence neither visible to modern instruments nor detectable via dissection.[4] Most practitioners therefore question the value to their practice of X-rays, magnetic resonance imaging (MRI), and similar diagnostic tools. Velayudhan claimed that one could not see a vital spot nor its affliction on scans, as these were not perceivable by the eye. He often refused to even take a look at X-rays which patients had brought from having been diagnosed elsewhere before their visit, stating, "Vital spots cannot be seen on that."

Despite the literal translation: "seeing the pulse," *nāṭi pār-ttal* is a hand-based, sensory diagnostic method, which does not draw on the visual faculty at all, but which consists of perceiving the pulsations of patients' radial arteries at the lateral aspect of the forearm below the wrist joint. Here, the three *tōcam* processes are felt by three fingers of a *vaittiyar*'s hand, respectively: the index finger senses *vātam*, the middle finger *pittam*, and the ring finger *kapam*. Examining all three at the same time, the condition of each should have a distinct weight (*eṭai*) and pace (*naṭai*) (*Varmakkaṇṇāṭi*, 310; Mariyajōcap n.d., 159). "Weight" in this respect means pressure felt at the artery, while "pace" means characteristics in comparison to animal movements. Thus, in a healthy patient, *vātam* should be one measure of weight and its pace like the stride of a swan, cock, or peacock. *Pittam* should be half the measure of *vātam*'s weight, exhibiting the characteristics of the walk of a tortoise or a leech. *Kapam* should be one-fourth of *vātam*'s weight and comparable to a frog's or snake's pace (Maṇiyaṉ 2012, 101–102). *Naṭai* animal descriptions thus appear as close to the similes of ancient Chinese pulse examination (Hsu 2000b, 321)—imaginative attempts to translate the tactile experiences of pulse reading into metaphors.

---

3. For an account of a siddha physician's display of pulse-reading skills, see Narayanaswami (1975, 30).

4. This is similar to other concepts of Asian medicines, a circumstance which forces practitioners to produce visible proof for their medical practices (compare Adams 2002).

Pulse examination in siddha medicine has been described as a state of equipoise between patient and physician (Daniel 1984b; Sujatha 2009). Not only is the vitiated *tōcam* detected, but physicians also have to become consciously aware of their own pulse while measuring that of a patient. *Ācāṉs* similarly attempt to modulate the pace and weight of their own pulse so that it will coincide with that of their patient, in order to experience a state of equipoise, by which they detect imbalances in the *tōcam* and the flow of life force within their patient's body. Increased *vātam* indicates an impact on a spot in the body's lower extremities. Prominence of *pittam* suggests an impact in the trunk or upper extremities, and an aggravation of *kapam* points toward an injury at the head (Chidambarathanu Pillai 2008, 56; Jekatā 2005, 22).[5] Yet there are also individual vital spots which, in the case of affliction, cause a particular *tōcam* to rapidly increase independently of the areas depicted above. Practitioners therefore have to attentively examine the pulse until they experience the state of *tōcam* and the flow of *pirāṇam* in a patient's body. I was told that in this way, *ācāṉs* conduct a thorough "scan" of the whole body, albeit a tactile one, thereby detecting even the most trivial abnormalities.

According to many accounts of siddha medicine, *nāṭi* pulse is felt in the right hands of male patients and in the left hand of female patients (Narayanaswami 1975, 31; Maṇiyaṉ 2012, 101). I observed however that *ācāṉs* are particular about checking the pulse in both hands of every patient, simultaneously or one after the other, so that they can compare both sides of the patient's body. The left hand represents the left side of the body and the right hand the right, and afflictions are diagnosed by noticing differences between the two. Similarly, *ācāṉs* probe with their thumbs the fleshy part of the hand between the root of the index finger and thumb of a patient's hand. This is done to check the blood circulation (*irattavōṭṭam*), a physiological process closely connected to the movement of *pirāṇam*.[6] If simultaneous pulsations and therefore a synchronized blood flow are felt in both hands, the circulation of life force is healthy. If not, persistence of problems must be assumed. An inhibited flow of *pirāṇam* or of blood can cause headaches, muscle

5. This is in accord with the "humoral anatomy" of siddha and ayurveda, attributing *vātam* as being concentrated in the body's lower portions, *pittam* in the digestive system, and *kapam* in the lungs and the head (Sharma 2002, 32).

6. Dharmalingam notes that *ācāṉs* may utilize "some varma natis on the back of the hand, near *kaulivarmam* [between index finger and thumb]" (Balasubramaniam and Dharmalingam 1991, 39) for diagnosis.

cramps, or back pain, or, in the long run, more serious ailments. Apart from the locations to examine *vātam*, *pittam*, and *kapam*, practitioners make use of *guru nāṭi*, palpated by the physician's little finger on a patient's forearm about three centimeters from the wrist joint. If a strong pulse is felt here, "life is strong," but if it is weak, "life is sure to depart," and I was told that in such a case, treatment is ineffective and therefore denied. At a fifth location, on the back of the hand, in the cavity between the root of the index finger and thumb, *pūta nāṭi*, literally "malignant spirit pulse," is examined by the physician's thumb. Whether a patient is possessed by the spirit (*pēy piṭi-ttal*) of a diseased person or by a malevolent god, for instance, is ascertained here.

Nāṭi pulse diagnosis is a highly complex process, requiring skill, concentration, and experience, as season, time of day, as well as the age and physico-mental state of a patient have to be taken into account (Maṇiyaṉ 2012, 101). It has aptly been remarked that "long practice is necessary, for this is more a subjective evaluation of the condition of the body than an objective one" (Narayanaswami 1975, 33). Pulse examination is therefore often said by hereditary practitioners of ayurveda and siddha to be too time-consuming to be taught in colleges. They accuse institutionally trained practitioners of being ignorant and incapable of understanding the subtleties of the technique (Langford 2002).

Sujatha understands pulse examination as an icon of an alleged fundamental difference of siddha vis-à-vis biomedicine with regard to their respective epistemologies or processes of knowing an ailment. According to her, biomedicine, being laboratory-centered and following strict disease categories, is comprehensible only to doctors; "the diagnosis, decisions about treatment and its evaluation take place in the language of experts" (Sujatha 2009, 77). This approach, she holds, excludes patients' experiences of their illnesses from the medical intervention in biomedicine. Pulse diagnosis in siddha, on the other hand, drawing on the experiences of both physician and patient, does not create a distance between patient and practitioner, nor between experience and knowledge or diagnosis, and hence not between illness and disease, according to Sujatha. Since the 1970s, studies in medical anthropology have distinguished illness from disease: the former describing sickness experiences of patients and laymen, the latter denoting doctor's or specialist's understandings and concepts relating to a condition (Kleinman 1980; Good 1996). Disease categories, however, have come to represent an objective fact, because they are scientific. Illness, on the other hand, is seen as expression of subjective experience, varying, and less reliable or constant. Because physicians may tend to neglect the subjective experiences, biomedicine has been charged with splitting off subjectivity from objectivity. Michael Taussig (1980, 8), for instance, has argued that the social relations that are signified in the symptoms of disease are concealed within the realm of biological signs. Biomedicine, he argues, denies the human relations embodied in ailments and their symptoms, thus neglecting the subjectivity of patients and creating a "phantom objectivity" of disease and biomedicine (3).

However, Mol (2002, 27) convincingly argues that it is time for social scientists to go beyond the illness-disease dichotomy. She stresses that diagnosis, in particular, is performatively produced between doctor and patient: in the consultation room, both physician and patient act together to jointly give shape to the reality of the patient's ailment. This diagnostic acting together of physician and patient can be well illustrated using the example of pulse examination in siddha medicine. In fact, this has been done before: *nāṭi* pulse examination, it has been argued, allows for a momentary merger of physician and patient, a state of "consubjectivity" (E. V. Daniel 1984b; cf. Sujatha 2009), since tactile experience is a mutual process, consisting of touching and being touched at the same time (Gibson 1966). In this sense, Sujatha (2009, 79) argues that in siddha medicine, "the patient is not merely an object of the physician's investigation through diagnostic equipment." The divide between physician and patient is neutralized and replaced with consubjectivity in *nāṭi* pulse reading as the siddha physician experiences the suffering and humoral imbalance of the patient, with the latter, according to Sujatha, being ultimately a "knower" of diagnosis and treatment (through what she calls "sensory knowing" [79]).

However, opposing patients of so-called traditional medicine to biomedical patients, with the former imagined as active, emancipated, and knowing, and the latter as passive, dependent, and kept in ignorance, does not much advance our understanding of the dynamics of the process of curing. Moreover, while it is true that siddha physicians try to gain in-depth understandings of patients' ailments by way of equipoise and skilled assessment of the pulse, the notion of emancipated, informed patients requires some examination.

Healing the Hidden

My first encounter with an *ācāṉ* was memorable. Acquaintances had directed me to Ramachandran, a practitioner living on the outskirts of Nagercoil. When I arrived at the dispensary, the *ācāṉ* was with a patient.

As I had not introduced myself yet, and since I did not want to interrupt the examination, I took a seat outside on the veranda. From here, however, I could overhear the conversation within. The patient, an adolescent boy, had been troubled by fever for thirty-two days, and his parents, who had come to accompany him, lamented that tests carried out in hospitals had not yielded any results. Therefore, they considered this ailment to be a "vital spot case," which was not unlikely since the young man had apparently been beaten up recently. Ramachandran physically examined the patient, who winced in agony under the palpation of his neck. The *ācāṉ* thereupon pronounced that it indeed was "[a] *varmam* [problem]" and that the fever would abate only after three successive treatments, for a total cost of 1500 rupees. The parents, surprised at this amount,[7] demanded to know what the treatment included. From here onwards, I cite from my field notes:

RAMACHANDRAN: Who is the *ācāṉ*? You or me? Are you going to treat the boy yourself? Why did you come to me, then? If you go to see a doctor in a hospital, will you ask him: "How will you treat?" or "What does this injection contain"? Certainly not!

PATIENT'S MOTHER: It is not like that, don't understand us wrong. My father was an *ācāṉ* too...

RAMACHANDRAN: Then let him cure the boy! If you know about this issue, then how dare you question me? The vital spots are a secret matter!

PATIENT'S MOTHER: We know about this, but would merely like to know how you will massage our boy, what you will do, and what it is that he is suffering from.

RAMACHANDRAN: Not possible. We are finished; now go [*pōṅka*]!

I was taken aback by the sudden and unexpected turn of events, and even more so by this practitioner's angry response to being questioned about his methods. A medical consultation had ended up as a dispute due to an offended ego, as I supposed. After all, the *ācāṉ* had virtually kicked out the parents together with their son, a patient obviously in need of medical attention. Besides, *pōṅka*, the imperative "go," is a form normally avoided when parting, as it does not convey the expectation of a reunion. Admittedly, in the setting of a physician-patient encounter this expression

7. At the time of my field research, 1500 INR equaled about $30 US.

might be considered less offensive, as neither party would desire a repeat visit, which a prolongation of the condition would necessitate. Hence, physicians may dismiss patients by telling them to go (*pōṅka*), rather than to go and come back (*pōyṭṭu vāṅka*), which is the standard, polite farewell expression in Tamil. This, on the other hand, would include a treatment. Ramachandran had not even attempted to attend to the patient, which appeared to me as utterly insensitive. However, the *ācāṉ* later told me that the parents' way of speaking to him simply had been wrong, and that it was not proper to enquire about the modalities of treating vital spot ailments. A patient had to obey and agree with him, otherwise treatment was not possible.

I must hasten to assert that uncompassionate behavior is an exception amongst *ācāṉ*s, who in general care well for their patients. Ramachandran in fact struggled to explain his reaction, saying that it was just not possible to tell patients, or me, what the ailment was, or how he would treat it. This he related to the nature of the vital spots, which, in his words, are a secret subject, potentially dangerous, and hence not to be revealed unnecessarily. Disclosure of locations together with stimulation methods of such vulnerable places might damage not only the patient but also the reputation of the practitioner. More importantly, there was no sense in explaining insights of his examination, the nature of the ailment, or the treatment, as these would never be understood. Vital spots, in this sense, are not only secret, because they are concealed by *ācāṉ*s, but also because they are delicately hidden aspects of life, graspable only by an experienced practitioner. Hence, in the words of Ramachandran, what *ācāṉ*s examine and treat is that which is both "kept concealed," and "[naturally] hidden" (*maṟaitta veccatum maṟaintappaṭṭatum*).

Radiography and Invisible Spots

According to some scholars, the development of diagnostic imaging devices has ensured the primacy of the sense of vision and of the eye and the image in biomedicine (Foucault 1973; Kember 1991). Soon after the invention of radiography by Wilhelm Röntgen in 1895, images of body structures and inner organs came to be considered as essential for traumatological diagnostics in Western countries. Usage of imaging devices moreover became important in distinguishing legitimate, trained physicians from unqualified practitioners, or "quacks" (Hinojosa

2004b, 268), and were therefore a reliable tool to discriminate orthopedics from bonesetters. But the use of such diagnostic tools in biomedicine "reveals attempts at making an 'objective' diagnosis through clinically isolating the medicalized site" (282), since it encourages "the idea that injury can be isolated, captured, and studied at a remove from the sufferer" (283). Michel Foucault (1973) famously termed this the "medical gaze." This approach has been noted to render patients' experiences, symptoms, presence, and even the patients themselves of secondary importance, subordinated to the images produced (Taussig 1980, 8). Biomedical procedure therefore determines disease and efficient cure by tests, "embodied in a techno-legal apparatus and situated entirely outside the felt awareness of the sufferer," as Naraindas (2006, 2662) writes.

Vital spot practitioners often dismiss radiography and imaging evidences, claiming that diagnosis of *varmam* ailments is an intricate and secret process graspable only by an experienced practitioner. Although they oppose the diagnostic use of images to their practices, *ācāṉ*s may use X-ray scans, which are frequently brought by patients who have been examined or treated by biomedical doctors before, to some extent. For instance, the black and gray insights into their patients' bodies can become documentations of the efficacy of an *ācāṉ*'s treatment. Before-and-after X-ray records of broken bones, subsequently mended after therapy, can serve a useful purpose, and often practitioners keep in their possession a number of such scans to testify to their healing prowess (compare Hinojosa 2002, 26). This happens as a way of archiving their therapeutic efficacy, as documents or proof of their medical legitimacy, not as supplementation of or surrogate for their diagnostic skills. Such techniques thus serve metamedical purposes, as is the case with social uses of diagnostic testing in India (Nichter 2002) and with the use of ultrasound in Tibet (Adams 2002).

Nevertheless, by emphasizing that vital spots cannot be seen, *ācāṉ*s tend to disparage the diagnostic value of imaging devices with regard to their practices. This is similar to Mayan bonesetters in Guatemala who, despite a partial utilization of X-ray scans, only moderately augment their diagnoses, which remain "hand-based," as Hinojosa (2004b) has pointed out. *Ācāṉ*s generally state that vital spots are hidden and that they can be detected neither by scans nor by the eye, since neither *pirāṇam* nor *varmam* is visible. Both categories can be felt only by vital spot practitioners through the use of their bodies.

Tracing the Secret: Palpating and Measuring Vital Spots

Palpation, *toṭu-ttal*, literally "touching," is another important diagnostic modality made use of by *ācāṉ*s. A practitioner's hands skillfully palpate the body surface, carefully sensing variations in the structure of tissues and vital spots. What *ācāṉ*s palpate is manifold, but it is generally stated that the surface of an impacted *varmam* feels cold to touch (Chidambarathanu Pillai 1995a, 69; 1995b, 12). This is because physical trauma at a vital spot causes a local blockage of *pirāṇam*, which in turn triggers an increase of *vāta tōcam*—the "wind humor"—or of pneumatic processes in the body. Externally, this can be felt as a localized coldness (*Varmapīraṅki Cūttiram*, 47; Nicivilcaṉ 2003, 50; Caravaṇakaṇēṣ 2009, 27). In fact, ayurvedic literature describes *sparśa parīkṣa* as examining the body's temperature. According to the *tōcam* deranged, a body feels cold (*cītala*) in the case of *vātam* being augmented, hot (*uṣṇa*) in the case of *pittam*, and wet (*ārdhra*) in the case of *kapam* (Sujatha, Aruna, and Balasubramanian 1991, 34). *Ācāṉ*s make use of parallel concepts: Fever may be caused if a *pittavarmam*, a vital spot predominated by *pittam*, is impacted. Cold sweat points to a *kapavarmam* being affected. As Velayudhan explained, if a lethal spot is injured, the place of injury feels cold to the touch. Neither patients nor unskilled individuals, however, are able to locate this. Only a skilled *ācāṉ* is able to detect such bodily changes, according to Velayudhan. As I myself experienced, discerning localized changes in body temperature is a difficult task indeed, a task that depends in turn on detecting *pirāṇam*, and with it vital spots, in patient's bodies.

In order to trace a particular vital spot after they have diagnosed an ailment, *ācāṉ*s may utilize different concepts to measure and palpate the body. Manuscripts mention several important measurement units for both diagnosing and treating *varmam*. These are thought to assist a practitioner in accurately locating a particular spot, since in many cases there is no mark of recognition on the body surface. The smallest commonly used unit is the measure of a grain of paddy, *nellaḷavu*. Two grains of paddy correspond to one "fingerbreadth," *aṅkulam*, or *viralaḷavu* (Jekatā 2005, 10; Shankar and Unnikrishnan 2004, 32). Next in size is *iṟai*, the length of the first joint of the index finger, which corresponds to one and a half fingerbreadths (Chidambarathanu Pillai 1995a). Ten fingerbreadths add up to one span, *oṭṭaiccāṇ* or just *cāṇ*, the distance between the tips of the thumb and forefinger when fully extended. Two spans correspond to one *muḻam*, the distance from the elbow to the tip of the middle finger, and four *muḻam* are equivalent to the height of a person (*Varmakkaṇṇāṭi*, 25; Mariyajōcap n.d., 14). The spot *koṇṭaikkollivarmam*, for instance, is situated at the top of the head, and practitioners, using combinations of spans and fingerbreadths, may set out from this spot to trace other loci, such as *carutivarmam*, situated eight fingers below. One span below *koṇṭaikkollivarmam* on the head's backside is *cīṟuṅkollivarmam*. The latter in turn is located exactly opposite to *tilartakkālam* on the forehead (Irājēntiraṉ 2006, 98). Some *ācāṉ*s can be observed to use these units and focus points to palpate patient's bodies. On the other hand, *pirāṇam* life force is the only reliable and ultimate guideline for tracing vital spots.

Kaṇṇaṉ Rājārām (2007c, 45) elucidates that there is not only a difference in the measurements used, but also conflicting views on the extents of these measures. *Iṟai*, for example, is defined in one manuscript as the breadth of a finger, while in others it is said to be the measure of the first joint of the index finger, or the breadth of the thumb; these constitute considerable differences in size. Many practitioners appear to have thoroughly internalized many loci, which they grasp without much scrabbling about. Velayudhan held that tracing a particular spot required long years of practice, and that an *ācāṉ* could never entirely rely on measurements alone, but rather had to "reach out and firmly grasp a spot." This is done by sensing *pirāṇam* concentration inside a *varmam*. In order to become aware of their own *pirāṇam*, and that of their patients, *ācāṉ*s practice different types of breath control or *pirāṇāyāmam* which makes this life force perceptible to them. This skill is required for palpating the skin, for sensing variations in temperature, and for detecting *varmam* loci.

Signs of *Varmam*

In the case of a vital spot affliction, a number of effects on a person can be observed. Velayudhan listed the symptoms of vital spot injuries to include:

> trembling of the torso; the Adam's apple pulls inside; shaking of the hands and foam formation around the mouth; profuse sweating, while fever spreads rapidly inside the body; the neck may pain and the head falters uncontrollably. Patients may roll on the ground; eyes staring, both hands clenched as if in agony. As soon as this subsides, both arms and legs will be moving; the mind will appear agitated. Then, the whole body cools down; the eyes turn red due to increased blood flow, yet remain closed. Blood or yellow-colored

mucus [*caḷi*] oozes from the eyes and nose. The ability to hear becomes defunct. Instead, the patient hears noises, like chirping crickets. The mouth will be tightly closed, but moving as if to chew. If the patient tries to speak, the voice will be soundless, the tongue swollen up and paling. The body droops, contracts, and shivers. The sensory organs [*jñāṉēntiriyam uṟuppu*[8]] become weak. While pain spreads through the body, the patient emits feces. Either he is insomniac, or drowsy.[9]

Judging from such signs, *ācāṉ*s detect the gravity of an injury, seriousness of a patient's condition, and possibly even an affected vital spot. Therefore, such symptoms are called "prognostic quality" or prognostic signs, *kuṟikuṇam* (also *kuṟivaṇṇam*), and are closely observed to understand the nature of the affliction. An affected *vātavarmam*, for instance, causes the body to pale, the limbs to swell up, the joints to pain, and patients to lose their appetite. In severe stages, flatulence, vertigo, hearing loss, and a gradual diminishing of respiratory functions may prompt fainting or fits. In contrast, if a *pittavarmam* is concerned, eyes blacken, limbs hang limply, and excretion of feces either happens involuntarily or, conversely, is obstructed. Tremors will trouble the patient's body, which will sweat profusely, accompanied by dryness of the mouth. Severe afflictions will, finally, cause delirium. If a *kapavarmam* is affected, patients tend to grind their teeth. At the same time, salivation increases, as does pain (Vasanthakumar 2004, 39). *Ācāṉ*s therefore carefully assess all symptoms to understand the nature of the ailment and possibly the place of the injury. Such can even indicate the chances of recovery, and inform about the curability or incurability of an ailment.

Curable or Incurable

It might be argued that a more fitting translation of *varmam* is "lethal spots" rather than "vital spots." Potentially dangerous to life, every *varmam* affliction has to be evaluated with regard to lethality or treatability. Thus, there are signs by which *ācāṉ*s estimate a condition to be curable, *cāttiyam*

8. The five sensory organs are: *mey*, "body" or tactile sense; *vāy*, "mouth" or taste; *kaṇ*, "eyes" or vision; *mūkku*, "nose" or smelling; and *cevi*, "ears" or hearing.

9. See Irācāmaṇi (1996, 26) for a similar account.

(Skt. *sādhya*), or incurable, *acāttiyam* (*asādhya*). Symptoms which point to incurability, that is, *acāttiya kuṟikuṇam*, are: heavy breathing, sweating and freezing of the whole body, rolling of the eyes, and emission of semen (*vintu*), feces (*malam*), and urine (*mūttiram*) (Irājēntiraṉ 2006, 318). The *Varmapīraṅki tiṟavukōl* (3; Nicivilcaṉ 2003, 52) mentions: "Eyeballs falling to one side, emission of urine, [and] feces" as "death signs," *cākuṟi*. Irācāmaṇi (1996, 28) adds that if memory is impaired, and if foam forms on a shivering patient's opened mouth, death is certain. One practitioner told me:

> Prognostic signs, from which we can understand if a disease is curable or not, can be seen in the way a patient behaves; he may make a grunting sound, or not be able to breathe. We can also ascertain from such signs how many days a patient will survive. If the pupils roll up, if only the white of the eyes is visible and the breath stagnates, then it is not only a sign of incurability, but of the patient's death being imminent! If water oozes from the mouth of a paralyzed [*pakkavātam*] patient, [the ailment] is incurable. If not [it is] curable. If the patient produces grunting sounds, it is curable. But if the eyes remain unmoved, it is incurable.

Some *ācāṉ*s hold that particular spots are by definition incurable, as will be any impact to them. Chidambarathanu Pillai (1994c, 46) points out that among the 108 spots, eighty-one are incurable, and only twenty-seven curable. For instance, *kapavarmam*, that is, vital spots related to *kapa tōcam*—the "phlegm humor" or unctuous processes in the body—are noted to be always incurable (*Varmakkaṇṇāṭi*, 313; Mariyajōcap n.d., 161). Further, after the expiration of the stipulated amount of time during which treatment of an affliction is promising, all vital spot ailments turn incurable, as described in chapter 3.

If an incurable situation is assessed by an *ācāṉ*, no treatment whatsoever is to be administered, but it is advised to send a patient away without administering medical treatment (Irācāmaṇi 1996, 25; Chidambarathanu Pillai 1995a, 69).[10] The *Varmapīraṅki Tiṟavukōl* (3; Nicivilcaṉ 2003, 52) cautions: "Do not venture to treat," and the *Varmakkaṇṇāṭi* (313;

10. But compare Dharmalingam, who states that "[e]ven an *asaadhya* injury can be treated successfully by an efficient *varma* specialist [whereas] if not taken care [of] properly even *saadhya* can be made *asaadhya*" (Balasubramaniam and Dharmalingam 1991, 45–46).

Mariyajōcap n.d., 161) gloomily states: "If [an ailment is] incurable, he is sure to die. Beat the death drum [*paṟai*] as his life is about to depart." To deny treatment to a patient is in stark contrast to the instructions of the *Aṣṭāṅgasaṅgraha*. This ayurvedic compendium advises physicians to treat *marman* spots even if recognizing an incurable situation (Fedorova 1990, 253). For *ācāṉ*s, however, an incurable case is not only one where treatment is futile, but also one in which a practitioner *must not* administer treatment. If treated nonetheless, Velayudhan explained, "in case a patient dies, this will be seen as the *ācāṉ*'s fault!" Relatives, in particular, often ascribe the death of a patient to malpractice, so to the *ācāṉ*, not to the actual injury. Regarding the reputation of a practitioner, no case at all might be a better reference than an unsuccessful one indeed and, as Sujatha (2009, 83) has noted, "in the event of death of the patient during treatment, there is a likelihood of the vaidya being beaten up by the aggrieved members of the patient's family."[11]

However, incurability does not necessarily mean certain death. An incurable ailment might still be manageable. Chidambarathanu Pillai (1995a, 76), for instance, relates that an injury to *uppukkuttivarmam*, located on the heel of the foot, will cause limping, irrespective of the severity of the impact and the treatment rendered. Thus incurable does not necessarily mean "fatal."

Signs of Death

Even signs which are not directly connected to the physical condition of a patient can indicate the nature of his or her affliction. These are called *laṭcaṇam* (Skt. *lakṣaṇam*), "symbol."[12] Manuscripts mention that if, for instance, a messenger, bringing a report of an accident, is seen "holding a post or pillar with his right hand or . . . the bar of the roof and standing on a single foot" (*Varmakkaṇṇāṭi*, 83; Mariyajōcap n.d., 39–40), an *ācāṉ* can ascertain even from afar that therapy is futile, and should refuse to treat a patient. Incurability of the ailment is also predictable if the people accompanying a patient carry tools, such as a spade (*maṇveṭṭi*). Likewise, a

11. Similarly, physicians in ancient China refused to treat patients whose conditions had been found to be terminal. Hsu (2000b, 323) assumes this as having been effective in maintaining a practitioner's credibility.

12. This aspect is not confined to vital spot treatment, but is found in many other prognostic/healing procedures in South Asia (Nichter 2008, 188).

buffalo (*erumai*) crossing the path of a patient when entering a dispensary signals imminent death, according to Velayudhan.[13] The same applies to a patient who is accompanied by his wife not wearing her *tāli* marriage ornament.[14] Such symbols are not recognized by all *ācāṉ*s, or may deviate substantially, since they are based not only on written lists or on *gurus*' teachings, but also on personal experience. In all cases, though, they are never communicated to patients, who may not be aware of such omens or their meanings.

While some practitioners refute the idea of dismissing patients on the basis of signs or symbols, I have witnessed *ācāṉ*s advising patients immediately upon entering a dispensary that they had "better go to the hospital and see a doctor." There, the ailment would be taken care of accordingly. I was surprised to hear this from one practitioner, who advised a patient suffering from a fractured ankle to go to a hospital in Nagercoil. I enquired if the *ācāṉ* honestly thought the patient was taken better care of in a hospital. The practitioner, Kanagaraj, was vague at first, but responded after the patient had left:

KANAGARAJ: Of course not! This injury cannot be cured.
ROMAN: Is it incurable?
KANAGARAJ: Exactly. Therefore I sent him away; you understand? No matter what treatment is given, there will be problems all his life. If I treat him and it does not heal, his family will scold me, thinking I am a bad physician. Therefore we should not treat such patients. If I treat him, he will rather blame me than his accident!
ROMAN: How did you find out it is incurable? You neither touched his ankle nor checked his pulse.
KANAGARAJ: Often this is not necessary. There are signs [*laṭcaṇam*], which tell if a disease is curable or not.

Upon further enquiry, Kanagaraj explained that he would never disclose a diagnosis regarding curability or incurability to patients or their families. "How is it possible," he asked, "to tell anyone that his ailment is not

13. This probably is the case because the buffalo is the mount of *Ēmaṉ* (Skt. *Yama*), the god of death.

14. The *tāli* is tied by the bridegroom around the bride's neck as marriage-badge (*maṅgalasūtra*), and is supposed to be taken off by a married woman only after the death of her husband.

curable?" Such an act would meet with neither comprehension nor acceptance, nor would it be in any way helpful, in Kanagaraj's opinion. For this and for similar reasons, *ācāṉ*s do not normally inform patients of their diagnoses regarding (in)curability of a disease, and this is largely true of most diagnostic insights regarding the vital spots.

Naming the Secret: Vital Spots and Biomedical Terminologies

Despite or, rather, because of such secretive behavior of *ācāṉ*s, patients often seek ways to comprehend and label what they are afflicted with. This is exemplified by the case of a young man who approached Velayudhan because of an ailment, from which he had suffered for several years. Already having been unsuccessfully treated by a variety of practitioners and medical systems, he had decided to consult the *ācāṉ*. The symptoms included a painful cough, and a constantly blocked nose, forcing him to breathe through his mouth, which he found very difficult. Velayudhan examined the patient's pulse and eventually pronounced that this was indeed a *varmam* (ailment), and accordingly treatable. The patient, relieved, asked the name of his disease (*nōyiṉ peyar*). Shaking his head in negation, the *ācāṉ* answered that this simply was "*varmam*." Obviously unsatisfied with this, the young man, mistaking me for a biomedical professional,[15] asked me to explain and name his disease, which, of course, I could not do. Velayudhan attempted to console the patient by describing that he had diagnosed excess *kapa tōcam*, which aggravated phlegm (*caḷi*) inside his body, causing a deficiency of *pirāṇam* circulation. Apparently still not satisfied with this, the patient continued consulting me, asking whether, among other things, this was a "sinus problem."

This case highlights several aspects: The youth with the mysterious respiratory problems attests to the fact that many patients turn to vital spot medicine as a last medical resort and in the case of chronic ailments, which biomedical treatment could not be cure. Nonetheless, the young man had not been content with the diagnosis of *varmam*, and reverted to lay biomedical categories rather than the one given by the *ācāṉ*. It appears that some practitioners recognize this and either concede and cater to the

15. Or, for a generic representative of the "West," or of Western concepts of health (see Trawick 1992; Nichter 2008, 169).

needs of their patients, or promote their practices in biomedical terms. With regard to ayurveda, Naraindas (2006, 2662) has noted that often in urban India "efficaciousness, and the very premises of the dialogue, are framed by the language of biomedicine or some pidgin version of it." There indisputably is an increasing deployment of biomedical terminology in order to address vital spot ailments and to promote related medical practices by *ācāṉs*. In particular, signboards of urban and semi-urban dispensaries depict lists of ailments treated by the practitioner. These often and increasingly include the nosological categories of biomedicine in addition to Tamil terms. The Tamil terms are often close or direct translations of biomedical diseases, such as: *taṭṭupitukkam*, literally "wheel protuberance," which appears to describe disk prolapse; *elumputēyvu*, "bone decay," referring to spondylosis; *elumpu tāpitam*, "bone heat," paraphrasing spondylitis; *taṭṭuvīkkam*, "wheel swelling," as translation of disk bulging; and so on. This may evidence a practice of promoting vital spot therapies in idioms borrowed from biomedicine. This may also be an attempt to provide options of verbalized explanations of vital spot ailments and treatments. Such processes of naming the secret in biomedical terms then are possibly aimed at patients, who seek to find alternative explanations of *varmam* than "that which is hidden." Moreover, in a field of diversified healthcare practices in India today, generally termed "medical pluralism" (Alter 2004, 182) the dominant frame of discourse, credibility, and legitimacy appears to be that of biomedicine and of its language (cf. Baer, Singer, and Susser 2003, 329). In fact, the term medical pluralism flattens out existing hierarchies between medical traditions (Lambert 2012, 1029). I suggest that "structured pluralism" (Mukharji 2007), "hierarchical plurality," or "stratified medical pluralism" describe the situation of hierarchies of credibility and negotiations of access in healthcare practices in India better than does "medical pluralism."[16] The dominance of biomedicine in this hierarchy is visible in biomedical nosologies, via which patients try to gain

16. Several researchers have observed the inequalities manifest in healthcare systems, especially with regard to plural medical systems (see Baer, Singer, and Susser 2003; Ram 2010). Frankenberg (1980, 198) even holds that "societies in which medical pluralism flourishes are invariably class divided." For India, Baer, Singer, and Susser (2003, 333) speak of a "dominative medical system." Broom and colleagues (2009, 207) note that "[t]hese romantic visions of plural medical cultures conceal social-cultural cleavages, overlooking (or even denying) the politics of human value and the restrictions placed on certain groups." Using the example of oncology in India, they demonstrate that health-seeking behavior depends largely on a number of sociocultural constraints and that the deployment of pluralism may act to conceal the structural impediments involved in healthcare.

agency and access to what their healers do. Practitioners, at the same time, partly subscribe to and perpetuate this dominance by adopting references understood in scientific and popular discourse, and by framing what they do in (what they understand as) biomedical terms.

This case is moreover interesting with regard to the fact that it points to patients as an important driving force in an attempt to produce a correspondence between biomedicine and other therapeutic approaches and in translating one system into another. Scholars have hitherto not acknowledged the role of patients to the same degree as they have emphasized the agency of professionals in this regard. Moreover, it is intriguing to note that, in order to gain a more involved and deliberate understanding, a patient receiving treatment from an exponent of a form of healthcare that has been described as empowering its patients seeks to resort to biomedicine, the therapeutic approach sometimes criticized as disempowering its patients. This case also cautions against perceiving biomedicine as a somewhat homogeneous practice or even system. In fact, what is generally described as biomedicine, and thus deliberately or unconsciously unified, may consist of widely divergent practices, techniques, and notions, of professionals and nonprofessionals, the world over (cf. Lock and Nguyen 2010; Mol 2002).

Healing the Vital Spots

If affliction of a vital spot is assessed and considered to be curable, treatment is administered. Siddha medicine knows two forms of therapy: *akamaruntu*, internal medication, and *puṟamaruntu*, medicines and techniques of exterior application (Subramaniam 1994, 128). Internal medication includes medicinal powders (*centūram, cūraṇam, paspam*), waxy substances (*meḻuku, lēkiyam*), herbal decoctions (*kaṣāyam*), and so on. External treatments consist of bandaging (*kaṭṭu*), bandaging of fractures using splints (*kompukaṭṭal*), ointments (*kaḷimpu*), medicated oils (*eṇṇey; tailam*), and massages (*taṭavu*).[17] Internal medicines are utilized by most *ācāṉ*s, yet external—mainly manual—techniques occupy a more prominent place in their therapies. These can be further divided into three categories: *iḷakkumuṟai, taṭṭumuṟai*, and *taṭavumuṟai*. *Iḷakkumuṟai* literally means "relaxing method" and

17. See Jekatā (2005, 27) for a list of internal and external applications. Suresh and Veluchamy (1983, 467) classify all the external applications mentioned here as part of *aruvai* or "surgery" in siddha medicine.

generally denotes emergency measures for reviving unconscious patients or for counteracting effects of a potentially lethal injury. *Taṭṭumuṟai*, literally "tapping method," designates a variety of manual techniques, by which particular spots are stimulated. *Taṭavumuṟai* denotes massage methods.

Emergency Treatment

Just as biomedical drugs and techniques are often understood as being highly effective in cases of acute diseases and injuries, Indian medicines are often thought to be of little value in emergency situations. Instead, they are regularly stated to be more suitable for "minor" ailments or chronic disorders (Nichter 1992; Naraindas 2006, 2663). Opposing this notion, *ācāṉ*s argue that they are not just able to treat long-term and chronic illnesses, but that they are equipped to deal with acute, severe afflictions (Irājēntiraṉ 2006). *Iḷakkumuṟai* indeed must be recognized as a kind of emergency treatment, which has to be administered as quickly as possible in vital spot injuries. This invariably includes stimulations of *aṭaṅkal* "therapeutic" or "relief spots." Etymologically, *aṭaṅkal* is derived from *aṭaṅku-tal*, meaning "to obey, yield, submit, to be subdued; to cease" according to the Madras *Tamil Lexicon*, and *aṭaṅkal* thus might be translated as "that which controls, represses, tames." Velayudhan explained such therapeutic spots in the context of a *varmam* injury:

> Sometimes a person falls, resulting in memory loss. But there are *aṭaṅkal*, which, when stimulated, bring back the memory immediately upon touching the right spot. Therefore, *aṭaṅkal* are places, which have the ability to subdue [*aṭaṅkiyirukkak kūṭiya iṭaṅkaḷṇā aṭaṅkal*]. The place which gives relief after a vital spot has been hit is an *aṭaṅkal*.

One *ācāṉ* referred to *aṭaṅkal* as a "main switch" (compare Maṇiyaṉ 2012, 180), which, after an injury, had to be flipped, so to say, as treatment measure; activating a specific *aṭaṅkal* subdues a vital spot injury.

The *Varmakkaṇṇāṭi* (5; Mariyajōcap n.d., 3) mentions several methods for reanimating unconscious patients, including use of medical substances, general body massage, chanting of *mantras*, and sprinkling of ritually purified water. But the most refined and effective method, this text holds, is revival through relief spot stimulation. Pressing such loci, using a specific hand and finger position (figure 4.6) or sometimes a small stick often quickly resuscitates unconscious persons. Velayudhan demonstrated several *aṭaṅkal*s on my foot, each causing excruciating pain. Revived by this method, the *ācāṉ* explained, a patient even regains memory and upon inquiry tells in which location a trauma has occurred. *Aṭaṅkal*s can furthermore be deployed for giving relief for various ailments, and particular spots may be stimulated according to very specific conditions.[18] Some spots, for instance, can be used to stop the blood flow in limbs; *maṇipantavarmam*, at the wrist, pressed for some minutes, inhibits blood flow in the fingers (Jeyrāj 2007, 78). Certain loci, some informants claimed, will mitigate the symptoms and severity of intoxication if pressed in the case of a venomous snake or scorpion bite. By decelerating the blood flow, such spots prevent poison from spreading through the veins, and thus provide time to administer serum, or to rush a patient to a snakebite specialist.[19] Govindan (2005) states that some families of practitioners specializing in dental treatments utilize *aṭaṅkal*s adjacent to the jaws, in order to suppress pain while extracting teeth.

Relief spot stimulation is at the core of emergency treatment, the general approach in which is to slacken—*iḷakku-tal*—or relax the body of the patient. Yet such relaxation refers for *ācāṉ*s to the body or parts of the body, but is not necessarily an aspect perceivable by the patient. It is rather inclusive of gross-physical and subtle processes, restorative of a state of equilibrium, which had been disturbed by the vital spot affliction. If a vital spot is traumatized, *pirāṇam* circulation gets blocked. Such a condition, and others associated with it, can be dealt with by "slackening" (*iḷakku-tal*) the afflicted vital spot, the blocked life force, and the whole body, by relief spot stimulation. This is the reason why this treatment is called *iḷakkumuṟai*, "slackening, relaxing method."

Velayudhan elucidated that symptoms of sprained muscles or numb limbs are sometimes due to incorrect positions during sleep. Nerves in unnatural poses were not straight but contracted. This inhibits blood circulation, which results in pain and reduced flexibility. Pressing the correct *aṭaṅkal* activates blood flow and straightens the nerves. Stimulating such relief spots has not only a direct effect on the blood circulation, but, with it,

18. Irājēntiraṉ (2006, 364) lists specific *aṭaṅkal*s used for different ailments such as: unconsciousness (*mayakkam*), fever or delirium (*jaṉṉi*), and for treating "insanity" (*paittiyam*).

19. Fedorova (1990, 349) reports that some specialists in treating poisonous bites use ayurvedic *marman*, since pressing these spots is believed to eliminate the poison via the body periphery.

also on the flow of *pirāṇam* and thus on sensation, mood, and so on. One day, Manikandhan, Velayudhan's student, massaged an elderly woman's hand, which was swollen and causing her pain. Under the pressure of the strokes the woman groaned and started to breathe shallowly, saying that she felt strange. Velayudhan stopped his student and ordered the patient to lie on her back. He stimulated a spot on the patient's left foot with circular motions, and this obviously had a relaxing effect, as the woman soon began to breathe normally, and finally continued having her hand treated.

In another patient consultation, a young man complained of chest and back pain. After having tended to and sent off the patient, the *ācāṉ*, Ilango, explained to me that *vilaṅkuvarmam*, located inside the clavicle notch, had been afflicted. He said: "This spot's connection is on its opposite side. After opening the spot on the opposite side, the problems abate." Both *varmam* and *aṭaṅkal* are "opened," *tiṟa-ttal*, which describes the correct stimulation of such loci. With the opening of a therapeutic spot, a corresponding, previously impaired spot is stimulated as well, and this effects the relaxation of this afflicted spot as well as the removal of *pirāṇam* blockage. Relief spots thus might be considered "keys" for opening particular loci and in fact are called *tiṟavukōl*, "keys." Often, when *ācāṉ*s stimulate such therapeutic spots, frequently using circular motions of their fingers, this is reminiscent of turning a key in a key hole. Just as in the case cited above, the spot opposite an afflicted *varmam* is the *aṭaṅkal* to be addressed in many cases.[20] *Naṭcattirakkālam*, located on the outer corners of both eyes, requires stimulation on its respective opposite sides in case of injury to either spot (Irājēntiraṉ 2006,116). *Tilartakkālam*, between the eyebrows, becomes a therapeutic spot in cases where *cīṟuṅkollivarmam*, on the back of the head, is affected. But not in all cases is the appropriate *aṭaṅkal* found on the opposite side of an afflicted spot. For instance, whereas *tilartakkālam* becomes an *aṭaṅkal* if *cīṟuṅkollivarmam* (on its backside) is hit, if *tilartakkālam* is affected, *cīṟuṅkollivarmam* does not qualify as a therapeutic spot, but stimulation of *paiyaṭaṅkal*, on the chest, is required.[21] Most emergency treatments require the opening of more than one *aṭaṅkal*. If, for instance, *kaṇṇāṭikkālam* is afflicted, spots inside

20. In *kaḷarippayaṭṭu* or *marmma cikitsā* therapies, relief spots are located on the opposite sides as well (Zarrilli 1989, 1295; Nair 1957, 22).

21. Opposing the notion of the opposite spot altogether, Dharmalingam maintains that "[t]he *varma* point nearest to, or those which are related to the affected part are stimulated" (Balasubramaniam and Dharmalingam 1991, 20–21).

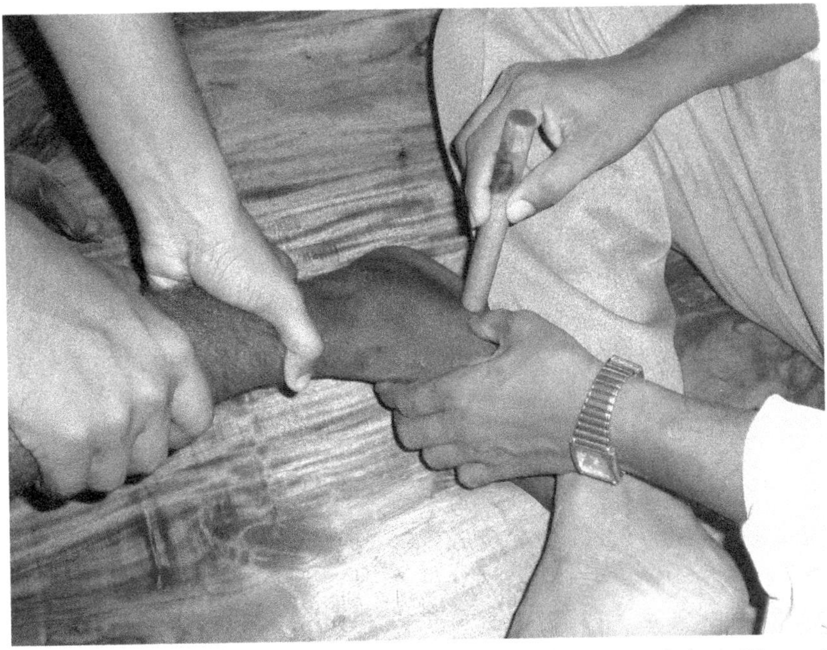

FIGURE 4.3 Localized stimulation of a vital spot using a wooden stick (*kaṭṭaikkampu*)

the protuberance of the ears and inside the armpits have to be pressed (Aleksāṇṭar Ācāṉ 1998, 59).

For each specific case of a vital spot being affected, one or several adequate *aṭaṅkal*s thus have to be known and correctly opened by *ācāṉ*s for counteracting the affliction. Practitioners hence cannot just press anywhere, as only the complete knowledge of vital spots and corresponding relief spots enables the therapy. Moreover, not all spots are opened uniformly, but have to be individually addressed by particular techniques of pressing, turning, or pinching, executed by hand (figure 4.6) or sometimes by instruments, such as wooden sticks or clubs (figure 4.3).[22]

It is important to note that relief spots are carefully concealed; their locations and usage are handed down within families or closed lineages of practitioners, who are reluctant to communicate any information about it to outsiders. Many *ācāṉ*s claim to know "secret therapeutic spots" (*irakaciyamāṉa aṭaṅkal*), considered to be most effective, yet unknown to

22. Some *ācāṉ*s claim to deploy needles or other tools for stimulating spots. Often, such practitioners argue that Chinese acupuncture originated from *varmakkalai* in South India. On the other hand, I have not come across any display of actual needling or any other kind of invasive stimulation of loci. Most *varmam* treatments largely consist of manual therapies.

other physicians (Jeyrāj 2007, 60). Even close relatives of patients are sent out of the treatment room when such relief spots are involved in therapy. The use of blankets or *saris* has been reported in cases of an *ācāṉ* having been called to the scene of an accident (Zarrilli 1992a, 40). Such covers are deployed to hide from the eyes of bystanders the location of the spots in combination with the particular way of stimulation.

When a patient is revived and saved from immediate danger through emergency spot stimulations, and blockage of *pirāṇam* is neutralized, *tōcam* processes and *tātu* body tissues still require restoration (Subramaniam 1994, 118). For this, therapy must be completed by internal medication and massages.

Vital Spot Massage

Continued treatment of vital spot ailments includes internal medication, but also, if required, bandaging alongside repeated manipulations of limbs, joints, and muscles. Such manipulation techniques take various forms and will be addressed here. Massage is called *taṭavumuṟai*, "massage method" (also *tokkaṇam*), and stroking and rubbing the body, skin, muscles, joints, and tendons is an important part of vital spot treatments, almost invariably conducted by using medicated oils (*eṇṇey*) or ointments (*kaḷimpu*).[23] These medicinal agents are spread over the whole body or the confined parts, to penetrate the skin and the vital spots (figure 4.4). This appears as parallel to the ayurvedic concept of massage (*abhyāṅga*), which aims to saturate body tissues with medicinal oil and to cleanse the body of toxins by reactivating the lymphatic system by means of friction (*utsādana*) and rubbing (*saṃvāhaṇa*). *Varmam* massage is furthermore intended to influence both the gross (*tūlam*), physiological structure of the body (bones, muscles, tendons) and the subtle (*cūṭcumam*) anatomy inclusive of vital spots and *pirāṇam*. Penetration of medicated substances and manual stimulations by the practitioner's hands or feet combine to relax (*iḷakku-tal*) a patient. For *ācāṉ*s, this means that both physiological, gross structures and transphysiological aspects recuperate to a healthy condition. Massages are offered as treatment for specific injuries or pathological conditions, bruises, dislocations, fractures, weakness of muscles and limbs, and also for restoring and preserving general health. Many patients regularly and over periods of several months keep visiting vital spot dispensaries for massages, designed to strengthen and straighten nerves

23. In a few cases medicated powders (*poṭi*) may be applied to the body.

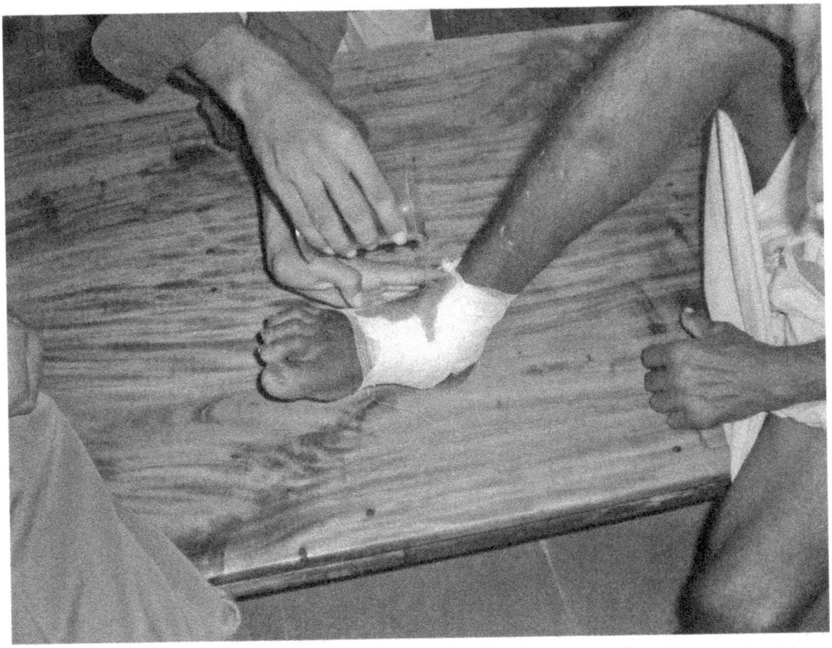

FIGURE 4.4 Application of medicated oil on a treated, bandaged fractured ankle

(*narampunīṭṭu-tal*)) and to relax vital spots (*varmattai iḷakkum*), in order to attain a "balanced" (*cīr*), normal condition.

Unless there is an immediate problem, like a fracture, in the area to be massaged, application of pressure is generally high, resulting in deep, intense massage strokes, which often cause patients to groan. The first time Velayudhan had me administer massage to a patient's back by myself, I was astonished at the amount of pressure I was ordered to apply. The *ācāṉ* directed my hands to spread oil all over the patient's back, and then to run my thumbs up and down the spinal cord, from the top to the patient's lower back.[24] After repeating this for some minutes, Velayudhan set me to execute the same strokes by myself without his guiding hands. Sensing that I was reducing the pressure, he urged me to use stronger, much stronger strokes than I deemed advisable. Velayudhan then realigned my hands and movements. Both hands flat, palms facing the patient, one hand on top of the other, I glided down along the spine from

24. Following Beattie (2004), I consciously avoid using Western massage terms such as "effleurage" or "petrissage" to describe these manual techniques in order to retain their distinct value.

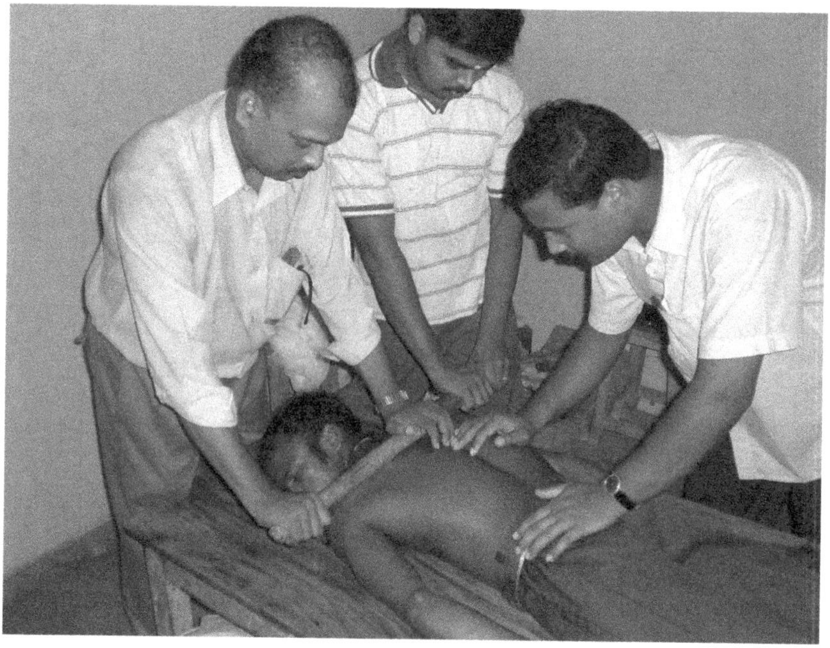

FIGURE 4.5 An *ācāṉ* and his students massage a patient's upper back using a wooden club

top to bottom. Next, in turning movements of the hands, my fingers spread wide apart, I was directed on how to massage down the back in a semicircular motion, exerting pressure in outward movements toward the sides of the back. Vigorous friction and the warmth generated over the whole back of the patient using both my hands ensured that the oil was fully absorbed. This kind of massage takes only about ten minutes, but is full of deep, intense strokes, focusing on the spinal cord, where many important spots are located.[25] Struck by the amount of pressure I was directed to use, I was surprised that Velayudhan complained of my "massaging like a woman," implying insufficient force in my strokes. I myself had experienced this massage, and had felt it hard to relax my muscles, which is often one of the prerequisites or positive effects expected by "Westerners" from massage. Rather, the force applied in vital spot massage causes receivers to wince or to tighten their muscles, sometimes in pain (figure 4.5).

25. Johari (1984, 17) emphasizes the importance of the spine for massage due to the presence of the *cakras* along this line.

Hausman (1996, 53) has remarked on the evidently painful vital spot manipulations, noting that children often start crying as soon as they are seated next to an *ācāṉ*. Painful sensations are involved in both localized vital spot stimulations and in massages. Patients frequently describe current-like sensations, triggered especially in several positions along the spine by such massages. *Ācāṉ*s explain the cause of the sensations as vital spots being touched and released (*varmattaitoṭṭu viṭu-ttal*), a process that stimulates *pirāṇam* life force. *Pirāṇam*, though invisible and normally not otherwise experienced, if activated by the stimulation of a vital spot, is made conscious and felt as a current-like sensation. Sambasivam Pillai (1993, 26) notes that,

> [*Pirāṇam*] is of the nature of the dynamic force of electricity and all life depends on it for its sustenance. It is the vital magnetic force absorbed by every human being in various ways; but it can be made flow forcibly under proper and favorable physical conditions. Susceptible persons will feel it as an electric current; because it is the life-giving energy in all things.

It is this very energy with which *ācāṉ*s are concerned. *Kaimuṭṭuvarmam*, "elbow vital spot," for instance, if opened, that is, stimulated correctly, causes a tingling sensation and bristling of the hairs. I found this experience similar, if not identical, to what I know as the effect of hitting the "funny bone" or "Musikantenknochen," in English and German colloquial usage, respectively.[26] On this background, it should be stressed that *pirāṇam* is more than "vital air" or "(vital) breath," though it is typically translated as such (Zysk 1993; Rao 1987), recently even as "oxygen" (Chidambarathanu Pillai 1994c, 12). Taking into account the explanations of practitioners and patients' experiences, it is better understood life force, or "vital energy."

In massage strokes, Zarrilli notes, *kaḷarippayaṭṭu* martial practitioners of Kerala transmit their own vital energy into the person being massaged. A requirement for this is an extraordinary control over one's own *pirāṇam*,

---

26. In anatomical terms, the "funny bone" is a nerve, "nervus ulnaris," not a bone. It is connected to tasks of hand and arm movement and to the sensations of the fingers. If this nerve is pushed toward the adjacent elbow bone, a nerve impulse is produced, felt in a kind of tingling sensation in forearm and fingers. Apart from *kaimuṭṭuvarmam*, where an analogy serves to convey the kind of sensation involved in vital spot stimulation, I have generally refrained from finding, or pointing to, Western anatomical correlations for vital spots.

which is acquired through austere physico-mental training of martial, medical, and meditative practices. When administering massages, this life force is experienced and channeled by skilled practitioners, and transferred through their own limbs into those of patients (Zarrilli 1995). Similarly, *ācāṉ*s direct this life force through massage techniques, using their hands, feet, or other body parts. They not only manipulate their own *pirāṇam*, but are at the same time susceptible to that of a patient as well. Controlling of one's own life force allows for powerful, effective massage strokes. Detecting life force in a patient facilitates an assessment of its circulation or blockage, by which an impacted vital spot can be identified, and an appropriate kind of massage chosen. Thus, *pirāṇam* control is an important therapeutic and diagnostic tool.

As Velayudhan reassured me, when I hesitated to put too much pressure into my initial massage strokes, even if patients groaned under the pressure of the strokes, this was no indication of wrong treatment. To the contrary, *pirāṇam* must be activated in such treatments, and current-like sensations or even pain are rather a sign of the correct application of manipulation than of wrong therapy. This mode of attending to ailing bodies demands some attention here.

A Somatic Mode of Attending to Ailing Bodies

Manual forms of therapy, such as bonesetting, though arguably underrepresented in the literature (Oths and Hinojosa 2004, xiii), have repeatedly been described as nonverbal, bodily engagements with ailing patients' distress. Servando Hinojosa (2002; 2004a; 2004b) speaks of "hand-based knowledge" and therapies in the case of Guatemalan Maya bonesetters, which allow for a coexperience of ailments and a bodily empathy between physician and patient. Such a mode of healing parallels what Csordas (1993, 198), drawing on Merleau-Ponty ([1962] 1996), calls "somatic modes of attention," which he defines as "culturally elaborated ways of attending to and with one's body in surroundings that include the embodied presence of others" (cf. Csordas 1990; 1994). For both Csordas and Merleau-Ponty, a person's presence and engagement in the world are primarily preobjective, preconscious perceptions that takes place in a multisensorial way. Conscious construction of any subject's world happens only after and on the basis of this multisensorial perception. For this reason, Csordas (1994) describes the senses and the body as "the existential ground of culture and self." Acknowledging such somatic modalities of attention and perception, Hinojosa describes how his informants physically engage with their patients. Maya bonesetters describe their healing knowledge as located in their hands, and claim that their bodies discover disorders by communicating with the bodies of others (Hinojosa 2004b, 265). Since the related knowledge is located in the bonesetter's hands, however, it is not subject to verbalization (Hinojosa 2002, 27). Diagnosis and treatment hence are a "body-based potentiality" (Hinojosa 2004b, 265), as patient's physical ailments are identified only via the bonesetter's body. This corresponds to how Elaine Scarry (1985) has described pain as an experience: it dispenses with any referent or object in the outside world. Precisely this "objectlessness, the complete absence of referential content, almost prevents [pain] from being rendered in language; objectless, it cannot easily be objectified in any form, material or verbal" (Scarry 1985, 162).

Moreover, Mayan bonesetters achieve "bodily empathy" (Hinojosa 2002, 28) with patients in various ways, as often practitioners are, or

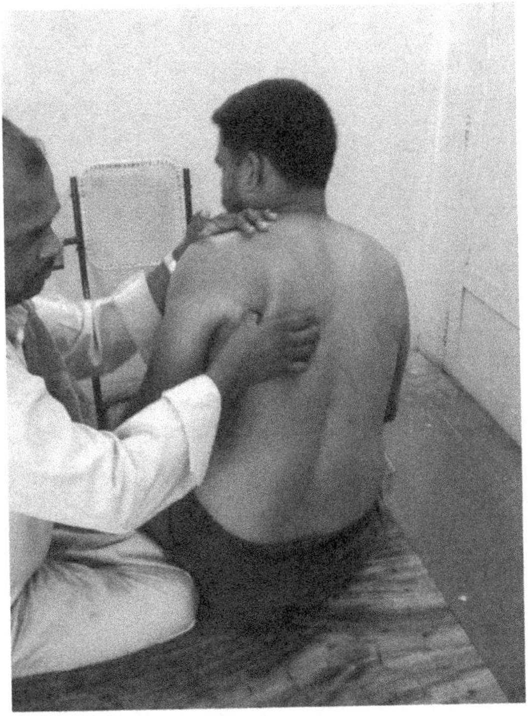

FIGURE 4.6 An *ācāṉ* opening a vital spot by indenture using his thumb

have been, suffering from ailments similar to their clients'. According to Hinojosa, bonesetters who coexperience their patients' conditions are better equipped to respond to bodily suffering. Similarly, Hsu (2005), writing on the infliction of acute pain in Chinese acupuncture techniques, argues that pain as a form of therapy causes an embodied experience of sociality. This contests the widespread biomedical explanations of the efficacy of pain inflictions as counter-irritation. Rather, pain creates a social and physical connectedness between patient and healer through sensory attentiveness, which, according to Hsu, can be therapeutically relevant. In contrast, practitioner-patient interactions in biomedicine, it has been argued, are characterized by distance and bodily noninvolvement; this particular relationship does not allow for reciprocity between patient and physician (Foucault 1965, 202). Biomedical doctors are said to avoid social involvement with their patients, and in the words of one of Taussig's informants (1980, 7), "don't feel the pain." Patients in biomedical hospitals therefore may be forced to interact more with copatients, who share each other's illness experiences (7). Patients, interacting with other patients, thus meaningfully tend to each other's illnesses, their subjective experience, while physicians merely care for patients' diseases, the allegedly objective aspects.

The observation of a sociality created through pain infliction may hold true for vital spot therapeutic practices as well. This is apparent from the induction of generally high pressure, which triggers *pirāṇam*, causing in turn pain, or a tingling sensation, strikingly similar to the painful, yet desired effects caused in acupuncture needling (Hsu 2005, 78–79). This is also seen in the way how "relaxation" is understood in vital spot therapy, which is different from its conceptualization in massages in the West. "Relaxation," *iḷakkum*, in vital spot treatments denotes a slackening of life force circulation and of vital loci. This kind of relaxation may even be combined with pain. If *ācāṉ*s manipulate spots, acute pain is caused, which, combined with its reduction and the ongoing care by practitioners, might be acknowledged as creating a physicosocial link between patient and healer. Voluntarily enduring pain at the hands of someone premises trust. Such trust forces patients into a close and intimate relationship with the practitioner, one that allows for the manual therapies administered, and also for enduring pain at an *ācāṉ*'s hands. Seen in this light, Ramachandran *ācāṉ*, the practitioner cited earlier, may have sent back a potential patient whose parents had queried his methods, not because of an offended ego, but because such questioning had jeopardized the treatment. Granting of trust might be seen as the social precondition for this kind of treatment, which involves physical intimateness, which in turn requires a kind of socializing and trust.[27]

An unwillingness on the part of *ācāṉ*s to discuss with their patients or with others the nature of an ailment, the position or importance of vital spots or of *pirāṇam*, or indeed any aspect of their therapy, stems from their own somatic involvement with their patients' bodies. They attend to ailing bodies while experiencing through a somatic mode the minutest aspects of the patient's suffering and its amelioration with their own therapy. These are aspects which preclude verbal communication. Without necessarily being able to communicate this verbally, *ācāṉ*s examine and attend to ailing bodies, experiencing how to treat, when, and when not through a somatic mode of attention.

When Not to Treat

As noted earlier, in emergency measures and massages, a patient's *pirāṇam* and with it the whole body is supposed to become supple and relaxed. Should this not be attainable, or if the patient's body is found to be too stiff, then massage and stimulation are not pursued, with the exception of emergencies. *Ācāṉ*s may deliberately administer massages during the morning and early noon but decline to do so in the afternoon and evening. During these times, patients are merely examined or prescribed medicines and advised to return either the next morning or after three days. Upon enquiry, Velayudhan explained this behavior thus:

VELAYUDHAN: Vital spot massage has to be concluded in the morning. From afternoon onwards, one mustn't massage. Of course, for any immediate danger to life, we have to treat immediately, no matter what time of day.

ROMAN: What happens if patients are massaged in the afternoon or evening?

VELAYUDHAN: For massaging a vital spot, the body has to be relaxed, which is the case in the morning, when the body and *pirāṇam* are relaxed. But in the afternoon both become stiff. Then we mustn't massage. This is so because in the morning *kapam* prevails and in the noontime *pittam*.

27. This is similar to the granting of trust as a prerequisite for a treatment and for an efficacious healing in the case of Nepali shamans as described by Pigg (1996, 185).

> During both times we can massage easily. In the afternoon, *vātam* dominates, making the body cool [*kuḷir*] and stiff [*muṟaikkum*].

In both siddha and ayurveda, the three *tōcam* are perceived to prevail in a person individually during particular times of day. During morning time, *kapam* dominates, during mid-day *pittam*, and during evening *vātam*. The first part of the night is again dominated by *kapam*, followed by *pittami*, and by *vātam* at dawn. In this way, the *tōcam* functions alternate every six hours (Rao 1987, 67; Chidambarathanu Pillai 1996, 40). *Ācāṉ*s hence have to be aware of the actions of a particular *tōcam* with regard to its effects on their therapies.

A patient's body can also be found too stiff or rigid regardless of the time of day. Such a state may be due to an imbalance among the three *tōcam*, on account of considerably aggravated *vātam*, for instance, which can render a body rigid. If practitioners diagnose this, they usually refrain from administering manual therapies, including massage. Instead, they may prefer to hand over medical preparations such as decoctions (*kaṣāyam*), generally of their own production, to patients, whom they advise to return only after consuming the medicine and observing dietary prescriptions (*pattiyam*) for three successive days. Due to the relaxing effects of medicine and diet, the patient's body is ready to be massaged after three days. In fact, when returning to the dispensary after three days, patients often feel relieved already, even before having received massage treatment, which is then administered to complete the cure.

Most patients, however, being aware that *ācāṉ*s mainly conduct manual treatments, only reluctantly accept being denied immediate massage therapy or stimulation of vital spots. Practitioners are often approached for their literal "luck of hands," *kairāci*. As patients perceive vital spot medicine chiefly as a form of manual therapy, they connect much of its efficacy to an *ācāṉ*'s hands and manipulations—to their "healing touch." Being sent off without having received a massage often disappoints patients who try to plead with *ācāṉ*s to relent and provide one. To one such patient, Velayudhan explained:

VELAYUDHAN: You need to understand that I cannot give you massage now. We have to treat your stiff nerves first, you see? Only after that will I massage.

PATIENT: But can't you massage me just a little bit now? At least apply some oil for me?

VELAYUDHAN: No, I can't, that's what I am telling you. Am I the physician or you? . . . Look, there's nothing I can give you except this decoction, which you must take for three days. After that your body will be ready for massage.

PATIENT: But if you only put some oil, wouldn't that be helpful?

VELAYUDHAN: No! Won't you listen? You have to take medicine first. If I massage now, your body might get damaged. We have to give medicine first, and massage only after three days. Do you understand? If there is anyone who treats you otherwise, then he is an idiot who doesn't know the vital spots. I will give you medicine now, come back after three days. You might experience strange feelings; that is normal, as your body and nerves relax. Don't worry, nothing will happen. Come back after three days and we'll cure you completely.

Frequently, like other practitioners, Velayudhan debated with patients who were denied an immediate massage and thus felt unattended, leaving the dispensary unsatisfied.

Conclusion

Of importance in siddha treatment and in vital spot therapy alike is the functional restoration of the whole body in the case of an illness. It has been stated that organic or physical processes, such as the balance of the *tōcam*, was more important in siddha medicine than the anatomical structure or particular organs (Narayanaswami 1975, 48; Sujatha 2009). Vital spot treatment modalities on the other hand show that physiological aspects of bones, muscles, and tendons are combined with transphysiological concepts of *pirāṇam* and *tōcam*. Vital spot therapy restores functions of the body by setting forth an anatomical structure of the body—albeit one which deviates from a "Western" anatomy—and by addressing it, combined with the *tōcic* balance, the circulation of *pirāṇam*, and the vital spots. For the same reason, these healing practices are hardly described comprehensively as "bonesetting." While *ācāṉ*s indeed frequently attend to fractures, various other ailments are treated by drawing on the detailed, theoretical system of the vital spots. Practitioners in Kanyakumari reflect this, by preferring the appellation *ācāṉ* over *elumpuvaittiyar*, "bone-doctor." They feel that their profession goes beyond bones and they take pride in reviving unconscious patients, anaesthetizing limbs, or regulating blood flow by stimulating vital spots.

This is not to mean that so-called "bonesetting folk practices" (Vedavathy 2003, 19) are fundamentally different from vital spot therapies, but rather that manual healing modalities in general are chronically underrated, misunderstood, and reduced to a few out of many current practices. This seems to be a global phenomenon. Touching in medical encounters and manual forms of therapy are much devalued in Europe (Van Dongen and Elema 2001) and North America, and are a reason for the lower status of practitioners than of physically uninvolved physicians compared with in other parts of the world (Hinojosa 2004a; 2004b). Human contact, especially in biomedical settings, appears to be particularly deprecated, and body workers, nurses, and manual practitioners are allowed merely for auxiliary status, not for medically authoritative opinions (Van Dongen and Elema 2001). Manual medicine does not enjoy a status that practitioners and some anthropologists (Oths and Hinojosa 2004) feel it deserves. It is far from being perceived as equal with other medical systems or procedures, its status being devalued by the authorities and scholarly research alike. Reasons for this include the prestige of the written word as against physical, embodied practices. Besides, the tactile nature of manual medicine partly impedes verbal and scholarly description and understanding. Furthermore, formal training provided in medical colleges and the use of technological devices are generally seen as more refined than manual practices, which are learned in a hereditary way and which do without expensive instruments. However, as this chapter has intended to show, such manual forms of medicine provide for a particular healing relationship between practitioner and patient—an important aspect which allows for reconsidering the concepts of patient and physician agency, and of the nature of healing.

Some scholars have argued that biomedicine alienates patients from their ailments, from the system of treatment, from their physicians, and from understanding or contributing to the treatment processes. But are patients of other forms of healthcare emancipated and actively involved in the medical proceedings? And is it legitimate to assume biomedicine to be a somewhat homogeneous entity on the one hand, and to lump together hugely diverse forms of healthcare on the other? Examination, diagnosis, and treatment of vital spot therapy are secretive processes. Neither diagnostic insights, nor disease categories, nor aspects of treatment are shared with patients. *Ācāṉs* claim to heal the "hidden"; *varmam* loci are not detectable by sight or modern imaging devices, but graspable only by an experienced practitioner. This serves to critique the romantic image of the "Oriental physician"—gentle and understanding—on the one hand, and of the corresponding patient—active and involved—on the other, clichés which have been expressed by scholars, healthcare personnel, and patients all over the world (Adams 2001, 558). Thus, the idea that the patients of (some) indigenous medicines are "knowing," "active," or "emancipated" is shown to be more ideological than actual.[28] Active patients of indigenous or alternative medicines may be a cliché, as may be the idea of the "passive patient" of biomedicine, bereft of autonomy. The fact that such clichés fail to distinguish the many different kinds of alternative medicine and assume that biomedicine is one monolithic entity should alert us to the fact that they are rhetorical, not descriptive. It is not justifiable to speak of biomedicine nor of "indigenous," "traditional," or even "complementary" medicine as generics when we know that these therapeutic ensembles vary from one geographical-cultural area to another, regarding the nature of medical practice, users, and patients, social policies, cultural practices, and so on.

Moreover, the binary of active subject or passive object exhibits a body-mind dichotomy with a strong mentalist bias, as conscious decisions, plans, or the resistance of patients and healers tend to be emphasized, while somatic circumstances, intersubjective and interactional healing procedures—conditions that transcend the actual healing encounter but nevertheless structure its proceedings—are neglected.

On the other hand, a crucial difference between biomedicine and vital spot therapy may be found epitomized precisely in the tactile, kinesthetic nature of techniques which *ācāṉ*s deploy and which appear to transcend verbal understanding and communication. While biomedicine treats and is concerned with static nosologies, with the "dead body," "the patient as an animated corpse" (Jonas 1981; Leder 1992; Sujatha 2009), vital spot medicine is concerned with patients' imbalances, and importantly tends to living, animated bodies. This is underscored by *ācāṉ*s being adamant on a *varmam* existing only if and where *pirāṇam* exists—*pirāṇam* being life itself. While, in contrast to an X-ray scan, the depiction of a broken bone or a lesion might theoretically exist without a patient, a *varmam* spot, or its affliction, never exists without living patients. Although I am aware of the danger of artificially unitizing both biomedicine and *varma maruttuvam*,

28. Some of the concerned studies are postcolonial ideological positions, and should also be analyzed as such.

in contrast to what has been argued about biomedical procedure, *ācāṉs* in general do not decontextualize their patients' bodies or ailments but rather attempt to grasp their very context. Ailments and patients are not being objectified, but subjectified, since *ācāṉs* do not look for universal norms or disease categories, but for individual states of health. Lastly, and essentially, while the professional understanding of the body of biomedicine is based on what has been termed "medical gaze" and is largely rooted in the sense of vision, the epistemology of the body in vital spot treatment could be described as a "therapeutic grasp," based on tactility.

Nevertheless, images of "active" or "passive" patients draw on clichés. The diagnosing or treating body of the *ācāṉ* and the diagnosed or treated body of the patient, allow for a more precise reflection of the particular type of agency involved, seeing the body as *body-cared-for* and as *body-caring* at the same time (cf. Van Dongen and Elema 2001, 150). The seat of this agency, both patient and practitioner agency, is the body. As argued by Marcel Mauss (1934), the body is at once object, tool, and agent. The mode of connection between all, and the object and subject of procedure is touch. While it has been argued that "the distinction between touching subject and touched object blurs" (Mazis 1998), this should not lead us to believe that there are no distinct agencies of healers and patients in vital spot medicine. As in other forms of healing, these are almost always asymmetrical and often shaped by influences outside the therapeutic encounter (such as health policies, licensing and registration laws, etc.). All vital spot techniques depend on highly intricate corporeal skills of practitioners, but also on the patients' physical presence. This does not mean, however, that vital spot therapy empowers patients or that it is an egalitarian exchange. There are distinct hierarchies involved. These are accentuated by specific techniques and diagnostic insights which *ācāṉs* (sometimes deliberately) withhold from patients and by the fact that practitioners often (have to) go against the wishes of patients, such as when pain is an indication of successful therapy or when *ācāṉs* abstain from treating. As this chapter shows, healing may not always involve the will and intellect of patients (or that of healers), but this need not lead to the conclusion that patients are unknowing, passive objects. Rather, as the analysis of diagnosis and therapy of vital spot ailments highlights, healing may take place to large degrees on somatic, multisensorial, and preconscious, nonverbal levels.

In the case of vital spot therapy, curing can be described as situational: this is seen in the diagnostic techniques, which in vital spot medicine are highly dependent on individual cases and on the specific situation of any ailment and patient. Curing is processual, as practitioners are concerned not so much with a general category, but with the state or process of an ailment, which drives the therapy. Curing is a somatically reciprocal intervention, as is highlighted by most diagnostic and therapeutic aspects of vital spot therapy, drawing as it does on *ācāṉs*' incorporated skills, tactility, and manual techniques and patients' physical presence and compliance. None of this is necessarily diverging from other forms of healthcare, but it is more informative than analyzing allegedly opposing and distinct agencies of physicians and patients.

Furthermore, as we see at the instance of naming *varmam* in biomedical terms and nosologies, such agencies can hardly be seen as isolated from broader phenomena such as the asymmetrically structured field of healthcare in India, which appears to be dominated by the credibility and language of biomedicine. We therefore need to understand subjectivity and agency as always socially embedded processes of intersubjective experience (Kleinman and Fitz-Henry 2007). As I have intended to show in this paper, this applies to the agencies of patients and physicians as well. Taussig (1980, 10) has emphasized the intersubjectivity of patient and healer: "Health care depends for its outcome on a two-way relationship between the sick and the healer. In so far as health care is provided, both patient and healer are providing it." The case of manual medicine in general and of vital spot medicine in particular draws attention to this interactive characteristic of curing as much as to its situational, corporeal, and processual aspects.

5

Virtue and Liability

THE VITAL SPOTS BETWEEN CONCEALMENT AND REVELATION

[In order] to be a secret, the secret cannot be disclosed as the secret it purports to be, but if the secret is not disclosed as the secret it secretly cannot be, it cannot be the secret it exposes itself not to be.

WOLFSON 2005, 2

FOLLOWING THE GERMAN philosopher and sociologist Georg Simmel, secrecy and concealment have been described by a number of scholars as a sociological technique, a fundamental social achievement and way social relations are built. Simmel (1907) understood secrecy as pivotal in developing, regulating, and dominating relationships through controlling the flow of information. Individuals or groups, according to him, always shape their status and relations through interactions defined by concealing, prohibiting, manipulating, or imparting information and knowledge. In this logic, secrecy has been dubbed variously as "society's way of explaining itself to itself" (Taussig 1999b, 161), as "ubiquitous" (Spitznagel 1998, 28), and as "as indispensable to human beings as fire, and as greatly feared" (Bok 1984, 28). Though apparently omnipresent in every society and relationship, the concept of secrecy is, where analyzed at all in scholarly writing, often poorly understood or remains as abstract as the above quotations (Marx and Muschert 2009). Scholars have rarely analyzed forms of performance and transactions of secrecy, that is, ways in which information is deliberately concealed, but also instances in which secrecy is communicated, enacted, or advertised.

In this chapter, I try to shed some light on acts of both concealment and revelation in vital spot practices. Some of the questions I address include: How is secret knowledge kept secret? How is it (if it is) sometimes revealed, communicated, or performed and why? What does such secret knowledge mean to its owner? And: What does it mean to those excluded from owning it? While I cannot answer all of them, posing these questions highlights the deeply ambiguous nature of secrecy itself, which, as I argue alongside others (notably Zempléni 1976; Bellman 1981; 1984; and Urban 2001a), is always characterized by a dialectic of concealment and revelation. Moreover, this somewhat paradoxical nature of secrecy inevitably constitutes simultaneously a source of power and liability for its owner.

Simmel (1906, 464) regarded ownership as the most important purpose that secrecy can fulfill. What is withheld from others appears as especially valuable, and the more restricted an object or knowledge and the less people possess of it, the more valuable it appears, he argued. According to Simmel, therefore, the *form* of secrecy, that is, its social expression and significance, can be analyzed independently of the *content* of a secret. The focus of the present chapter is this form of secrecy, and demonstrates that restriction of knowledge attains importance with regard to authority, legitimacy, social position, status, and hierarchy in the case of the vital spots. Secrecy may therefore be described as a source of power, or as a form of symbolic capital, to use the terminology of Pierre Bourdieu (1986). Such symbolic capital is translatable into other forms of capital as well. Into social capital, for instance, in the form of social prestige and a title, *ācāṉ*, as only a practitioner who maintains secrecy is considered a "true" *ācāṉ*. This, in turn, might be translated into economic capital, as only a "true *ācāṉ*" is considered efficacious in healing and therefore frequented by paying patients. As will become apparent, secrecy must be understood as crucial in practitioners' endeavors for legitimacy and authority, and evidently even with regard to (therapeutic or martial) efficacy.

Although secrecy may be acknowledged as a source of power, this always premises a partial revelation of secrets. Simmel (1950, 337) in this regard wrote that "what recedes before the consciousness of others and is hidden from them, is to be emphasized in their consciousness," an aspect termed the "paradox of secrecy" by Bellman (1981). *Ācāṉ*s too engage in a kind of advertisement of secrecy, a dialectical process of "lure and withdrawal" (Urban 2001b, 101). Although all practitioners emphasize the need for concealment, and secrecy is exhibited in restrictions regarding what to display openly and what to communicate to outsiders or even to patients or students, different "transgressions" in the form of public displays are frequent. Often, the same practitioners who stress concealment also dare to make certain alleged secret aspects public, including through martial arts shows, vital spot demonstrations, and straightforward disclosure of these alleged secrets. In fact, these transgressions are so frequent that they may be speculated to be a way of emphasizing that there *is* a secret.

Secrecy therefore appears to always only exist in partial disclosure. However, this oscillation between concealment and revelation produces an inherent and constantly reproduced ambiguity relating to vital spot knowledge and its practitioners. This influences the status of *varmakkalai* and of *ācāṉ*s, for whom secrecy is as much a source of virtue as it is a liability.

"Varmam Means Secret": Concealment of the Vital Spots

Practitioners frequently state that their knowledge is dangerous and therefore has to be kept hidden, concealed. The Tamil term *varmam* itself, like the synonymously used *marmam*, can be translated as "secret." A "*marma* novel" in Tamil is a detective story, full of mysteries and riddles. The Madras *Tamil Lexicon* ([1924–1936] 1982, 3506) translates *varmam* as "malevolence, spite, malice," and refers to *marmam*, which it interprets as "vital part, as of the body; ... secret" (3095). The Monier-Williams *Sanskrit-English Dictionary* (1899, 791) translates *marman* similarly both as "mortal spot, vulnerable point" and "anything which requires to be kept concealed, secret quality, hidden meaning, any secret or mystery." For my informants, *varmam* and "secret" were synonymous. Illustrating this, *ācāṉ*s often recite the *mantra*-like formulation: "The vital spots are [a] secret" or "*Varmam* means secret," *varmamṇā marmam.*

Why is this so? Irājēntiraṉ (2006, 28) describes the vital spots as "more dangerous than poison itself," by which he suggests that the related practices, if learned or used incorrectly, can cause many problems both to individual health and to society. It is for this reason that practitioners have kept this art hidden, from time immemorial, to foreclose potential misuses, most accounts state (Subramaniam 1994, 140). The author of the *Varmakkaṇṇāṭi* proclaims: "We have hidden [the art of *varmam*], so that it is [of help] to none but the worthy and does not become public. To prevent it from [falling into] evil [hands], do not give away this treatise" (2; Mariyajōcap n.d., 1). By the same token, many contemporary *ācāṉ*s are reluctant to transmit their knowledge except to the most trusted persons. The vital spots are kept within families: often teacher and student are in a filial relationship. Alternatively, the concerned knowledge is passed on only within lineages of succession, that is, intimate knowledge of vital spots is handed down exclusively from a teacher to a student, while the latter lives with and observes the former by way of an apprenticeship. Fortunate individuals who have become apprentices of an *ācāṉ*, are required to undergo a formal initiation, which includes vowing to the *guru* not to reveal the vital spots to anyone else (Jeyrāj 2000, 3; see chapter 6).

The Hidden Practice: Concealing Treatment and Martial Activities

We have already seen that concealment of practices finds a spatial expression in the layout of both dispensaries where vital spot afflictions are therapeutically addressed, and the training spaces for vital spot martial arts. Even in the smallest dispensary, at least a curtain separates a space in which treatment is conducted. Vital spot medicine is thus not conducted publicly, and observers, apart from patients and students of *ācāṉ*s, are only rarely allowed inside the treatment space. This space, which may be situated behind a curtain, inside a back-room or *séparée*, is called *uḷḷē*. *Uḷḷē* (*uḷ*) means "inside; interior," but also translates as "that which is private, secret, esoteric" (*Tamil Lexicon* [1924–1936] 1982, 470). This term thus parallels the Greek *esôterikos*, which literally means "inner," and which is the root of the English word "esoteric" (Stuckrad 2010, 45).

Textual sources on vital spots, such as the *Varmakkaṇṇāṭi*, advise practitioners to conduct treatment either after having sent every last bystander away, behind a screen, or in the confines of a separate room (7; Mariyajōcap n.d., 4). Emergency methods in particular, which involve the manipulation of therapeutic spots, should be done "without people witnessing" (6; Mariyajōcap n.d., 3). In the times of the Siddhars, notes Jeyrāj (2007, 7–8), when therapeutic spots had to be stimulated, "four students on all four sides had to hold blankets like a screen and turn their heads to all sides." Only then did the practitioner inside the blanket ring proceed to stimulate the patient's therapeutic spots. Contemporary *ācāṉ*s have been reported to utilize veils such as *saris* or bedcovers to shield their treatment techniques from the eyes of outsiders in the case of revival methods being conducted in public after an accident, for instance (Zarrilli 1992b, 3; Langford 2002, 214; Vasanthakumar 2004, 143). Consider an anecdote which Krishnan Vaidyar, one of Zarrilli's informants, recounted. This practitioner claimed that after several ayurvedic and biomedical physicians had tried their remedies to no avail, he managed to successfully revive an unconscious boy, who had fallen from a coconut palm:

> I asked for a sari and a bronze vessel. I covered [the patient's] body with the sari so that no one could see the revival technique I was performing, applied pressure to one nerve and the boy urinated into the bronze vessel. The boy immediately regained consciousness and I was given a gift of 101 rupees.
>
> (Zarrilli 1992b, 3)

Concealing Knowledge Toward Students

*Ācāṉ*s are known to carefully select their apprentices, and many practitioners decline to accept students or teach only their own kin, thus making transmission of vital spot knowledge, at least partly, a system of filial or kin apprenticeship. *Ācāṉ*s withhold their knowledge from those other than their own students. Often, however, even apprentices may deliberately be prevented from observing a particular technique or loci by being sent away—sometimes under false pretenses (Chidambarathanu Pillai 1995b, 27). One informant, Palani *ācāṉ*, narrated to me how, during his apprenticeship, his *guru* had repeatedly sent him off, apparently with the intention of concealing a particular technique or recipe from him:

PALANI: One time I was assisting my *guru* in treating a complicated arm fracture. After he had set the fracture and massaged the patient's arm, he told me to quickly run to the village and obtain bandage material, as the cloth for the bandages had run out. Back then, we were not using cotton bandages like today, but cloth. So I hastened to the village and back, bringing cloth as he had told me. But when I arrived, the *ācāṉ* was sound asleep, taking a nap.

ROMAN: What about the patient?

PALANI: The patient had long gone! Of course, treated and fully bandaged. When I later asked what had happened, my *guru* simply told me he had eventually found enough material for the bandage. But I am sure that he never had run out of cloth in the first place.

ROMAN: Do you think he wanted you to be away while he was tying the bandage?

PALANI: I am sure of that! It was a technique I had not seen before and he didn't want to show me. He frequently did things like this.

Krishnan Vaidya, Zarrilli's informant quoted above, in a similar vein elucidated that he would part with the secret of the revitalization technique he had applied only to his most trusted student and that, too, only on his death bed (Zarrilli 1992b, 3). Some observers have noted with regret that it is the habit of not revealing certain secrets even to the most trusted students which has led to a decline in the overall knowledge and efficacy of vital spot practices (Jeyrāj 2007, 7). Velayudhan explained that most practitioners had special skills for which they were famous, but which they often refused to share, even taking their secrets to the grave. In particular, the locations of spots or, more importantly, the particular methods of opening, that is, of penetrating vital spots, are transmitted only in a restricted way. According to Velayudhan:

> Most practitioners don't know all the 108 points. They will however pretend they do, but will teach to students only a part of what they know. Suppose someone knows 80 vital spots; he may teach only 20. The student is unsatisfied with this and goes to another teacher, who might himself know 70 *varmam*, but teaches only 40. Thus, the student has learned 60 vital spots. Like this, students try to increase their knowledge, while *gurus* carefully guard theirs.

Vital spots are subjected to a particularly high degree of concealment in all aspects related to vital spot martial training. Zarrilli (1998, 186) has observed that, philosophically, an *ācāṉ* is not supposed to attack at all and that for this reason all practice movements in *varma aṭi* start with a blocking posture, rather than with offensive techniques. Further, while practitioners teach their students various martial exercises, such as bare-handed blows, blocks, throws, locks, and weapon techniques, such as staff fencing, the actual utilization of vital spots is not part of most of the training, but reserved for instructing advanced and trusted students. Thus, instruction of vital spot martial arts consists of several successive stages, or forms (*muṟai*), in which a student has to excel before being allowed to proceed to the next stage, and *varma aṭi*, the actual instruction on attack and defense of the vital spots, is the last and final stage (Aleksāṇṭar Ācāṉ 1998, 5; see chapter 3). Hence, ideally, application of *varmam* loci in combat situations is revealed only to the most advanced students. Moreover, students are strongly discouraged from penetrating vital spots for offensive or defensive purposes. They often learn numerous defensive techniques which avoid any vital spot penetration. Such techniques, which are in the foreground of combat training, include locks, blocks, and throws, all of which are suited to circumvent vital spot applications and thus serious injuries.

All these behaviors indeed function to preserve secrecy related to vital loci and to the methods of their penetration. However, there is another layer and effect to such rhetoric. Secrecy regarding vital spot practices may, for instance, help to assert an individual mastery of *varmakkalai,* while it effectively impedes any scrutiny as to its truthfulness at the same time. Presumably, such concealment may not only be used for preventing a dangerous practice from falling into the wrong hands, potential incompetence of practitioners may be concealed as well. While I will return to this point later, it is important to note this particular kind of power which secrecy confers.

The Virtue of Secrecy

Several scholars have pointed to a connection between concealment and power. Elias Canetti (1963, 290) postulated that "secrecy lies at the very core of power," and he is not alone in doing so. Taussig (1999b, 7) has paraphrased this as "Wherever there is power, there is secrecy," and, according to Foucault (1990, 101), "[s]ilence and secrecy are a shelter for power, anchoring its prohibitions." Concealment has been asserted to convey advantages—economic and political ones, in particular. For instance, most scholars have described secrecy as a peculiar tool and privilege of the powerful, expressed in the *arcana imperii,* the secrets of the ruling, most often translated as "secrets of the state." As such, concealment has been acknowledged to protect forms of administration and governments, but also (intellectual) property.

Furthermore, scholars have considered the mysterious character of secrecy as something that has an awe-inspiring effect on others (Luhrmann 1989, 161). In the words of Simmel (1950, 338), secrecy is an "adornment" of the person who possesses secrets or claims to do so, and invests a person with a special authority. Such adornment, or covering, "gives the person enshrouded by it an exceptional position[,] heighten[s] it by fantasy, and . . . distinguish[es] it by a degree of attention that published reality could not command" (Simmel 1907, 465). Secrecy in this sense,

> [l]ike precious jewelry . . . or expensive clothing . . . is *a covering,* something which *conceals or obscures* aspects of the physical person; but it is also an *ornament,* something which accentuates the person, and so serves as a mark of distinction and prestige. The secret, like

a piece of fine jewelry or clothing, "radiates" a kind of aura of good taste, honor, and status.

(Urban *2001a*, 5)[1]

Such considerations link secrecy with power and legitimacy, somewhat similar to Foucault's (1988, 16) notion of a technology of power.

In this regard, Richard Weiss's recent study of siddha medicine, *Recipes for Immortality: Medicine, Religion, and Community in South India*, is of interest. Weiss argues, inter alia, that many forces, which transcend therapeutic relevance, shape the practice, legitimacy, and status of contemporary siddha medicine. This includes the rhetoric of Tamil identity and science, but also a discourse on the usage of secrecy. Siddha is known for its difficult-to-understand manuscripts, which promise long life or immortality through medical panacea, jealously guarded by contemporary practitioners who claim to be able to utilize the recipe. Weiss argues that regardless of the substantiality of such obscure recipes or siddha physicians' claims to hold the secret of immortality, the mysterious texts and concealments fulfill crucial tasks. Secrecy, according to him, is a means to put the claims of siddha physicians beyond the scrutiny of science and the scope of biomedicine, by utilizing an independent sphere of influence, that of tradition and the secret—being unfathomable and conferring a separate domain of authority (Weiss 2009, 161). This aspect is further explored in the following sections, as the vital spots may be viewed in this light as well: as being concealed and hence protected from the scrutiny of "science" and biomedicine.

X-ray Scans and "Seeing an Ailment"

Vital spot *ācāṉ*s in Kanyakumari describe their therapeutic practices as opposed to conventional biomedical theories and procedures. Their perspective is that the latter are costly and dangerous, often requiring risky surgical interventions. Vital spot medicine, on the other hand, is cheap, without side-effects, and often obviates invasive operations, they argue. According to most *ācāṉ*s, the reasons for such shortcomings of biomedicine are found precisely in its neglect of the subtleties of the vital spots (Chidambarathanu Pillai 2008, 57). This can be best described using the

1. Or, as Johnson (2002, 4) puts it: "Secrets are to religion what lingerie is to the body; they enhance what is imagined to be present."

example of vital spot diagnostics. *Ācāṉs*, due to the manual modes of diagnosing and treating vital spots, draw largely on somatic or sensory techniques. Many practitioners completely dispense with X-ray scans. More important is the discourse in relation to imaging devices, in which *varmakkalai* is portrayed as unknown to biomedicine, anatomy, and the allied sciences, and the vital spots as undetectable by the auxiliary diagnostic tools on which the former rely, but only graspable by a skilled *ācāṉ*. In this way, *ācāṉ*s place their practice above the grasp and scrutiny of science and of biomedicine. Vital spot practitioners precisely attend to that which is hidden, secret, and therefore eluding the clinical gaze of biomedicine.

Vital spot practitioners frequently express their view that biomedical doctors do not understand vital spot related ailments. Velayudhan one day received a ten-year-old boy, accompanied by his parents, who complained about knee pains:

VELAYUDHAN: Come, sit down. What is it?

PATIENT'S FATHER: Our son has pain in his legs, he can barely walk. We don't know why.

VELAYUDHAN: (*while examining the patient's pulse*) When did the pain first appear?

PATIENT'S MOTHER: About one month ago.

VELAYUDHAN: When does it hurt the most?

PATIENT: When riding a bicycle.

VELAYUDHAN: Here, in the knee is a big vital spot. If there is any problem, it'll cause pain and limping.

FATHER: Yes, he does limp. They told us to have an operation.

VELAYUDHAN: "They" means in a hospital, right? I tell you: no operation is needed. Above all, any operation would be wrong! Where does it hurt, in both knees?

PATIENT: In both knees.

VELAYUDHAN: Does it hurt here? (*pressing slightly on the knee with one finger*)

PATIENT: It hurts.

VELAYUDHAN: (*presses further around the knee*) Is the pain less now?

PATIENT: Yes.

VELAYUDHAN: I will give you some medicine and after a few days, we will start massages. Don't worry, if you strictly observe the dietary prescriptions you will be fine—without operation.

When the patient and his parents had left after having agreed to try Velayudhan's treatment, the *ācāṉ* explained to me that typically, and too often, patients were told to undergo surgery in biomedical hospitals, even for ailments where this was not required at all. Such operations were even dangerous to the vital spots and many of his patients saw him precisely for past malpractices or surgical complications. Velayudhan lamented:

> You know what a [biomedical] doctor does? He takes an X-ray [scan]. Of course, he can see nothing there. Without detecting the disease, he orders an operation, because he doesn't understand what the cause is! That is not medicine. And how expensive it is: scans, surgery, and so on! Even though the patients always say, "He [the biomedical doctor] took care of me very well!" But they come to me afterwards with a stiff leg or hand.

One vital spot practitioner writes that vital spot ailments are "a blind area for the modern medical world" (Citamparatāṇuppiḷḷai 1991, 35). Despite all instruments biomedical doctors were neither able to detect, nor find effective remedies for, vital spot inflictions, this author suggests. Most *ācāṉ*s ascribe this to the fact that "the impact of Varmam . . . and diseases arising therefrom are beyond the reach of scientific knowledge" (Chidambarathanu Pillai 1994b, 18).

One *ācāṉ* informant, evidently addressing me as a representative of the West,[2] said, "Your science does not see *varmam*." Seeing, in this sense, is not to be understood in its restricted form as visual perception, but rather as a faculty of comprehension. This, in vital spot diagnostics, is exemplified in pulse examination, *nāṭi pār-ttal*, literally "seeing the pulse." Despite its name, pulse diagnosis is a tactile process of palpating a patient's pulse with the fingers, during which a physician is said to comprehend the nature of an ailment and how to treat (E. V. Daniel 1984b; Sujatha 2009, chapter 5). The practitioner was adamant that *varmam* was neglected by "science," as it was secret. He stated, "In every body, there are secret circulations [*marmamāṉa iyakkaṅkaḷ*]. Connected to these are the vital spots. But these do not exist for your science!" Indeed, I was repeatedly told by *ācāṉ*s that vital spots were hidden and could neither be detected by means

2. Nichter (2008) and Trawick (1992) have similarly observed how the ethnographer may be addressed as a representative of the "West."

of the eyes, nor depicted by images, and that was why *varmam* loci did not appear on X-ray scans. The cited practitioner therefore concluded that vital spots did not exist for such a science.

*Ācāṉ*s are engaged with precisely these loci, which exist in a nonvisible sphere, being elusive to the eye, and which can be grasped only in its physical sense. For this reason imaging devices and scans are deemed useless by many hereditary practitioners of the vital spots. Velayudhan often replied to patients who brought radiographic images of fractures from biomedical practices by saying: "I can see nothing on that! Vital spots cannot be seen." *Ācāṉ*s stress that no auxiliary device or instrument other than their tactile sensations can detect an affliction of the vital spots. Not even the most advanced methods and technical innovations of CT scans or MRI scans had the slightest chance of conveying a picture of the *varmam* loci, which are, in this sense, hidden, secret.

The development of graphic methods of diagnostics such as radiography may have ensured the primacy of the sense of vision and the image in biomedicine (Kember 1991; Stafford 1991), or the "medical gaze" (Foucault 1973). Soon after the invention of radiography by Wilhelm Röntgen in 1895, body images came to be considered as essential, especially for traumatological diagnostics. X-rays became, moreover, an important tool for distinguishing legitimate, trained practitioners from unqualified practitioners or quacks—orthopedists from bonesetters, to be precise—in Europe and North America (Hinojosa 2004b, 268). The use of sophisticated diagnostic technology, especially that drawing on the visual faculty, is still regarded as one of the hallmarks and indication of "qualified" practice (Hinojosa 2004b; Prasad 2005). Biomedical doctors in Kanyakumari may criticize *ācāṉ*s on the ground of their disregard of imaging devices, or their incompetence in understanding them. Comprehensive utilization of radiography in South India still largely divides institutionally from noninstitutionally trained medical practitioners. In contrast to biomedical doctors, *ācāṉ*s essentially rely on their hands, and examine ailments mainly by sensing a patient's *nāṭi* pulse, and by palpating the body surface, through which the state of vital spots and *pirāṇam* life force are discerned. It may be speculated that the idiom used to express their diagnostic faculties has been influenced by the biomedical emphasis on the visual and technological: Hinojosa (2004b, 278) has described Mayan bonesetters, who liken their hands to X-ray machines. *Ācāṉ*s similarly compare their examination to "scan or scanning," or claim that their hands are better than any X-ray machine.

However, while orthopedic professionals have interpreted the neglect of imaging devices as a lack of formal education on the part of vital spot practitioners (Shah et al. 2003; Onuminya 2004; Salati and Rather 2009), *ācāṉ*s turn the tables in this regard. According to them, it is biomedicine which lacks efficacy and competence with regard to the vital spots, since it ultimately fails to diagnose and treat *varmam* afflictions in spite of refined techniques and instruments. *Ācāṉ*s achieve what doctors cannot: detecting vital spots and curing diseases associated with them (Irācāmaṇi 1996, 38). Such a notion, it should be noted, is typical for siddha medicine in general:

> Everybody wonders how it was possible in those primitive days when modern science had not developed. Without any laboratory or microscope [the Siddhars] had invented [*sic*] several facts about human organism, its ailments and their remedy. It was possible only due to their super human powers attained through yogic practices. A yogi through his "gnanam" [*ñāṉam*, wisdom] can penetrate into anything and know everything about it.
>
> (Natarajan 1984, 117)

As in the case of the ancient Siddhars, *ācāṉ*s claim that only austere learning and meditation generate the ability to understand the subtle connections of the vital spots, an ability that cannot be achieved through formal instruction in medical colleges. Therefore, practitioners argue that vital spot diagnosis and therapy transcend the efficacy and realm of biomedicine altogether. In contrast, *ācāṉ*s highlight their own therapeutic efficacy, which is characterized by being quick, cost-effective, and ultimately refined, without having to rely on any techniques or instruments. Following this logic, it is the very ignorance of *varmam* which makes biomedicine expensive, invasive, circuitous, and dangerous to patients' health.

Weiss (2009, 71) writes that "Vaidyas [physicians] often speak of the siddhar's skills of intuition in physiological terms" and that "[t]he deficiencies of science are exposed in the superior faculties available to the siddhars, faculties that enable knowledge of the universe beyond the imagination of scientists." One such physiological skill available to *ācāṉ*s, which is perceived as exposing the deficiencies of science, is the knowledge of how to detect the vital spots, which elude the clinical gaze of biomedical analysis. But it is important to emphasize that secrecy plays a crucial role for *ācāṉ*s in claiming this skill. Only an *ācāṉ* is enlightened to the locations, intricacies, ailments, and treatment modalities of *varmam*, while these remain a mystery and secret to biomedicine and other medical systems. To the latter, the vital spots have not been revealed. One practitioner laments: "Modern scientists do not know this secret [of the vital spots], and yet they dare to [criticize] the indigenous system of medical treatment as unscientific" (Chidambarathanu Pillai 2008, 57). As such, secrecy can be a powerful tool in the struggle for the therapeutic legitimacy of *ācāṉs*.

Ācāṉs, who relinquish most auxiliary devices but rely on their somatic skills, must respond to the criticism from biomedical doctors, who appear to be suspicious of the nonstandardized and exclusively manual practices. It is thus the highly competitive medical field in contemporary South India, characterized by a plurality of healthcare modalities, that governs discourses on healing legitimacies. Especially the "hegemony of biomedicine in modern India," asserted by Alter (2004, 182; 2005b; also Sax 2009, 243; Sax 2010; Sax and Quack 2010), and related notions of science, must be seen as conditioning the discursive importance of claims of secret spots for *ācāṉs*, in helping to remove their practices beyond scrutiny. In arguing for the imperceivability of *varmam*, its locations, diagnostics, and conditions, by modern technical equipment, and especially by imaging devices, *ācāṉs* manage to raise their practices beyond the very comprehension of science and biomedicine. This is done by explicitly noting the vital spots to be "secret," and therefore invisible from a biomedical point of view. In the words of one practitioner, science does not see *varmam*. This is similar to other regions and to other forms of indigenous medicine, such as ritual healing, where often a struggle occurs over not so much the efficacy of a particular form of healing, but over whether it is "modern" or scientific (Sax 2009). It appears that *ācāṉs* answer this question by asserting a distinct "scientificity" to their practices to which only they have access.

Perceiving the Secret

The aspect of seeing the unseen, or controlling that which eludes the control of others, is further exemplified by the concept of the "gaze spot," *nōkkuvarmam*. Differing notions abound, but generally, practitioners describe "gaze spots" as a category of vital spots which are not stimulated by touch, but by the mere gaze of an experienced *ācāṉ* (Balasubramaniam and Dharmalingam 1991, 29–30). Whereas there is a tendency to emphasize the combat uses of gaze spots in contemporary, popular publications on *varmakkalai* (Rājēntiraṉ 1998; 2009), most *ācāṉs* acknowledge their therapeutic aspects. Velayudhan explained *nōkkuvarmam* to be a set of spots which can cause an injury, but which can also cure, merely by visual perception. Gaze spots are thus the subject of many cheap booklets in Tamil, often available in small bookshops or at railway stations. They only vaguely describe techniques, but accentuate the magical, supernatural skills of *ācāṉ*s by extolling their martial prowess. Such booklets report exciting stories of fights and the incapacitation, without touching, of a superior number of ferocious attackers, or *ācāṉ*s causing milk to become sour, or even glass, mirrors, and stones to burst, merely by the power of the gaze (Rājēntiraṉ 2008, 45).[3]

Though many practitioners eschew such esoteric practices (Zarrilli 1989, 1297), some *ācāṉ*s claim to possess the skill of *nōkkuvarmam*, which requires a particular combined power of the mind and body achieved only through the most austere meditational practices, combined with yogic exercises and breath control (Zarrilli 1998, 197; Balasubramaniam and Dharmalingam 1991, 29–30). Rājēntiraṉ (2008, 47) even holds that such a skill cannot be attained by just anybody—even through the most austere efforts—but rather is an accomplishment attained in former births (*uḻviṉai*). One practitioner explained that every look communicates energies and therefore has an effect. A person entertaining thoughts of envy, disgust, or jealousy while looking at someone or something, is likely to negatively affect whoever or whatever receives such a gaze, which might influence health and well-being.[4] Conversely, a gaze laden with positive thoughts, like affection, has beneficial effects. In a similar way, for a skilled *ācāṉ*, the gaze emerges as a powerful tool, and a mere look at a vital spot can be enough to incapacitate an attacker, or alternatively, to revive incapacitated opponents and effectively cure ailments.

Jean Langford, in a brief discussion of ayurvedic vital spot practices called *marmma cikitsā*, concludes that its therapies achieve the precision of

3. Such mostly cheap paperback booklets bear thrilling, promising titles, such as *Decree [of the] Deadly Vital Spots* (Rājēntiraṉ 1998; also 2008; 2009), *Secrets of the Art of the Vital Spots* (Caravaṇakaṇēṣ 2009), *Secrets of the Art of the Vital Spots as Discovered by the Siddhars* (Jekatā 2005), or *Even You Can Learn the Art of the Vital Spots* (Rācā [1997] 2002).

4. This idea is closely related to the concept of *kaṇṇuttiruṣṭi*, literally meaning "eyesight," but generally translated as "evil eye," to which both persons and objects may be vulnerable (Woodburne 1992). For instance, being flawlessly beautiful or apparently perfect is a state which causes jealous glances, and hence a black dot is generally anointed on the cheeks of small infants in India, in order to make them look less cute and to avert jealous looks. This is true for houses as well, and masks of abominable faces adorn construction sites and finished buildings.

high-tech facilities with "rustic tools" or by a practitioner's control of sensory perception and motor skills. A practice, notes Langford (2002, 214), "that, for modern observers, seems to draw its authority from the mystery with which it cloaks a sophisticated esoteric knowledge in apparently 'primitive' practices." In a similar vein, Weiss (2009, 195) writes that, apart from compounding and prescribing medicines, a world that modern science can describe and understand, siddha physicians "also imagine a second world that exceeds the possibilities of a limited science." This second world includes esoteric practices like the gaze spots, which epitomize the claim of *ācāṉs* to be able to perceive and penetrate merely with their eyes what lies beyond the scope of biomedicine, and, indeed, that of modern science. By highlighting their own ability to diagnose physical trauma and diseases, by claiming to be able to detect and handle what eludes the biomedical gaze and knowledge altogether, *ācāṉs* profess to be better physicians than the biomedical doctors, despite the help of auxiliary devices. The practice of secrecy, in this context, must be viewed as crucial, since it "cloaks" the vital spot practices and makes them less transparent and conveys authority at the same time.

Secrecy in this sense is not the *arcana imperii* of old, the "secret of the powerful" for upholding the status quo. Much as Elizabeth Hsu (1999, 53) asserts, "a secret can also be a weapon of the weak." Rather, it may be recognized as a tool in the hands of the subordinate or marginalized, in order to subvert, challenge, or undermine established hierarchies. In the case of the vital spots, the struggle appears to be defined by the hierarchies of the pluralistic medical field in India today, which is controlled by the hegemony of biomedicine.

But, importantly, no secret simply remains concealed. In this regard, Simmel (1950, 337) wrote that "what recedes before the consciousness of others and is hidden from them, is to be emphasized in their consciousness." Beryl Bellman (1981) termed this the "paradox of secrecy," by which she described the fact that every secret is always only a secret through partial disclosure of what is supposed to be concealed. The remainder of this chapter will explore this paradoxical yet integral nature of secrecy, that is, its (partial) revelation, transgression, and display.

The Secret on Display: Performing and Transgressing Secrecy

Despite all assertions that the art of the vital spots must be kept secret, there are frequent deliberate displays or transgressions of secrecy, often by the same persons who state the reprehensibility of doing so. This highlights the intriguing circumstance that revelation appears to be an integral aspect of concealment and secrecy in general. In fact, it has been argued that "true secrecy is a virtual impossibility" (Taussig 1999b, 58). Etymologically, the English term *secret* is derived from Latin *secretus*, which means "set apart, withdrawn, hidden," as is the verb *secrete*, which, as Paul Johnson (2002, 3) points out, can denote "to hide" and "to release." In his influential article *La Chaîne du Secret*, Andras Zempléni concludes that secrets are always *meant* to be eventually revealed. A secret thus begins with a *détenteur* or "possessor," who confides in a *dépositaire*, a "custodian" or depositary. But the focus of the secret, according to Zempléni (1976), is ultimately its *destinataire*, its "addressee." However, this addressee is the very person or group meant to be excluded from a secret!

This is an important aspect, according to which a secret, in order to be a secret, always requires those who possess it and those who are excluded from it. In other words, a secret of which no one knows that it is secret is no secret at all. Thus, every secret, writes Taussig (1998, 355), has "to be not only concealed but revealed as well," and indeed, intentionally or unintentionally, secrets are constantly being revealed, at least in parts (Spitznagel 1998, 24). This, in the words of Bellman (1981, 21), is the "paradox of secrecy," as "secrecy is constituted by the very procedures by which secrets get communicated." This paradox grapples with the fact that every secret to some extent always *has* to be known; the fact that there is a secret has to be communicated. Secrecy thus only exists in a dialectic between concealment and revelation or, as Urban (2001b, viii) in his study of the *Karthābhajā* tantric tradition of Bengal has put it, in "a back and forth movement of . . . advertisement, partial revelation, and general obfuscation of elusive hidden truths" (see also Gray 2005, 433). Likewise, Robert Levy (1990, 298–299) has noted in his study of Nepali tantric rituals that veilings and obfuscations can be recognized as "advertisements." Such concealing behaviors and techniques advertise "that there is, in fact, a secret that is being hidden" (see also Khan 2008). It is not merely essential that there *are* secrets, but also for others to *know* that they exist. This may be recognized as "secretism," a term which Johnson (2002) coins as an analogy to what Simmel in German called "Geheimnistuerei." Johnson speaks of secretism in the case of practitioners of Brazilian Candomblé, who actively promote the reputation of their secrets, with the outcome of circulating and spreading its reputation and prestige. As Herzfeld (2009, 151) points out in an exploration of Southern European negotiations of privacy, secrecy must be performed in a public fashion in order to be understood to exist.

There is, of course, an important difference between advertising the fact that there is a secret and revealing its contents. In the case of the vital spots, however, a partial or momentary display of related loci, of martial or medical techniques, appears to be a powerful and frequently deployed method of advertising its secrecy. Practitioners in Kanyakumari frequently both demonstrated the importance they accorded to secrecy and deliberately breached such secrecy for self-promotion. One informant, even after I had introduced myself and my research by pointing out that I respected the traditional concealment of knowledge and that it was not my objective to discover or reveal the contents of his practice, countered by saying, "*Varmam* means secret, yes. But don't worry. I can give you [full information on] all the 108 spots. I can tell everything to you . . . ; I can teach you everything." I will come back to this and similar statements shortly.

Publishing the Vital Spots

An increasing number of publications, largely in Tamil, with a few Malayalam and English exceptions, address the vital spots in various ways. These tend to focus on the more mysterious aspects of *varmam*, like the ability to penetrate loci by the mere use of the gaze, or the miraculous revival of near-dead or even deceased persons.[5] Interestingly, a feature shared by many of these publications is the solemn promise to publish all secrets of *varmakkalai*. Authors may claim to "detail all the secrets" (Jeyrāj 2007, 12) and to explain every last intricacy of the vital spots. In a small booklet titled *Varmakkalai rakaciyam*, or "the secret [of] the art of the vital spots," the author Caravaṇakaṇēṣ (2009, 3) declares his intention to break with the tradition of keeping the spots rigidly concealed, maintaining that "[a]nyone can easily learn the vital spots through this book, which is written lucidly and clear[ly]." Another practitioner-turned-author, writing on therapeutic spots, notes: "With the help of photographs I have published and presented in this book all *aṭaṅkals*, which hitherto have remained like hidden rubies" (Jeyrāj 2007, 5).

Another genre of publications, which in its character is different from those described above, attempts to concisely depict the system of vital spots. Such works may contain anatomical charts showing *varmam* locations.

5. Dharmalingam, for instance, maintains that, earlier, *ācāṉs* were able to reanimate dead persons, albeit only for a short time. The practitioner claims this was widely practiced to enable deceased sovereigns to spell out their last wish (Balasubramaniam and Dharmalingam 1991, 40).

The authors of such treatises, mostly practicing *ācāṉ*s and college-trained siddha practitioners, nearly always claim that they are revealing what has previously been kept secret so as to counteract an alleged threat of extinction faced by *varmakkalai*. The secrecy surrounding the vital spots, they suggest, impairs and endangers the related practices. The general tone adopted by those engaged in purportedly demystifying and making the knowledge accessible to all, is one of scientific research and pragmatic dissemination of knowledge. All such publications emphasize that their contents now reveal the secret knowledge of the vital spots. In doing so, the value of the contents is also emphasized, characterizing it as rare and valuable (see Chidambarathanu Pillai 1994b, 3).

Paradoxically, these publications maintain an aura of mystery, and depict the vital spots as something that deserves to be kept concealed, despite claiming to reveal all its secrets. In one of his numerous books on *varmam*, Chidambarathanu Pillai (1995b, 64) cautions that "the reader should not divulge the contents of this rare text to all and sundry. The recipient should have the quality of submissiveness and be ever dutiful and indebted to his teacher"—this is despite the fact that anyone can purchase the book. The same author further writes: "There is no other better book than this, for those who want to learn. No one will tell you about *varmams* including the description of its physiological organs. This book may seem to be simple. But no other teachers in the world know the subject perfectly" (35). The author manages to exalt his expertise far above that of others and to esotericize his subject at the same time. Such affirmations of the secret nature of the subject on the one hand, and of the uniqueness of its revelation on the other, are not only common, but far from being a recent phenomenon. A premodern vital spot manuscript states: "What is explained in this treatise can be found nowhere else. [Only] he who understands this book is worthy of being called *ācāṉ*" (*Varmakkaṇṇāṭi*, 136; Mariyajōcap n.d., 64).

Anaesthetizing a Chicken: Live Demonstrations of the Vital Spots

Despite all caution against revealing their locations or applications by practitioners, demonstrations of vital spots and their effects are not uncommon. A book published by the hereditary practitioner Aleksāṇṭar Ācāṉ bears the title *V(m)armakkalai kaḷañciyam*. This is a pun, which, depending on whether *v* or *m* is read, means the "treasury of the art of vital spots," or the "treasury of the secret art." Though noting repeatedly that the vital spots are secret and must always be kept concealed, this book shows the author anaesthetizing and reviving a goat and a chicken by pressing particular spots. Black-and-white photographs back descriptions of the loci, which the *ācāṉ* stimulates for numbing and reanimating the animals. Irrespective of whether animal or human vital spots were stimulated, the author concludes, the effect was the same (Aleksāṇṭar Ācāṉ 1998, 29–30).

Vital spot practitioners have often been reported to publicly demonstrate their skills by similar presentations. Usually animals are used for such performances: chickens or goats that are held tightly, temporarily paralyzed, and subsequently reanimated by pressing one or several loci.[6] Langford (2002, 213) mentions that the Kottakkal Arya Vaidya Sala in Kerala was known for demonstrating effects of *marmma cikitsā* by making a rooster unconscious and revitalizing it, though such a demonstration had been refused in her presence. The video documentary *Ayurveda Art of Being* by Pan Nalin has had a greater public impact. One sequence in this movie shows how a practitioner benumbs and revitalizes a goat to the barely suppressed amazement of the audience.

A similar display was offered to me by an *ācāṉ* in Kanyakumari district; I will call him Kumaran. When I first met this practitioner, he told me that he had already heard of my research and me and wanted to know what I had learned about the vital spots. He asked, "You have spoken to many *ācāṉ*s in the last few months. But has anyone taught you anything at all?" Kumaran subsequently assured me that whatever I had been told hitherto had been trickery and fraud, performed by swindlers and quacks. After he had finished denouncing most practitioners in the area in this manner, he consoled me; for now I had finally found a truthful *ācāṉ*, who would let me in on some real vital spot secrets:

KUMARAN: You have come all the long way from Germany, so you should learn some true [*uṇmaiyāṉa*] facts about *varmam*. I will show [you]. Come, catch my fist and open it! You can use both hands (*I try to open*

6. Some manuscripts are said to separately deal with vital spots of animals. A *kukkuṭa cāstiram*, "treatise on fowls," was mentioned to me by Thomas *ācāṉ*, a practitioner who also elaborated how he had brought to perfection the catching of wild animals like lizards (*uṭumpu*, Lat. *varamus bengalensis*) or even snakes, by stunning them through *varmam* stimulation (compare Rājēntiraṉ 1998, 3). Dharmalingam and Balasubramaniam (1991, 70–72, 43) report that *mahouts*, persons directing elephants, knew of a number of points for controlling their mounts, and that similar spots were equally applicable in horses or oxen.

his tightly closed fist, but in vain). Now, I will show you *varmam*! But you have to promise me that whatever I teach you, you should never show it to someone else. Promise!

ROMAN: I promise I will not show it to anyone.

KUMARAN: Good. Now make a fist yourself; keep it tightly closed. (*Though I am tightly keeping my fist closed, he opens it with astounding ease by pressing a spot between the knuckles of the small and the ring finger. This produces stinging pain, forcing me to open my hand*) You see? This is *varmam*!

ROMAN: I see. And it does hurt a lot.

Kumaran continued with similar demonstrations. Just as he had forced my fist to open, he effortlessly bent my arms and legs against my will by stimulating various spots. The *ācāṉ* then had me deliver punches to different parts of his body, which he effortlessly blocked or averted by catching my punching arm or fist in an interlocking technique. Holding my arm behind my back in a twisted position, leaving me immovable and in pain, Kumaran all the while asserted me that this was the "real *varmam*."

The *ācāṉ* then told me to follow him into his little garden in the back of his house. A flock of chickens were roaming freely here. Grabbing one skillfully, he turned to me and said: "Now, I will show you what only very few can do. But no photo[s], understand?" After I had consented not to use my camera, he held the chicken on the ground, while it squawked in terror. As the practitioner pressed a spot on its neck, the resistance and voice of the animal slowly abated until it finally appeared to be sleeping, completely motionless. Kumaran said, "Did you see that? Now it's like dead [*cāvatu pōlirukku*]. It does not matter whether it's a chicken or a dog or even a human being, this always works." Feeling sympathy for the chicken, I urged Kumaran to revive it, which he did by pressing the same spot. Awakening with a cry, the chicken hopped away after briefly reorienting itself. The *ācāṉ* addressed me again:

> Now you have seen *varmam*. This is something that no one else will show you. Many boast, saying, "I can show you *varmam*; I know all [vital spots]." But they do not show anything because they don't *know* anything. Others say: "I won't teach you anything." But that is because they don't know anything either! If they give [information], it's only lies. Though they call themselves *ācāṉ*s, in reality they are only *kaḷḷaṉ*s [deceivers].

Although Kumaran assured me that his demonstrations of *varmam* loci were unique, my research in Kanyakumari was punctuated by similar displays. In fact, I grew relatively comfortable with vital spot stimulations, which forced my hands to open or which produced tingling sensations. Most of these applications were far from extravagant or unique, but instead paralleled those described by Gary Hausman (1996, 25–26, 52), who, in his dissertation on hereditary siddha medical practices in Kanyakumari, relates how one and the same spot near the knuckle of the hand was pointed out to him by five different individuals. Each of these practitioners affirmed that this *varmam* was strictly secret, not to be revealed to anyone else and that no one else would ever know or reveal this spot. Like in the instance cited above, most *ācāṉ*s thus demonstrating their skills not only had Hausman promise not to give away techniques they had demonstrated, but insisted that there was no one else who would demonstrate them, or who would even be capable of doing so. This is reminiscent of Bellman's discussion of "telling a secret." According to her, telling a secret always includes a preface, which clarifies that:

> (1) the speaker is telling information that is concealed, (2) the occasion of telling the information is not an illegitimate exposing, (3) the teller is trusting the respondent not to reveal the information or its source, and (4) the teller can still be trusted as one who can keep a secret even though he or she is engaged in the activity of telling the hidden information.
>
> (Bellman *1981, 9*)

Consequently, the revelation of secrets invariably contains an essential contradiction, or paradox, as something is communicated that is not supposed to be communicated. At the same time, the act of communication is characterized as no breach of proscriptions to communicate a secret.

This is an almost ubiquitous concomitant phenomenon of *varmam* displays as well. However, it ultimately jeopardizes the integrity of what is communicated or demonstrated and of the individual who conducts the revelation of secrets. Whereas the (partial) revelation of something concealed thus emphasizes the possession of a secret and may serve to heighten the position of its holder, the act of disclosure always renders the person disclosing vulnerable to scrutiny and criticism.

"These Boys Only Learn *Cilampam*": A Martial Arts Tournament

Shortly after I had established contact with the *ācāṉ*, he told me that if I was interested in vital spots and in *viḷaiyāṭṭu*, literally "play" or "sport," a term often deployed in describing various martial practices, I should accompany him and his students to a *cilampam* staff competition (*cilampāṭṭappōṭṭi*). A few days later, we boarded a bus to Teppankulam village, where such a *cilampāṭṭappōṭṭi* was about to take place. The program was to start around 7:30 p.m. and go on until late into the night. Having reached the village, we took a footpath, crossing thick coconut groves in order to reach the spot of the tournament, a squarish area of about 15 square meters, which had been leveled and covered with smooth, sandy earth in order to prevent possible injuries to the contestants from falls. Like an oversized boxing ring, the square was fenced by a rope on all sides. Bright neon lights had been installed in all four corners on surrounding coconut trees to provide sufficient visibility, yet immediately upon our arrival at the venue a power cut blacked out the place. For most of the event only two of the lights were powered by a diesel generator, which hummed loudly. Even noisier was a music group, consisting of two elderly men who played drums, and a young boy playing small cymbals. This trio maintained driving, rhythmic beats throughout the competition, energizing the competitors as well as the cheering audience.

Upon arrival, Velayudhan was respectfully welcomed and led to a table on the side of the arena. On it a golden goblet was placed, which was to be awarded to the winning team together with a cash prize of 2000 rupees. The winning team was to be chosen by a jury, which consisted of respected *ācāṉ*s of the area, including Velayudhan. About 300 spectators had shown up, standing behind the fencing of the square to witness the competition. Within the arena, six groups were sitting on the ground, each group surrounding an elderly person seated on a chair. As was explained to me, these were the *ācāṉ*s of the participating *kaḷaris*, surrounded by their respective students, who were going to participate in the tournament. The all-male competitors appeared to be aged from approximately fifteen to forty. Their dresses, which displayed some uniformity within teams, ranged from neat, all-white short pants and undershirts, to long, black sweat pants and white shirts. Before the event started, a presenter introduced via loudspeakers the participating teams by calling out the name of their *ācāṉ* and their place, such as "[from] *Kaliyakkavilai*, Jeykumar *ācāṉ*."

The program started off with the competitors bowing before the audience, which cheered wildly in expectation of the show. Each group, taking turns, performed saluting exercises (*vaṇaṅku-tal*), consisting of short sequences of moves and choreographed hits, kicks, and defensive moves, and of the competitors finally bowing down to and touching the feet of their respective *ācāṉs*. This was followed by individual performers displaying various bare-handed body moves, speedy series of kicks, punches, turns, and jumps. Choreographed partner performances were featured next, utilizing similar techniques. After this, performers introduced weapons, and exhibited their skill in handling short bamboo sticks called *ciramam* (about one meter in length), in choreographed partner fights. *Cilampam* long staff forms swiftly swirled around a practitioner's perpendicular and horizontal axes were up next. Again, practitioners displayed *cilampam* solo performances first, exhibiting their individual skills in rapidly twirling one or two staffs. More weapons were featured in choreographed fight sequences afterwards. This included weapons made of the horns of deer or oxen (*māṉkompu*), small knives (*katti*; figure 5.1), machetes (*veṭṭikatti*), and axes (*kōṭāli; kaṇṭakōṭāli*), all of which were featured in one-on-one performances of the individual

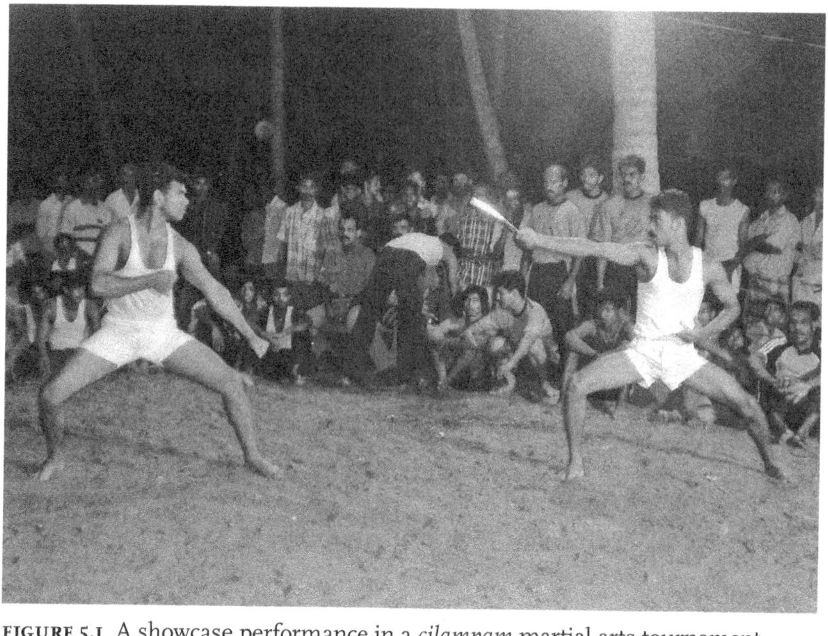

FIGURE 5.1 A showcase performance in a *cilampam* martial arts tournament

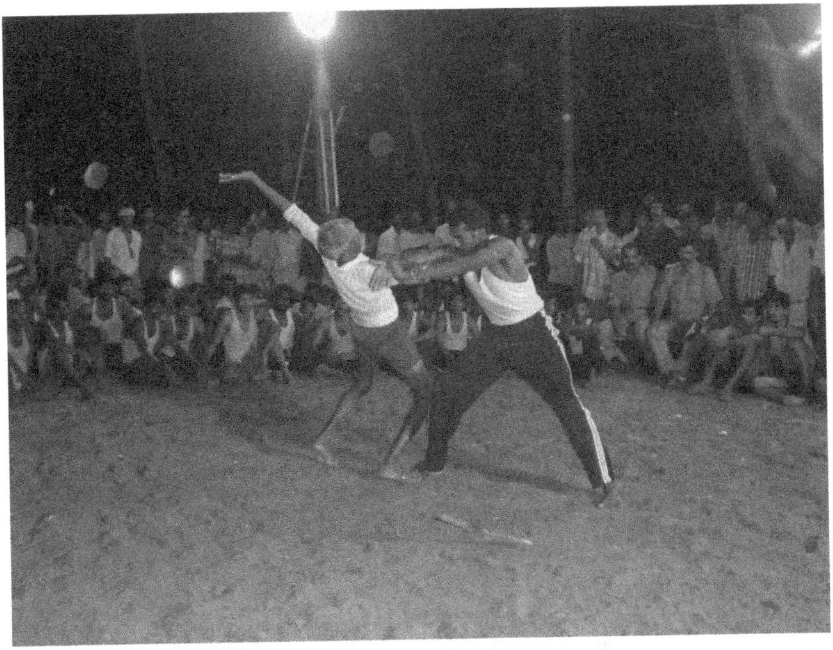

FIGURE 5.2 A showcase performance in a *cilampam* martial arts tournament

teams, displaying skills to disarm an opponent by one unarmed practitioner (figure 5.2).[7] Each team also presented choreographed partner performances with swords (*vāḷ*) and shields (*kēṭakam*).

These preliminary performances took from 8:00 p.m. to about 11:00 p.m., during which time Murukan and Manikandhan, Velayudhan's students who were sitting next to me, repeatedly told me that all this was just "show" and that the actual competition was only to start later. Indeed, it was only after 11:00 p.m. that staff-fighting matches commenced. From each team, five contestants fought one-on-one against opponents of the other teams. These fights only took about five minutes each, during which the combatants tried to direct their staffs in such a way as to touch their opponent's body, while simultaneously blocking strikes directed toward their own body. Velayudhan explained to me later that he, as a member of the jury, had to decide upon the weightage of each individual fight, by assigning "points" to the contestants. Touching an opponent's legs with

7. Weapons used in competitions and most *kaḷaris* are training weapons and not actual combat weapons; blades of knives or axes are not sharpened, but blunt, to prevent any serious cut injuries.

one's staff was rewarded with one point, the torso with two points, and head contact with three points, as was causing the opponent to drop his staff. Points awarded could also be upgraded in cases of difficult or outstanding blows, such as those delivered out of a turning movement, without seeing the opponent or while jumping.[8] Rather than an individual contestant winning the competition, the victory was adjudged team-wise. At the end of this tournament, around 3:00 a.m., after about twenty-five one-on-one fights were complete, a winning team was announced and the audience dispersed.

Thrilled from the impressions of the fights, I asked Velayudhan on our way back to what extent vital spots were important for these competitions. I was eager to know whether points would be awarded by the jury with regard to specific *varmam* penetrated by a contestant. But Velayudhan dismissed this idea, and held that vital spots had not been involved at all. If this had been the case, if a *varmam* had been impacted, severe health problems could have resulted. But the *ācāṉ* further maintained that vital spots were not found in such "games" (*viḷaiyāṭṭu*) owing to the deadly nature of the loci, as even a slight penetration of a vital spot could under certain circumstances cause a person to die. If vulnerable loci had been affected tonight, Velayudhan held, it would have happened by chance, and not by intention. The present contestants, he added pejoratively, did not know *varmam* at all. I was surprised, as I had expected the opposite, and enquired whether learning vital spots was not part of these practitioners' practices of vital spot martial arts. The *ācāṉ* responded:

> These boys only learn *cilampam*! And to someone who only learns *cilampam*, you cannot teach the vital spots. One can teach the vital spots only to someone who has learned everything. One can never learn how to hit [the vital spots] without learning [vital spot] medicine. These boys are not learning *varmam*! What they know is staff-dance [*cilampāṭṭam*]. They learn how to swing the staff and how to hit and parry and all that, but not where vital spots are. Vital spots cannot be found at such games, and, to tell you the truth, neither can *ācāṉ*s. Those who perform there are never real *ācāṉ*s, you know.

8. The system of point allocation is not regulated or fixed, but rather discussed before most competitions by the members of the jury. At other tournaments, varying systems have been applied. The same is true for the duration of fights, the size of the ground, and the organization of each tournament.

Velayudhan explained that some of these performers might learn medical applications as well, but most did not. If they did, and did so with an experienced *ācāṉ*, one deserving the title *ācāṉ*, they would eventually be taught the vital spots as well. Others surely did not. However, the so-called *ācāṉ*s at the competition did not know *varmam* themselves and, hence, were not *ācāṉ*s at all; if they were *ācāṉ*s, they would stay away from such "shows" or "games," Velayudhan asserted.

Secrecy as Liability

This kind of argumentation was soon to become very familiar to me, and must be recognized as a central aspect of the discursive dialectics of secrecy. Most *ācāṉ*s I visited would denounce the abilities of nearly all other practitioners, who did not deserve being called *ācāṉ*, but were rather quacks (*vīmpuvaittiyaṉ*) and swindlers (*poykkāraṉ*). Practitioners who argued in this way would then often go on to set themselves apart from such an inept lot and, to prove their claims, offer demonstrations of their skills. These were almost invariably conducted only after making me promise not to reveal any spots or methods of stimulation to anyone else. By way of conclusion, practitioners might add that what had been revealed to me was secret and that no one else would ever reveal it or anything similar.

On the other hand, practitioners would often denounce precisely such demonstrations on the grounds that only quacks conducted them. Velayudhan, for instance, frequently condemned demonstrations using animals or, even worse, human guinea pigs. For him, such performances, inclusive of martial art tournaments, were rather a sign of the immaturity of a practitioner and should be taken as an evidence of his or her ignorance of the vital spots (compare Zarrilli 1998, 158). Velayudhan asked: "What good is it if you prove that you can put a rooster to sleep? What is that good for? If you are skilled in *varmakkalai*, would you not rather treat patients? If you run a dispensary, treat diseases, and if you are successful in that, why put some animal to sleep?" With this logic, those who demonstrate vital spot knowledge run the risk of being criticized by fellow practitioners, and expose themselves to the scrutiny of other *ācāṉ*s. Any person divulging *varmam* secrets in public displays might be denounced as either morally depraved, or, even more likely, as ignorant, that is, not *really* knowing the vital spots correctly. Many practitioners criticize others for boasting unnecessarily and for publicly paralyzing chickens or goats, maintaining that this was done only by frauds and charlatans to boost their ego and make others believe they were skilled *ācāṉ*s. This might be seen as an attempt to cover up deficiencies, as knowing how to mesmerize poultry might be said to be entirely different and ultimately less refined than stimulating a vital spot in a human being.

However, as we have seen, those who make such displays tend to argue the reverse, and claim their own demonstrations as proof of their knowledge and skill! Those who refrain from displays, such practitioners might claim, do not demonstrate their knowledge, precisely because they lack comparable skills, since they are incompetent in *varmam*. Kumaran, who had demonstrated his mesmerizing of a chicken, explained that if others had the ability to achieve the same effect, they would certainly do so. The criticism and condemnation of others, following this logic, are merely signs of defensiveness and envy. In this way, every *ācāṉ* is prone and susceptible to critique and scrutiny. Indeed, most tend to doubt the abilities of their fellow practitioners. One question always appears to surround the justification of vital spot practices and the hotly debated and contested authenticity of their practitioners: who *really* is an *ācāṉ*?

Who Is an *Ācāṉ*? Another Double Bind of Secrecy

Murukan, a practitioner living close to Tirunelveli town, north of Kanyakumari district, related to me that it was crucial for *ācāṉ*s to pray daily to their *gurus*, or preceptors, before commencing to perform any martial or medical techniques. If this practice was followed regularly and conscientiously, many forms of therapeutic manipulations would not be required at all or, alternatively, would be highly effective, just as any combat application would be very successful. Reverence for one's *guru*, according to Murukan, was characteristic of a "true *ācāṉ*." And such a true *ācāṉ*, he held, could cure any ailment. Importantly, this requires asking, "Who is a (*true*) *ācāṉ*?" This question involves uncertainty, and this uncertainty or ambiguity defines the status of vital spot practitioners as well. This means that *ācāṉ*s and their practices are critically scrutinized not only by biomedical doctors, but also by copractitioners and siddha physicians. Concealment and secrecy as discursive and performative elements characterize an *ācāṉ*, on the one hand, but on the other they might jeopardize his or her claims to such a status.

Velayudhan frequently lamented that in the whole district of Kanyakumari, which is home to numerous vital spot practitioners, only about six or seven *ācāṉ*s were to be found; that is, persons who *deserved* to be called *ācāṉ*. He judged practitioners in his area according to whether they were "proper" (*cariyāṉa*), "true" (*uṇmaiyāṉa*), or "sincere *ācāṉ*s" (*cattiyamāṉa ācāṉ*). Such were only very few, whereas others, described as "quacks" (*vīmpuvaittiyaṉ*), were legion. Velayudhan did acknowledge that some had sufficient knowledge for treating minor diseases. Serious cases of vital spot afflictions, on the other hand, were beyond their ability, and hence such persons did not deserve to be called *ācāṉ*. It is thus quacks who literally have to "cover up" their incapacity:

VELAYUDHAN: Those who use a *sari* to cover patients before treating are not proper. If they were true physicians, they wouldn't do this. But they don't know *varmam* at all. That's why they use *saris* to cover their treatment of unconscious patients!

ROMAN: But if they don't know *varmam*, what then are they doing?

VELAYUDHAN: Well, I think they cover themselves and the patient, because they produce some awfully stinking medicine from their pocket and rub it under the patient's nose. This way, the patient may regain consciousness, albeit only in minor cases. No one can observe this, and because of the cover, even the smell is suppressed. I tell you, son, there are many similar tricks and deceit [*cūṭcam*], as many as there are people undeservingly claiming to be *ācāṉ*s.

Another time, Velayudhan stated that too many persons were "faking" *varmam* practices. In this logic, concealment may be recognized not so much as a means to hide the vital spots, but rather as a method to hide the fact that a practitioner does not know vital spots, or to hide the amount of knowledge he or she really commands. It is interesting to note, therefore, that Velayudhan, who on one day had criticized any public display of vital spot practices, was not averse to condemning deliberate acts of their concealment on another; or that he had criticized the very martial arts performance, discussed above, that he had indirectly contributed to.

Such a discourse on vital spot practices reveals an intriguing double bind. Many practitioners tend to justify their own knowledge and techniques as true, while judging those of others as deceit or quackery. Now, what is important for the discussion of secrecy is that vital spot practitioners reveal a discourse on efficacy and authenticity, which is framed by secrecy. This may be abstracted in the following way: those who reveal can never be true *ācāṉ*s. Those who conceal, on the other hand, are not necessarily accepted as *ācāṉ*s either, but are prone to be criticized precisely for allegedly concealing what they do not know. Practitioners of *varmakkalai* are trapped in a most intriguing position of ambivalence as secrecy is both power and liability at the same time. As Herzfeld (2009, 153) has observed, the "performance [of secrecy] is both its enabling condition and the source of its destruction."

I would argue that this is intrinsically connected to a postulated double bind of secrecy. Secrecy might easily be recognized as one of the most intricate and complicated topics for any researcher, "one of the most tangled methodological snarls," in the words of Hugh Urban (2001b, 15). For anybody describing and analyzing social, cultural, and political secrets or secretive traditions, at least two interrelated problematic issues can be identified: one is of an *epistemological* nature, the other of an *ethical* nature. How, on the one hand, is it *possible* to penetrate and analyze secret practices, characterized by restricting information about themselves? How, on the other hand, is it *ethical* to analyze and publish secrets (if indeed given access to alleged secrets)? This two-tier problem has been termed the "double bind of secrecy" by Urban (2001b). This includes the perception that those who know a secret do not reveal it, and, in the reverse of this argument, those who reveal a secret do not really know the whole truth. In Urban's words, "if one knows, one cannot speak; and if one speaks, one must not really know" (15). This double bind of secrecy has been largely described in the case of researchers facing the predicaments entailed: whether to share and publicize hitherto secret knowledge, and whether such shared knowledge really is authentic. But this predicament is paralleled, or better, mirrors the fact that an analogous double bind applies to the nature of the secret and to the status of persons dealing with concealed knowledge. While the double bind which secrecy poses to researchers has been self-reflectively analyzed (Bok 1984; Urban 1998; 2001b; Wolfson 2005), the predicaments of concealment and revelation or of secrecy as discursive and performative elements still require further attention.

Being a source of both power and liability, such an analysis may profit from acknowledging secrecy as a form of symbolic capital, by following, to some extent, the insights of Pierre Bourdieu on social strategies and practice.

Secrecy as Capital

> Secrecy . . . is better understood, not in terms of its contents or substance—which is ultimately unknowable, if there even is one—but rather in terms of its *forms* or *strategies*—the tactics by which social agents conceal or reveal, hoard or exchange, certain valued information. In this sense, secrecy is a discursive strategy that transforms a given piece of knowledge into a scarce and precious resource, a valuable commodity, the possession of which in turn bestows status, prestige, or symbolic capital on its owner.
>
> (Urban 1998, 210)

The French sociologist Pierre Bourdieu has influentially argued for acknowledging other forms of capital than purely economic ones. Defining capital as "all goods, material and symbolic, . . . that present themselves as *rare* and worthy of being sought after in a particular social formation" (1977, 178), Bourdieu recognizes instead several forms of capital, *economic capital*, "which is immediately and directly convertible into money" (1986, 47 248), being only one among these. He further describes *cultural capital*, which exists in an embodied form as education and learning and in an objectified form as objects of art. Another category is *social capital*, "made up of social obligations ('connections'), which is convertible . . . into economic capital and may be institutionalized in the form of a title of nobility" (248). Further, Bourdieu speaks of *symbolic capital*, which can be any of the above mentioned, but which is "unrecognized as capital and recognized as legitimate competence, as authority exerting an effect of (mis)recognition" (1986, 245). All of these forms of capital can be obtained, possessed, and transformed into other manifestations of capital. Their possession and transformation is a process of social alchemy, which arises from, and is constrained by, agents' engagement in a given social field (1990, 125).[9]

Secrecy might be viewed as a form of symbolic capital, keeping in mind that already Simmel (1950, 332) has asserted that what is restricted "attains a characteristic value accent through the form of secrecy" or that "[s]ecrecy gives the person enshrouded by it an exceptional position" (1906, 465). In tantric rituals in Bhaktapur, Nepal, as Robert Levy (1990, 337) has observed,

9. Bourdieu (1984, 101) uses the following equation: "[(habitus) (capital)] + field = practice," where "habitus" is embodied dispositions and "field" is the social setting of the actors.

"the possession of secrets is equivalent to the possession of economic and political force in the 'material' realm." Urban (1998, 210), who heavily draws on Bourdieu, has elucidated this further, noting that "secrecy is a discursive strategy that transforms a given piece of knowledge into a scarce and precious resource, a valuable commodity, the possession of which in turn bestows status, prestige, or symbolic capital on its owner." In this sense, concealment may be recognized as intended to allow for exclusive use of resources, such as by "allowing clever underdogs to hedge advantages opposite more influential and/or superior persons" (Burkert 1995, 79).

Secrecy is a means for *ācāṉ*s to protect a valuable resource, a form of capital: their knowledge of the vital spots and their capacity for dealing with it. But, furthermore, in maintaining a social order of connoisseurs and of people ignorant of *varmam*, of those within practitioner lineages and those without, of healers or fighters and patients or opponents, secrecy is indeed a form of symbolic capital. This symbolic capital of secrecy can be converted into social capital—the social obligations toward and relations with patients or other practitioners—and this is expressed in the status of an *ācāṉ*. Vital spot social capital can be acknowledged as institutionalized in the form of a title, *ācāṉ*, which confers respect and authority. This social prestige, together with considerable amounts of cultural capital in the form of incorporated vital spot therapies, in turn can be transformed into economic capital: a practitioner, who is famous for being an *ācāṉ*, that is, a good, "real *ācāṉ*," is consulted much more than other practitioners. Some practitioners in Kanyakumari indeed earn exceedingly well with their occupation and, in some cases, are in a position to charge substantial fees for the therapies which they offer. Velayudhan, for instance, during the time of my stay with him, was able to buy a used car—a modest form of luxury, which, however, only few practitioners of Indian medicine at that time were able to afford. The symbolic capital of secrecy thus can be transformed into other forms of capital—social, cultural, and economic—and hence confers authority, legitimacy, and possibly therapeutic efficacy, which in turn can be transformed into economic wealth and power. Recognizing secrecy as a form of symbolic capital allows us also to focus less on the content of secret knowledge, which may be information difficult to attain, and of a status difficult to assess, but on the very fact that such knowledge is claimed (Stuckrad 2010, 55). Following Urban (2001b, 213), secrecy can thus be described as "a unique type of *discursive strategy* . . . integral to the ongoing construction and deconstruction, support and subversion of the greater social order."

In the case of vital spot *ācāṉ*s, several uses of such a capital can be observed. These are deeply connected with the nature of their practice and with the character of the field of health care in contemporary India, which is generally termed "medical pluralism," but which is more accurately described as a hierarchically structured plurality of healing modalities. Manual forms of medicine have been reported as disrespected and the work of manual healers is often considered as having a lower status vis-à-vis other healing specialists all over the world (Huber and Anderson 1996; Van Dongen and Elema 2001; Hinojosa 2002, 30). In South India, biomedical doctors often show their contempt toward vital spot medicine, a largely manual practice that eschews most modern technologies and which is practiced by allegedly untrained individuals, that is, not trained in accepted, institutionalized ways. In view of a highly competitive field of healing practices in contemporary South India, expressions of secrecy must therefore also be interpreted as ways to argue for and communicate legitimacy, and to answer to critical enquiries, especially from biomedical practitioners. Indeed, many *ācāṉ*s argue that the vital spots remain secret, hidden to the gaze and understanding of science and biomedicine, as we have seen (figure 5.3).

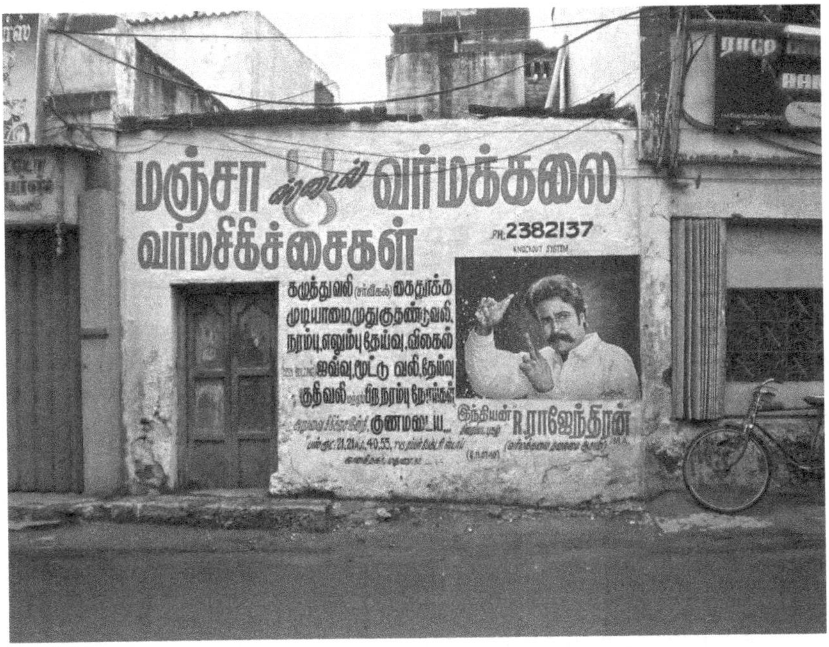

FIGURE 5.3 Advertisement for a vital spot practice painted on the façade of a house in Madurai

Amongst manual healers in Mexico, it has been observed that those who performed fewer physical manipulations, but other, especially divinatory actions, were considered by patients to have superior status (Fabrega and Silver 1973, 42). Hinojosa (2002, 31) speculates that the "implementation of religious or magical elements in an otherwise manual therapy can upgrade the status of a person performing massage." This is an interesting observation with regard to the case at hand and the relation of *varmam* to secrecy. Comparing magic and secrecy, Luhrmann (1989, 137) speaks of the "magic of secrecy," by noting that secrecy empowers particular actions, even therapeutic ones. Veiled acts or performances are fuelled with authority, it appears. Frederik Barth (1975, 219) has expressed this circumstance by noting that "concealing information about a subject can reinforce the belief in its claims." It is in this sense that we may describe, at least partly, some of the meanings of secrecy for *āċāṉ*s and its form of symbolic capital—maybe even with regard to a kind of *therapeutic capital* (see chapter 6).

Yet, being a powerful form of capital, secrecy remains deeply ambiguous, as its exchange is never open, but more of a kind of black-market symbolic capital, a term coined by Urban (2001b, 22). It is a capital which is "only . . . exchanged behind closed doors" (22). The tactics of secrecy, and the claim to be in possession of hidden truths, Urban concludes, "very often function as a potent source of symbolic power, status, and prestige—though a rather ambivalent and dangerous one, which is always a potential liability for its owner" (viii). This is so, as secrecy is always open to criticism and the accusation of being "immoral, scandalous, and politically or morally subversive" (26). Secrecy and its exchange are hence never conducted in public, open spheres, but rather in the environment of a black-market economy, in which secret knowledge is exchanged almost like illegitimate goods or contraband. But since secrecy itself, as we have seen, exists always only in a partial revelation, those who claim to possess a secret, and draw authority from this fact, are likely to be criticized exactly on this aspect. This we see in the circumstance of *āċāṉ*s always being subjected to scruples among copractitioners regarding whether they deserve the title *āċāṉ* or not, whether they are unique, authentic, and good *āċāṉ*s, or, conversely, cheats, fakes, quacks, or swindlers. Moreover, the ambiguity secrecy holds reflects on the way vital spot practices are viewed by biomedical practitioners as well, namely as an obscure, misguided, and illicit practice. The power that secrecy conveys in some regards is a highly delicate and vulnerable one. In this oscillation between concealment and public display, exchange and restriction, secrecy is as much a form of capital and power as it is a source of insecurity and social and professional liability. While practitioners may profit from secrecy, this is always an ambiguous, delicate profit that comes at a price.

Regarding the secretive behavior and methods of instruction in vital spot practices, it is not only hard for a researcher to tell how much an individual practitioner knows (Zarrilli 1998, 157). Among *ācāṉ*s, the apparently all-embracing secrecy involved in all their practices may be a cause for insecurities about the (in)capability of fellow *ācāṉ*s and even about their own knowledge. We have earlier seen Velayudhan reporting that, although every practitioner universally claims to know all 108 vital spots, most do not. Zarrilli cites one of his informants saying that a "student today is very lucky if he is given 70% of one master's knowledge. At least 30% will always be left out" (159). This may force students to seek out more and more practitioners in order to receive instruction, to widen their professional network in order to overcome the restricted flow of information. Indeed, most if not all *varmam* practitioners in Kanyakumari have learned from more than just one *guru*, and many *ācāṉ*s list thirty or more preceptors. The practitioner Irājēntiraṉ (2006, xi) lists in a publication thirty-five (!) *ācāṉ*s as his *gurus*. This is a strong indicator of the highly ambiguous, but also insecure nature of the knowledge, practices, and status of *ācāṉ*s. Moreover, it is practically impossible to judge whether a practitioner is an *ācāṉ*, that is, a real, or good, authentic *ācāṉ*, or whether this is an unresolvable question, inextricably linked to the double bind of secrecy. In this aspect, every vital spot practitioner is prone to criticism, and the line between an *ācāṉ* and a quack is a delicately fine one.

Conclusion

Vital spot practitioners, alongside vital spot manuscripts, argue that their practices are secret and have to remain concealed. By investigating the secretive behaviors and discourses on secrecy, we have seen that *ācāṉ*s, who constantly shift between concealment and revelation, move in an ambiguous and often contradictory sphere, which on the one hand emphasizes and amplifies, but on the other hand potentially compromises their practice and status.

"To tell a secret," notes Bellman, "is to do secrecy" (1981, 9); Taussig (1999b, 51) speaks of "unmasking" secrets in a "drama of revelation." Thus, parallel to the power of transgression, as argued by Georges Bataille

(1986), the power of secrecy might be acknowledged to lie precisely in the dialectical interplay between restrictions and their nonobservance, in taboos and transgressions. Secrecy, in other words, derives its power largely from its (partial) revelation. In this regard, Taussig's comment, noting the importance of the relation between secrecy and healing is notable:

> The real skill of the practitioner lies not in skilled concealment but in the skilled revelation of skilled concealment. Magic is efficacious not despite the trick but on account of its exposure. The mystery is heightened, not dissipated, by unmasking and in various ways, direct and oblique, ritual serves as a stage for so many unmaskings. Hence power flows not from masking but from unmasking, which masks more than masking.
>
> (Taussig *1999a, 273*)

Secrecy seems to incite, or already include, its transgression. In the words of Taussig (1998, 355), secrecy is likely to be "defaced," that is, unmasked. But, importantly, the unmasking of secrets does not equal its dissolution; it may even ensure continuing concealment. The display or performance of secrets hence must be described as a "skilled revelation of skilled concealment" (Taussig 1999b, 356), an act, which adds to the value of a secret, but which does not (fully) reveal it. When *ācāṉ*s display their techniques, they are sure to do so only when the display is connected with the claim to actually reveal something of value—something that no one else is capable of achieving, knowing, or revealing—and with administering an oath from the observer not to impart the object of the revelation to anyone else. In this way, though actual secrets may be disclosed, an overall secrecy and mysterious nature of a subject and of the person owning it is heightened, not reduced. In this sense, "to tell a secret is to do secrecy" indeed.

Using Bourdieu's terminology of "capital," we may recognize the power, status, and prestige that lie in this performance of secrecy. It allows us to recognize secrecy as a possible strategy to accumulate capital: social, cultural, and economic; it allows us to recognize secrecy itself as a form of symbolic capital. It is here that secrecy is closest to its etymology, "that which is secreted" or "set apart" (Zempléni 1976, 313), which can be of major importance in a competitive market such as the pluralistic field of healthcare in contemporary India. Deploying different forms of secrecy, *ācāṉ*s discursively connect secrecy with right conduct, as *varmam*, a potentially dangerous practice has to be kept concealed. Also, secrecy is connected with medical efficacy, and legitimacy of practices, as *ācāṉs* claim to be able to detect spots, invisible and unknown to science, and thus place their abilities in the precise realm which is impenetrable to biomedicine. To *ācāṉs*, as practitioners of a medical practice that is in a limbo of not being fully recognized and authorized, secrecy confers on vital spot medical practices a certain "alternative source of status in an alternative social hierarchy" (Urban 2001b, 214), which defies the general hegemony of biomedicine and of science in contemporary India. In this sense, secrecy is deeply related to authority, performing an "authority effect," as Bruce Lincoln (1994) has put it.

In more than one way, secrecy not only poses as an at times powerful tool for negotiating the status and authority of vital spot medical practice vis-à-vis other medical practices, but may also attain therapeutic capital. In a potentially similar case, traditional specialists on poison bites in Kerala have been reported to keep the ingredients of medicines secret, as patients, if familiar with a substance or recipe used, would not regard it with the same seriousness (Shankar and Unnikrishnan 2004, 146). In Micronesian Yap society, secrecy is closely tied to the idea of a medicine's potency; the more people know a recipe, the less powerful a medicine is assumed to be (Throop 2010, 144). Secrecy as a healing device may confer mystery on a healer, and thus increase his or her personality, as Hsu (1999, 56) has argued. Extending this insight, we might acknowledge the importance of secrecy with regard to the therapeutic efficacy of *varmam*.

Ācāṉs engage in this particular exercise of power via a negotiation and deployment of concealment and controlled or partial revelation of their knowledge. Those who keep their knowledge as concealed as possible are most powerful, and of a high status compared to others, an instance that has been observed in other contexts as well, for instance in doctor-patient encounters in Europe (Fainzang 2005, 43). Sharing knowledge means sharing power and status, whereas withholding knowledge means defending one's power and one's status and place in social hierarchy. Thus, secrecy is as much a form of symbolic capital as of symbolic violence, as outlined by Bourdieu (1977). But like all the technologies of power which Foucault (1988, 16) describes, secrecy has not only productive, useful sides, but it can be restraining: the authority that secrecy conveys comes at the price of partial revelation. Vital spot *ācāṉs* must therefore engage in dialectical processes of "lure and withdrawal," that is, a kind of "advertisement of secrecy" (Urban 2001b, 101). But this is not the only liability involved. Not only is revelation connected with immaturity and wrong conduct, highlighting the incompetence of practitioners who give demonstrations, rather than prove their skill. Practitioners putting vital spots on display run the risk of being condemned as fakes and quacks by those who claim not to indulge in public demonstrations or revelation of secrets. But secrecy itself becomes a liability, as even concealment may be interpreted as deliberate hushing up of incompetence. Thus evolves the double bind of secrecy, a predicament of vital spot practitioners, who are always subject to ambiguity and scrutinized regarding their sincerity and authenticity. With a growing awareness of incidences of alleged quackery, the establishment of a Medical Central Bureau of Investigation (MCBI), which conducts regular "antiquackery" efforts, and the planned formulation of an "antiquackery bill," according to which alleged quack practitioners could be sentenced to maximum punishment of life imprisonment (*Times of India*, July 29, 2010; *Deccan Chronicle*, March 30, 2013), this is becoming a matter of increasing concern for contemporary hereditary vital spot practitioners in India.

In this chapter, I have analyzed some expressions of secrecy, its *form*, rather than its *content*. This is tempting and has its value. On the other hand, it may lead to reducing the actual contents of what is concealed to an inferior position compared with its social form. Let me explain this by pointing out what I perceive to be yet another predicament of secrecy: its "capacity for dissimulation" (Johnson 2002, 4). This means that the possible discrepancy of what is purported to be real and what in fact is real, renders secrecy prone to criticism. Academic research is no exception in this regard. Simmel understood secrecy not only as a kind of social cloak, with which actors hide aspects of their life from others, but also as an adornment, a social ornament that awards its owner mysteriousness and distinction, but also status. But Simmel tended to overemphasize this latter aspect of secrecy, so much that for him the actual contents of secrecy, that which is being concealed, receded before the cloak, that is, the practice of secrecy. This is expressed by Simmel's (1906, 465) dictum that from "secrecy, which throws a shadow over all that is deep and significant, grows the logically fallacious, but typical, error, that everything secret is something essential and significant." This notion also implies that secrecy might be empty: any secret behavior, regardless of whether it serves to hide and protect actual contents or not, Simmel argues, is structurally similar and "quite independent of its casual content" (464). In a similar vein, Walter Burkert (1995, 94) has postulated: "nur das Geheimnis akzentuiert das Besondere [only the secret accentuates the significant]; the medium is the message." Yet while it might be tempting to look for the meaning of secrecy exclusively in its sociological form, this ultimately is a limited and limiting approach. To view secrets as empty, then, is to ignore the inherent ambiguity and the delicate power of secrecy. After all secrecy, as the case of *varmakkalai* highlights, does not merely convey symbolic capital, and thus power, but is also a liability to its owner.

This raises the question of why secrecy is such a central aspect in *varmakkalai*. Answering this question by reference to the form of secrecy and with it to its function of imbuing the vital spots and their practitioners with a unique, awe-inspiring status alone, neglects the frailty of the status and the ambiguity that *ācāṉ*s suffer from because of it. Furthermore, I argue that there is an ethical problem involved in neglecting the nature of the contents of secrecy, while focusing only on its form. Assuming, like Simmel, that the content of secrets is secondary, leads to the suspicion that secrets are empty. Alternatively, secrecy has been described as merely a strategy for economic well-being and for gaining authority and legitimacy. Such notions have, moreover, cast a dark shadow over secrecy: restriction of knowledge tends to be viewed as immoral, and is publicly disapproved of by most people. Simmel (1906, 463) depicted immorality as one of the intrinsic values pivotal in triggering secrecy, noting that "the immoral hides itself," and that "secrecy is not in immediate interdependence with evil, but evil with secrecy." As I highlight in the next chapter, however, it can be precisely moral, ethical values that give rise to restrictions of knowledge. As will become apparent, moral considerations and a tacit nature of the contents of vital spot secrets account to a large degree for the vital importance of secrecy for *ācāṉ*s.

6

Embodying Secrecy

A MORAL ECONOMY OF LEARNING AND THE TRANSMISSION OF TACIT KNOWLEDGE

Do not give away the powerful treatise;
if the student learns for twelve years,
and is knowledgeable and devoted,
[only then] accept the gift, my son, and hand over the knowledge.
Varma Cūttiram (Treatise on the vital spots),
verse 3; from Subramaniam (1994, 14)

If you behave as I have laid out,
you will be reputed as a mighty man in this world;
even among your enemies many will respect you,
if you know the shining spots with inmost thought.
Varmakkaṇṇāṭi, verse 150
(Mariyajōcap n.d., 71)

What is "learned by body" is not something that one has, like knowledge that can be brandished, but something that one is.
BOURDIEU (1990, 73)

ASKED ABOUT THE vital spots, many practitioners resort to such *mantra*-like phrases as "the *varmam* are secret" (*varmamṇā marmam*), or "the vital spots are a secret subject" (*varmamṇā oru irakaciyamāṉa viṣayam*). As described in chapter 5, concealment to prevent a leakage of knowledge to persons outside their lineage is of utmost importance to most *ācāṉ*s. This present chapter constitutes an attempt to come to terms with protestations by practitioners that they "cannot talk about" and "are not supposed to talk about" the vital spots or, in the words of Gary Hausman (1996, 71), the "litany of *colla muṭiyātu* and *collak kūṭātu*." Like Hausman, who has described the elusiveness of many siddha practitioners and their constant refusal to part with information, I too was frequently confronted by phrases like "this is a subject not to be talked about," and "this is a subject which cannot be talked about," implying both a censure and the impossibility of communicating the vital spot knowledge.

A study of secrecy as an important aspect of *varmakkalai* and its transmission yields insights into hereditary practices and into the nature of the philosophical concept of secrecy itself. This chapter draws on my personal experiences of learning *varmam*, which mostly happens in an intimate learning relationship between teacher and student, called *guru-śiṣya-paramparā*. Through a detailed analysis of this mode of knowledge transmission, it is recognized that vital spot–related practices are indeed ineffable because they simultaneously pertain to a *nonverbalizable* and a *not-to-be-verbalized* sphere. Thus, *ācāṉ*s indeed *cannot* talk about vital spots as the related knowledge transcends verbalized and verbalizable thought: it is of a tacit nature, experientially learned and *embodied*. At the same time, practitioners indeed *must not* speak about the vital spots or put them on display out of moral considerations; vital spots are prone to misuse, and are also potentially deadly. *Ācāṉ*s appear to embody Wittgenstein's famous dictum: "whereof one cannot speak, thereof one must be silent" ([1922] 2003, 156). As this chapter highlights, the *guru*-student educational system is ideally suited for the purpose of teaching the martial and medical intricacies of vital spot practice, which require sensual incorporation and experiential learning due to the tactile, kinesthetic, and hence tacit nature of knowledge. Furthermore, the close relationship between *guru* and student allows for a careful selection of trustworthy persons, a strong lineage of descent, and an education, which conveys moral and ethical values, which are of a primary importance, since related practices are potentially dangerous.

Taking both the tacit and the moral, ethical dimensions of secrecy into account is not only crucial for understanding the hereditary transmission of *varmakkalai*, but it also throws new light on the social functioning and meaning of secrecy, esotericism, and the transferal of secret knowledge. As I hope to show, learning the art of the vital spots is an embodied process whereby secret knowledge is communicated by a teacher to a disciple in an intimate relationship. Secrecy here is not just a function of deceit or of deliberate and cunning repression of information, but a dynamic mode of learning that has moral virtue unto itself as a process of empathic communication based on and enabled by the bond of the relationship between *guru* and student. Moreover, secrecy is the outcome of moral behavior, and both must be recognized as crucial aspects of vital spot efficacy.

Knowledge Transmission as Moral Economy and as Embodied Learning

As mentioned earlier, Simmel emphasized the sociological importance of secrecy with regard to possession: possessing secrets excludes others, a fact that, according to Simmel (1906, 464), defines the nature of possession itself—the fact that others forego possession of it. Furthermore, what is withheld from others appeared to him as imbued by a special value, and the more concealed an object and the fewer the people who know it, the more value it has. Simmel went so far as to claim that this was true even if no real secret existed at all, that is, in case of an empty secret, void of significant content. He therefore emphasized that not only the *content* of secrecy is important, but even more so is its *form*, or its sociological expression, which could be analyzed independently.

This idea has been taken up by several scholars working on occult, secretive traditions (Urban 1998; 2001b, 16; Johnson 2002, 8), and Richard Weiss (2009) has reproduced the distinction between the content and form of secrecy in his recent exploration of siddha medical practitioners' discourses on secrecy encountered in siddha manuscripts. Siddha manuscripts are characterized by *paripāṣai*, an ambiguous, coded language, difficult to unravel even for siddha practitioners.[1] Nevertheless, the latter claim to be able to decipher and utilize medical preparations encoded in this encryption—often alchemical transmutations or panacea, promising long life and immortality. Weiss, on the other hand, suggests that the most secretive recipes are indeed all about the (*form* of the) secret, and cannot be unraveled at all, as there allegedly is no *content* to unravel (Weiss 2009, 161). Rather, obscurity fulfills the role of conveying authority, and at the same time makes siddha medical practices immune to criticism and critical inquiry (151).

Weiss is not alone in advancing such a view of secrets in which content is seen either as receding before the form of secrecy or as ephemeral or empty (Simmel 1950, 332). Disclosure of tantric Buddhist texts, for instance, has been argued to be a "truly empty signifier, devoid of

1. In fact, there is a long tradition of tantric, mystical cults in South Asia that make use of cryptic, esoteric language (Skt. *sandhābhāṣā*) to express their mystical teachings. Some scholars have traced this back to the Buddhist *Caryāpadas* (texts composed between the eighth and twelfth centuries; Mojumdar 1973), a tradition that may have informed Bengali tantrism (Urban 2001b, 34) and North Indian *Nāth*-siddha cults (White 1996).

fixed referent" (Gray 2005), similar to Jewish mysticism (Wolfson 2002), on which Jacques Derrida (1986, 49–50) has written that the secret of Judaism was "finally discovered as an empty room, [as] not uncovered, [as it] never ends being uncovered, as it has nothing to show." Johnson's (2010) study of Brazilian Candomblé is largely concerned with the replacement of secrets by what he calls "secretism," the circulation of the pretense and reputation of secrecy, which he describes as quite independent of actual secrets. Frits Staal's (1979; 1996) assertion of the "meaninglessness of ritual" must also be mentioned in this regard. Writing on tantric *bījamantra*s, Staal concludes that ritual is full of rules, but barren of meaning, and therefore all rules, although structuring every ritual, are empty.

Such notions of secrecy as being empty or as concealing the fact that there is nothing to be unraveled might be explained by a general conception of the nature of secrets and esotericism. As highlighted in chapter 5, secrecy's "capacity for dissimulation" (Johnson 2002, 4), that is, the apparent possibility of a discrepancy in secrecy between what is purported to be real and what in fact is real, renders secrecy prone to criticism. Scholarly research is no exception in this regard. Both secrecy and esotericism have generally been connected to immoral or illegal information and behavior, such as crime and reprehensible conduct (Warren and Laslett 1980; Kippenberg and Stroumsa 1995, xii; Nedelmann 1995, 1). Secrecy has been largely understood as reflecting the "dark side of man" (Spitznagel 1998, 28), dreading the light of day and publicity. Simmel (1906, 463) himself defined immorality as one of the intrinsic values pivotal in triggering secrecy, writing that "the immoral hides itself," and that "secrecy is not in immediate interdependence with evil, but evil with secrecy." For him, secrecy is "the sociological expression of moral badness" (463). Alternatively, it has been argued that secrets serve entirely purposes of assuring the power of the powerful: *arcana imperii* (Spitznagel 1998, 31). The concealment of knowledge or techniques in this view has been regarded as maintaining economic prowess. By keeping a particular formula secret, it might be claimed, medical practitioners merely try to protect their economic well-being (23). With regard to apprenticeship learning and artisanry, scholars have interpreted an often observed reluctance of master craftsmen to reveal their skills or trade secrets to apprentices as originating from a fear of competition from their own apprentices (Herzfeld 2009, 151). In this regard, secrecy is often understood as "individual self-interest," an expression of social competition, and thus as the "oppositional force" of trust and communal concerns (Fine and Holyfield 1996, 24, 29).

The objective of the present chapter is twofold: on the one hand, I describe the modes of knowledge transmission of the vital spots, information of which is restricted and ideally passed on only from master to pupil in an intimate relationship. On the other hand, and with this relationship in mind, I intend to demonstrate that concealment can neither be comprehensively and justifiably explained in merely economic terms, nor in the suspicion that secrets are empty or necessarily of an immoral nature. To do so, the practice in scholarly studies of neglecting the *content* of secrecy, while emphasizing merely its *form*, has to be questioned, as it may be a limiting approach, likely to render truncated depictions of secret traditions. Luhrmann (2010, 212) has argued that anthropologists in general tend to concern themselves more with forms and less, if at all, with content. They describe the representations and symbols of kinship, but shy away from biological relatedness; they describe the ways of local shapes of madness, but shy away from an exploration of the nature of madness. In a related move, I argue that in order to understand secrecy in vital spot traditions (and most likely in other esoteric traditions as well), it is crucial to understand both their form and their content.

The knowledge of the vital spots transcends in large ways textual frameworks, and while transmission of knowledge and knowledge itself are largely experience-based, "embodied," and nontextual, secrecy in *varmakkalai* addresses the ineffability of vital spots. The related knowledge transcends realms of the verbal, and pertains to spheres of sense and experience. Accordingly, a highly sense-based, experiential, "hands on" approach to learning characterizes the hereditary mode of knowledge transmission of the vital spots. The tacit nature of the knowledge involved has to be inscribed into the body of a student—embodied—not verbally or textually communicated.

Further, *ācāṉ*s transmit to their students moral values and ethical directives, altruistic conduct, obligations, and ethical codes, which most *ācāṉ*s regard as inextricably connected to their practice. I argue that knowledge transmission of vital spots is a "moral economy" in the widest sense of the phrase. A moral economy is, according to Thompson (1991, 188), "grounded upon a consistent traditional view of social norms and obligations, of the proper economic functions of several parties within the community." Admittedly, I am using this concept in a modified and narrower form than that represented in the studies of Thompson (1991) or

Scott (1976), in order to fit the case at hand. Nevertheless, transmission of vital spot knowledge is not a one-sided flow of information or knowledge, but based on an exchange between teacher and student. Several social ties prevent both from misusing their respective positions, which are connected to ethical values, altruism, and a common relational bond. Thus, *gurus* convey knowledge and techniques after receiving not only necessarily monetary transferrals and so on, but rather after students have actively participated in the knowledge transmission by proving themselves worthy in the eyes of their teachers. This is done by gradually progressing, while learning *varmakkalai*, not only in the techniques related to vital spot martial and medical practices, but also in underlying notions of ethics and morality. This is epitomized in the act of initiation, since it enacts and manifests a relationship based on moral values, familiarity, and mutual responsibility. My description of the transmission of vital spot knowledge is thus similar to Sayer's (2004, 2) understanding of a moral economy, as "the study of how economic activities of all kinds are influenced and structured by moral dispositions and values."

The concepts of secrecy as nonverbalized and nonverbalizable, and the aspects of morally invested learning and embodied learning, are shown to be not only closely linked in the case of hereditary vital spot instruction, but pivotal to what practitioners regard as a correct, successful practice.

Hereditary Transmission of Knowledge

Traditional forms of education in South Asia have been the topic of numerous studies (Subramanian 1986; Crook 1996b; Scharfe 2002). As Zvelebil (1973, 14) has accurately noted, various arts, scholarly knowledge, and crafts in South Asia, "one does not learn by oneself; the guidance of a master, or a guru, is necessary." This relationship between a preceptor, *guru*, and a student, *śiṣya*, is generally referred to as *guru-śiṣya-paramparā*. The word *paramparā* denotes the lineage of descent from *guru* to *śiṣya*, the succession and transmission of knowledge from master to disciple. This has been described as an intimate relation between both, who live together in common residence in the house or family of the *guru* (Skt. *gurukula*; Steinmann 1986; Neuber 2006). Such learning allows for observing a practitioner by living with him or her in close contact, and similar modalities have been described as structuring apprentice styles of learning the world over (Coy 1989; Singleton 1998). Milton Singer (1968, 117) evaluated the particular relationship between *guru* and disciple as so crucial in the Indian context that he postulated it to "operate as the very lifeline of the culture and social structure."

In indigenous Indian medicine, *guru-śiṣya-paramparā* and classroom-style mass education are regularly contrasted (Brass 1972; Crook 1996a; Gurumurthy 1979; Wood 1985; Subramanian 1986). Contemporarily, the term for lineage, *paramparā*, has attained the meaning of "tradition," and hereditary siddha practitioners use both words interchangeably. Though one has to carefully avoid simplified categories and an unreflective tradition-modernity dichotomy, contemporarily, *guru-śiṣya-paramparā* is the education mode used by hereditary or "traditional" practitioners of siddha, or *vaittiyar*s, while mass education is utilized in institutionalized frameworks of colleges, which produce professionalized, "modern" siddha practitioners, or "doctors." Rajamony (1983, 473) claimed as early as 1983 that vital spot therapies, considered a branch of siddha medicine, were "now being taught and practiced as part of the siddha system in [government] institute[s]." Despite numerous attempts to integrate the vital spots into the siddha curriculum and, in a parallel fashion, to practice and instruct vital spot applications in private institutions, this is yet to be implemented; we will come back to this in the epilogue. Still, at the present time, hereditary *ācāṉ*s are the main exponents of *varmakkalai*, and they conduct instruction through *guru-śiṣya-paramparā*.

According to the Madras *Tamil Lexicon*, the term *ācāṉ* denotes, amongst other things, a "teacher, preceptor" ([1924–1936] 1982, 211; see also Pillai 1986, 62). This emphasizes the fact that most *ācāṉ*s are, almost by definition, teachers, who instruct disciples into vital spot intricacies. This is an aspect in which *ācāṉ* is not only phonetically but also semantically close to the Sanskrit term *ācārya*, "teacher."[2] Regarding the proper pedagogy for instructing the vital spots, *ācāṉ*s generally denounce classroom style education on many accounts, downplaying its efficiency in knowledge transfer in contrast to the "traditional" (*pārampariyam*) method of education. Rather, they stress a close, personal contact between teacher and student in an intimate relationship, and indeed, disciples are often relatives of teachers. The *gurukula* system of education has thus been described as "a secret and sacred process, for the reason that the process of an individual growth ... can only [be] achieved by a close and constant touch

2. On the other hand, it is not clear whether Tamil *ācāṉ* is in any way linguistically related to Sanskrit *ācārya*.

between the teacher and the disciple in their personal relationship from which the whole world was excluded" (Krishnamurthy and Chandra Mouli 1984, 227).

Generally, however, in describing *guru-śiṣya-paramparā*, scholarly literature has in the past emphasized texts and verbal learning as crucial modalities of instruction (Thakkur 1965, 168). The contributors to *Heritage of the Tamils: Education and Vocation* (Subramanian 1986) stress that ancient education was language-based, and that "[k]nowledge received through the ear was considered best" (Pillai 1986, 60; Pitchai 1986, 140). Referring to the *Naṉṉūl*, a Tamil grammar of the early thirteenth century, Pillai (1986, 64) notes "reciting-listening, questioning-answering, narrating-repeating, thinking-reflecting and investigating-discussing" as crucial techniques of instruction. However, I believe that in focusing on texts, several important aspects of this intimate relationship have remained overlooked. This is not to say that *ācāṉs* do not possess or utilize textual resources. Rather, we need to analyze the role of texts in practice. Several scholars have recently emphasized that texts are always practiced. Hindu scriptures, for instance, are recited, uttered, learned by heart, chanted, and witnessed, and thus always produce their most considerable effect via these practical aspects of texts (Flood 2006; Wilke and Moebus 2011).

Text and Context

There certainly are a number of manuscripts which deal with *varmam*. In Tamil, these are called *ōlaiccuvaṭi*, since they are inscribed on palm-leaf (*ōlai*) bundles (*cuvaṭi*).[3] Today, some published versions of these even exist in book form. They deal with various aspects: descriptions of theories of life, anatomical elucidations, enumerations and locations of vital spots, and explications of symptoms, diseases, and treatment methods, and some include combat techniques and oral commands for martial exercises.

Just as in the case of other so-called literatures or texts of South Asia (Hiltebeitel 1999), vital spot manuscripts indicate that their contents were supposed to be transmitted orally—being sung and listened to—rather than through writing and reading. Transmission of Vedas and Upaniṣads, today perceived as texts or books, has been an oral process for centuries, passed on by word of mouth and listening, *śruti*. In

3. Irājēntiraṉ (2006, 11–15) lists 116 such vital spot manuscripts.

the case of vital spot manuscripts, this becomes clear from the recurrent phrase *ceppuvēṉ/colluvēṉ*: "I am telling/speaking" (*Varmakkaṇṇāṭi*, 2; Mariyajōcap n.d., 1). Moreover, vital spot manuscripts, like siddha compendia in general, not only deploy a colloquial language, but frequently address the recipient as *appā*, which means "father" in Tamil, but which is also used to address a young man, boy, or son by adding the suffix *-ppā* to words in colloquial parlance. Manuscripts mirror this in the ubiquitous phrase: *keḷuppā*, "listen, [my] son." This might be interpreted as the author addressing his own son, indicative of a filial relationship between *guru* and student. It also serves to demonstrate that a close relationship between teacher and pupil is established or assumed.[4] Further, it shows how such "texts" are supposed to be transmitted: orally, through a teacher speaking to a student.

Velayudhan explained that what makes a good practitioner is having learned from an accomplished *guru* and having attained experience. Learning from books was not sufficient to achieve this (compare Jekatā 2005, 3). He devalued "mental lessons," *maṉappāṭam*, that is, something learned by heart and retained in the memory, as against experience, *aṉupavam*. The translators of the manuscript *Varma cūttiram* similarly stress the importance of practical experience of vital spots over text-book reading:

> Practical [instructions] remove confusion arising out of textual reading. Learning each varma [spot] becomes complete only when the student observes the process of a patient being treated. This makes it a difficult thing to master all the varmas in a short period of time. Thus the student-teacher interaction has to be spread over a period of time comparatively longer.
>
> (Subramaniam 1994, 92–93)

While hinting at long periods of learning, this quotation also asserts that intricacies of the vitals pots have to be observed or demonstrated by a practitioner. Many of the manuscripts themselves repeatedly note that a particular aspect or technique had to be taught only by a good or experienced *guru* (*Varmakkaṇṇāṭi*, 156; Mariyajōcap n.d., 75–76).

4. See also Weiss (2009, 166) for a similar discussion of colloquial language of premodern siddha texts.

One reason for this might be the complicated language used in most manuscripts, which makes them difficult to understand by the uninitiated. They consist of poetic verses (*pāṭal*), some of which are hard to comprehend even by practitioners themselves. One of Zarrilli's (1998, 159) informants on *kaḷarippayaṭṭu*, for instance, though willing to share his texts on vital spots, was unable to explain them, as it had been so long since he had used the manuscripts.[5] Zvelebil (1973, 229) has described such texts as "a closed mystic treasure-box bound by the Lock of ignorance, and only a practising Siddha yogi is able to unlock the poems and reveal their true meaning." Siddha poetry is said to use a codified language, through which certain aspects have allegedly been kept concealed (Jekatā 2005, 9). If a student has not been initiated into a text, its contents can either appear as incomprehensible or be open to a variety of interpretations. As Wood (1985, 115) points out, the explanations of a knowledgeable teacher are required to understand these manuscripts, which are fairly meaningless without such a teacher who knows the practical skills and techniques himself. For example, a vital spot may be described in a text as located two named measures below the nipple, but the lack of a standard measure corresponding to the name in the text would mean that an experienced practitioner would be required to interpret the text and point out the spot.[6]

Furthermore, as we have seen in chapter 2, manuscripts exhibit considerable deviations regarding many aspects of vital spots, including names, locations, or treatment methods. Practices of contemporary *ācāṉ*s also show vast variations, regarding both the manuscripts and fellow practitioners' practices. Importantly therefore, one needs to acknowledge Zarrilli's (1989, 1291) observation that "different lineages of practitioners have always existed, each possessing its own interpretation and techniques . . . [yet] the authoritative text in the living tradition is the master's embodied practice." This is not to mean that textual learning does not figure in the transmission of vital spot knowledge. Students may learn certain manuscript passages by heart, especially regarding numbers of vital spots or their names.

---

5. Also, oral commands (*vāyttāri*) for fighting exercises often require much practice. Therefore, despite the fact that the *vāyttāri* commands still exist in text form, several techniques in *kaḷarippayaṭṭu* are said to have been virtually lost since they are not found in practice (Nair 2007, xvii).

6. Eliade (1970, 53) similarly has remarked that most *yoga āsanas* in *haṭha yoga* treatises are described only in outline, "for āsana is learned from a *guru* and not from descriptions."

Meaningful Names

Most vital loci bear names (*peyar*) which make sense, or which have been given for a reason (*kāraṇam*), a *kāraṇappeyar*. Some vital spots are labeled according to their location, such as *uccivarmam*, situated on top of the head (*ucci*). Likewise, *tilartakkālam* is located at a person's forehead, where in India the *tilaka*, a round mark in red, white, or black, is anointed with ash or sandalwood, as ornament or sectarian distinction. Some appellations point to an appearance of a particular spot. This is the case for *muṭiccuvarmam*, on the neck, where a bundle (*muṭiccu*) of nerves is said to be found (Subramaniam 1994, 170; Kaṇṇaṉ Rājārām 2007c, 412). Other names may relate to effects which particular spots cause in case of an injury, descriptive of symptoms observed. An affliction of *uṟakkakālam* thus causes drowsiness, *uṟakkam* (*Varmakkaṇṇāṭi*, 155; Mariyajōcap n.d., 74). Another spot, *uṟumikālam*, causes a patient to grunt, *uṟumu-tal*, like a pig (*paṉṟi*), and hence is also known as *paṉṟivarmam* (*Varmakkaṇṇāṭi*, 214; Mariyajōcap n.d., 112). Explaining to me the meaning of *aṭappavarmam*, a spot located near the lowermost bone of the rib cage, Velayudhan pointed out its tasks of protecting the inner organs, by way of shutting, closing, *aṭaippu*. *Kaiviralmaṭakkivarmam* describes both location and effect together, as it literally is "the vital spot [which causes a] bending [of the] fingers."

Most names therefore, hinting at a location, the outcome of an affliction, or appearance, assist practitioners in locating spots, and in diagnosing and treating an affliction. As such they can be considered valuable mnemonic aids, together with oral commands for combat techniques and the memorizing of passages from manuscripts. Importantly, on the other hand, *ācāṉ*s emphasize concepts for instruction, which only very rarely integrate such mnemonic techniques or manuscripts.[7]

Experiencing the Vital Spots

The particular nature of apprenticeship learning required for *varmakkalai* benefits precisely from the close relationship between *guru* and disciple (figure 6.1). A particular mode of teaching and learning is possible and

7. Production of palm-leaf manuscripts has become virtually extinct, not least because the use of paper and pen is cheaper, faster, and easier. Most *ācāṉ*s store their manuscripts in cupboards, where the brittle leaves eventually fall prey to ants and the ravages of time.

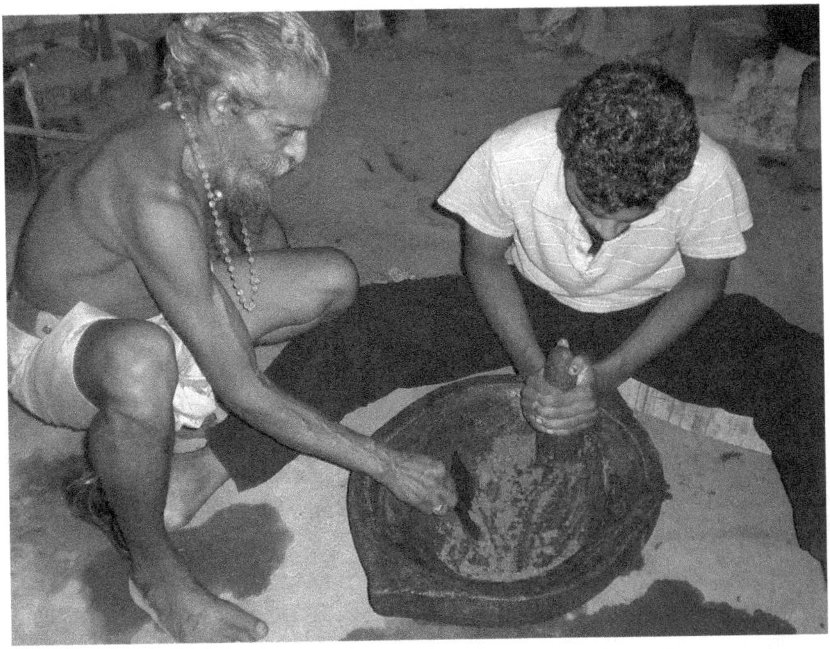

FIGURE 6.1 A siddha practitioner with his student preparing medicine

ideally develops in the transmission of vital spot knowledge from teacher to student. Verbalization of knowledge in this education plays only a minor role, whereas a somatic understanding, an experiential incorporation, or embodiment of vital spot practices is of primary importance.

While interviewing Velayudhan regarding his instruction, which I knew he had received mainly from his father, I was surprised when the *ācāṉ* laughingly responded that his father had not taught him at all. He stated: "My father would not teach me [*collit tara māṭṭār*]. Although he did not teach me, I watched him." It is important to note that the word for "teaching," that I had used in my query, *collittaru-tal*, is a compound word which translates as "giving by way of speaking." Velayudhan, on the other hand, stressed that instruction had taken place not so much by way of communication, but that his father had been teaching him through "giving-by-showing." In Tamil this is conveyed through *kāṭṭikkoṭu-ttal*, another verb meaning "to teach," with the sense of "showing the method of doing something."

Students of the vital spots are neither expected nor entitled to ask questions, similar to what has been observed by Zarrilli (1998, 159) in *kaḷarippayaṭṭu* training. As Goody (1989, 252–254) has pointed out, asking questions in apprenticeship learning environments in West Africa may be interpreted as an attempt or indication to question the authority of a master (see also Marchand 2010, 9), and this may be the case in transmitting vital spot knowledge as well to some extent. While an absence of verbal asking-answering initially seemed to affect my ethnographic research—often I did not receive the reply I had expected, or not a verbal reply at all—I soon recognized that many aspects of *varmam* are not easily put into words, questions, and answers. Again, Zarrilli (1998, 160) has observed a similar pattern for *kaḷarippayaṭṭu* vital spots, accurately noting that "knowing the vital spots is not a 'knowledge' that can be taught, but only intuited experientially, as a mode of 'revealed' knowledge."

The "*guru*'s method," *gurumuṟai*, is the proper method for instructing vital spots, one informant named Satyamurthi *ācāṉ* explained to me. This, he stated, was in opposition to education in colleges and schools, which conveyed "book knowledge," *nūlaṟivu*, through textual sources of instruction. Sathyamurthi said: "One can listen and learn which vital spot is in which place. But without the *guru*'s method, one cannot do anything with such knowledge! Even if you hear and see all points, you cannot do anything with it." Zarrilli (1998, 160) cites one of his informants as explaining the experiential nature of such knowledge, which cannot be communicated by texts or words: "Even thousands of volumes and talks of the masters cannot explain or give knowledge about the sweetness of sugar. One can experience the sweetness of sugar only when some sugar is put on his tongue."[8] Indeed, vital spots and related practices pertain to large degrees to a kind of *experiential knowledge*, which is difficult, if not impossible, to be described by words, and which must be observed and incorporated to be understood. This is elucidated by its instruction methods.

Knowledge, Skill, and Lucky Hands

The concepts of *ceypākam* and *kaipākam* characterize different forms of therapeutic knowledge and skill in siddha medicine. Both concepts are important in the preparation of medicines, treatment of patients, and transmission of knowledge. The term *ceypākam* jointly incorporates *cey*,

8. Suśruta, the ancient authority on ayurvedic surgery, is quoted thus: "An ass carrying a load of sandalwood feels the burden but not the fragrance thereof; similar are those who study many a text sans understanding" (Valiathan 2007, 9; Thakkur 1965, 169).

"deed" or the verb "to do," with *pākam*, "cooking, dressing food." The *Tamil-English Dictionary of Medicine, Chemistry, Botany, and Allied Sciences* of T. V. Sambasivam Pillai (1991–1998) explains *ceypākam* as "process or method of preparation as per rules" contemplated in Indian medical texts, and explicitly contrasts *ceypākam* with *kaipākam*, which the dictionary translates as "practical experience, skill" (Sambasivam Pillai 1991–1998, 5:527). A word composite of *kai* and *pākam*, *kai* means "hand," and can also denote "that which is fit to be done." In short, *ceypākam* denotes a formula or recipe, and *kaipākam* denotes having internalized how to correctly apply this formula or recipe (Weiss 2009, 16).

Amongst other things, important concepts for the instruction in *varmakkalai* include the location of spots, symptoms in case of an injury, stipulations of time limits for treatment and amount of pressure for both attack and treatment. These aspects can be said to pertain to *ceypākam*, and could all be formulated. *Kaipākam*, on the other hand, denotes the state of an accomplished *ācāṉ*, who is able to combine all the aforementioned functions in order to treat patients or fight opponents; in other words, to put the theory into practice. While *ceypākam* is related to the general understanding of a system and its theory, *kaipākam* is seen by practitioners as an aspect which can be achieved only with time, in most cases long periods of time, spent with observing and practicing. *Kaipākam* is therefore deeply experience-related. According to Velayudhan, *kaipākam* includes knowing how to "open" (stimulate) a spot. This is illustrated by the fact that in contemporary Malayalam, *marmmam* denotes "secret," but also "special knowledge of the particular knack necessary to do something" (Zarrilli 1998, 157). Indeed, stimulation of a vital spot always incorporates a particular movement, or "knack." How this is done can be learned only through hands-on instruction.

Another important concept worth mentioning here is *kairāci*. Subramaniam (1994, 137) states that for learning the vital spots, "training and wide reading alone are not adequate, but one should possess the in-born healing touch." With this, the author means *kairāci*, literally "luck of the hand." This denotes dexterity but also a kind of natural skill to achieve something with one's hands, especially with regard to healing. According to some *ācāṉ*s, this is often found in families of hereditary vital spot practitioners. Velayudhan highlighted this concept with regard to therapeutic applications, saying that "only one who has 'luck of the hands' will treat successfully." Yet, while it was true, he admitted, that some persons had an inborn skill, a person's healing effectiveness could not be ascribed fully to it. Rather, apprenticeship with an experienced *guru* was crucial, and hence *kairāci* was as much innate as acquired. But just like *kaipākam* knowhow, acquiring "lucky hands" requires a long, experiential learning process, which employs and triggers a student's senses—first and foremost the sense of touch, as both these concepts suggest.

Grasping the Vital Spots

> When a patient consults an *ācāṉ*, a student sees the ailment, its symptoms, and how to treat. This way, he must discover it [by himself]. Otherwise, it won't enter the mind [*maṉacule ākātu*]. You can learn all *varmam* locations, but if it hasn't entered the mind, you won't understand. The kind of knowledge, which you have learnt comes from books. But on *varmam*, there exist no books. Even if you read all the manuscripts, you won't be able to grasp the vital spots. (Velayudhan *ācāṉ*, personal communication)

Velayudhan pointed out more than once that the direction of an experienced *ācāṉ*, necessary for acquiring practical knowledge of vital spots, resembles a "key," *tiṟavukōl*. This is an important term in *varmakkalai*, as "key" may be used synonymously with *aṭaṅkal* relief spots. Such spots have to be opened (*tiṟa-ttal*) in case of an injury, and hence allegorize the key to vital spot emergency treatments. Manuscripts on these therapeutic spots are themselves frequently called *tiṟavukōl*.[9] With these, a practitioner could also "open the secrets of vital spots," in the words of Velayudhan. However such "key texts" are themselves locked, and have to be opened with yet another key. This key was none other than an *ācāṉ*'s experience, the *ācāṉ* elucidated. In this notion, manuscripts have to be seen as mnemonic devices, aiding a practitioner in understanding their art and refreshing their memory. But without prior knowledge and experience, their locks cannot be opened. The key is a *guru*'s direction, a student's observation, and an apprentice practitioner's developing experience.

Once I presented Velayudhan with a bilingual publication on vital spots in Tamil and English, including names and locations of spots. The *ācāṉ* attentively flipped through the pages of the book, before he confided, "This is just what is mentioned in our manuscripts." Mistaking his statement

9. This includes *Varma tiṟavukōl*, *Caracūkṣattiṟavukōl*, and *Varmapīraṅki tiṟavukōl*.

for an appreciative remark regarding the book's authenticity, I asked him if he felt it was possible to learn *varmam* by using it. He responded,

> Not at all possible! What I meant is that this author himself does not know the vital spots! Would he merely copy what is written in manuscripts if he had learned it? He would not *write*, but *practice*! He translated a manuscript, but he didn't understand it. Otherwise he might have explained it in detail. Otherwise he would not have written a book at all, you see? Did I write a book? No, I do not write *varmam*, I practice it! Manuscripts help to teach students. If memorized, they help remembering. But one has to learn with an *ācāṉ*, stay with him, observe him, and obey his orders [*atikāram kēṭṭu*]; if one only reads, the vital spots won't enter the mind.[10]

The *ācāṉ* thus despised the knowledge gained from books, which conveyed theoretical knowledge, but which had no bearing on practical vital spot applications. This is not an individual notion of Velayudhan alone. Mentioning to a different *ācāṉ* that I had gathered from a book the existence of 108 spots, he responded agitatedly, "You've read it in a book? What a waste! If you want books, I can give you books! I bought a full shelf: all useless. They tell you that this is one spot, that another. All wrong. Not a single spot is correct. Books can't teach about *varmam*."

Learning by Touching: Nonverbal Vital Spot Instruction

During my stay in Kanyakumari district a recently set-up, private *varmam* college started offering the certificate of Diploma in Varma and Massage Science, DVMS, during a one-year course. One young alumnus of this institution confided in me that although the college had provided "excellent material," he had not learned much of "practical use," recalling the lessons as text-based. Let me quote Velayudhan on the matter of the same institution:

VELAYUDHAN: You know, there is this *varmam* college (*his facial expression implying a low standard of teaching*).

ROMAN: What about it? The instruction is not good there?

---

10. Compare this incidence with a very similar account by Hausman (1996, 45).

VELAYUDHAN: Not at all! One boy who I know has studied there. He even got a diploma. Although they award degrees, they are not teaching the truth [*uṇmai*]. One earns a certificate for reading about points displayed in books. But they are not demonstrating the exact locations.

ROMAN: They aren't even teaching that?

VELAYUDHAN: Well, locations are not everything. One also has to know how to grab and pull [the spots], but they are not teaching that! They copy books and hand them [out]. They declare: "This is one spot; that is another." That's all. I'm not like that. Look: this is the way one has to show and give (*he grabs my arm, stimulates a spot, which causes a painful sensation in my arm and makes me wince*). One has to grasp the place! They say that "only if you turn your fingers, you will understand" [*kaiviral tiruppiṉāltāṉ teriyum*]. There is another proverb [which goes]: "A science, which is not shown by touching, will not become a science." This means that only what is taught by touching will become memory [*ñāpakamākum*], and only what we perceive with our fingers will enter our mind. Only if I take your finger, place it on a certain spot and thus show it to you, you will know it.

In this statement, Velayudhan expressed many of the intricacies of the embodied mode of learning that is utilized by *ācāṉ*s. First, he deals with the two Tamil terms for teaching, "giving by saying" (*collittara-ttal*) and "giving by showing" (*kāṭṭikoṭu-ttal*). Whereas the recently founded college allegedly teaches the vital spots by means of books and tables, deploying numbers and pictures, he himself makes his students *feel* the locations. This mode of instruction triggers physical sensations in students, such as in the above quotation. Grabbing my arm with his left hand, slightly lifting it away from my torso, Velayudhan had pinched my skin near the armpit with the index finger and thumb of his right hand. A sudden, unexpected, and painful current-like sensation caused my fingers to twitch for a second. As I had known before, this spot is called *kaiviralmaṭakkivarmam*, the "finger-bending spot." But only the demonstration on my own body had revealed to me where this spot is located and how it has to be penetrated; that is, the particular knack required for this, and the effect it causes.

The proverb that Velayudhan recited is decisive in this regard: "a science, which is not shown by touching, will not become a science" (*toṭṭukkāṭṭāta vittai vittaikkākātu*), a common phrase among *ācāṉ*s.[11] To be sure, before I got to know exactly how to use my fingers to perform the particular action of stimulating this spot myself, I had to practice the step numerous times. I discovered that names and pictures can be helpful in this regard, yet are ultimately dispensable as opposed to *experiencing* a location, effect, and knack pertaining to a particular spot. The sense of touch in this regard featured constantly, and must be seen as the most crucial of senses in the context of learning the vital spots. Even manuscripts, such as the *Varmapīraṅki tiṟavukōl* (11; Nicivilcaṉ 2003, 55), state that to learn the subtleties of the vital spots, and other sense-based techniques such as pulse examination, "it needs a *guru* who shows by *touching*" (compare *Varmakkaṇṇāṭi*, 156; Mariyajōcap n.d., 75–76).

Whenever Velayudhan instructed his students in any new aspect, this happened in a "hands on" manner, both in martial training and therapeutic methods. For instance, massage techniques were shown to me, but not verbally communicated. Unfortunately, as a result, I find myself at a loss for words to describe many techniques in that category. It should be noted that other scholars have similarly remarked on the difficulties of writing about learning and practicing manual medicine (Hinojosa 2002, 22; Walkley 2004, 33). Instead of verbal explanations, Velayudhan would place his hands on mine, carefully directing my movements along a patient's body exactly as intended, using my hands as he would use his. During such instructional sessions, the student's hands are guided by those of the *guru*.

In learning massage techniques, for instance, students have to follow their *gurus*' action closely. Any hesitation—such as would be suggested by a dragging of the hands, when brisk, energetic movement is called for, to keep pace with the *guru*'s own movement—even merely holding the hand passively, would weaken the power of the massage strokes. Sensing the guidance which Velayudhan offered, I would instantly adapt and modulate my own hand movements and the pressure administered accordingly. After a student has understood a particular technique, the *ācāṉ* removes his or her own hands, and observes whether the student can continue and sustain the required technique. Whenever I was left to conduct the massaging by myself, I could feel the reduction of pressure at the very moment

11. I have encountered this or similar proverbs repeatedly, both in oral statements of *ācāṉ*s and in published accounts. See, for instance, Rājēntiraṉ (2008, 79) and Irājēntiraṉ (n.d.), who both cite variations of the phrase.

Velayudhan had removed his guiding hands. Almost reflex-driven, I strove to maintain the indentation, having somewhat internalized the required pressure. I had understood by having experienced for myself how much pressure was required, or how much pressure would be too forceful—concepts that can hardly be expressed verbally. Brigitte Jordan (1993, 192–193) has given strikingly similar descriptions of the embodied instruction of Yucatan midwives, for whom verbalization is only a secondary tool of education as compared to the acquisition of bodily skills, which are transmitted through a teacher's hands. She concludes that such embodied knowledge is in a real sense located in and transferred by the hands. Similarly, Servando Hinojosa (2002, 27) speaks of the "hand-based knowledge," which Mayan bonesetters exhibit, who claim that it is their "hands that know" how to set fractures.

Intricacies of a Learning Relationship

Carefully Choose, Test, and Conceal

One hot afternoon in May, I joined Velayudhan on the veranda of his house-cum-dispensary, reposing from a rush of patients. A young man entered the compound and introduced himself as a student at Munchirai Siddha College.[12] He expressed his interest in *varmakkalai* and his wish to spend his holidays of one month to learn from the *ācāṉ*. Velayudhan summarily refused this proposal, saying: "One month? Not possible. One has to learn for twelve years! Finish your studies and if you are still interested then, come and we will think about it. But one month will never do!" After the young man had left, obviously disappointed, Velayudhan explained to me that all manuscripts and *ācāṉ*s most steadfastly agreed on the prescribed apprenticeship period of twelve years (*Varma cūttiram*, 3; Subramaniam 1994, 14); this was a hard and fast rule. Each year of instruction, he said, corresponded to learning one *paṭuvarmam* "lethal spot," and to eight *toṭuvarmam* "touch spots," or less vulnerable loci.[13] According to

---

12. ATSVS Siddha College and Hospital of Munchirai in Kanyakumari district.

13. A period of twelve years appears frequently with regard to South Asian learning traditions. In musical instruction, for instance, a period of twelve years may be stipulated for comprehensive learning, as each year one of the twelve major notes is said to be taught. The duration of twelve years of education is furthermore mentioned by Vedic and Sanskrit texts for various eruditions (Thirugnanasambandhan 1986, 123). For instance, Glaser (1912, 16) describes that the period for entirely learning a Vedic compendium is stipulated as twelve years.

this logic, the overall number of 108 spots is apportioned into twelve years of apprenticeship.

As most manuscripts emphasize, students are required to remain with a *guru*, and learn by assisting and observing during this period. Jeyrāj (2007, 7), a hereditary *ācāṉ*, writes that "[u]sually those who had learned the vital spots used to teach ... those, who showed the right conduct, and who were devoted to god and master." Although the selection of a student should be done disregarding caste, religion, or other differences (Irājēntiraṉ 2006, 18), manuscripts frequently advise that none other than a *Śivayogi* was fit for learning vital spots (Subramaniam 1994, 140; Mariyajōcap n.d., xii; Maṇiyaṉ 2012, 13). This, I would argue, means that a student has to be spiritually inclined, an aspect which may transcend faiths. Kanyakumari, being one of the major concentrations of Christianity in South India, with almost half of the population subscribing to one of the Christian churches, is also home to a large number of Christian *ācāṉ*s. They just as frequently deploy concepts like devotion (*teyvapakti*), sympathy (*urakkam*), and compassion (*irakkam*) as prerequisites for a student. Velayudhan explained that he would teach only students who believe in god (*teyva nampikkaiyuṭaṉ*), as only those individuals "possess divinity themselves," and hence show sympathy to other beings and nourish righteous thoughts. The *Varmakkaṇṇāṭi* describes a student as one who "is without any mistakes and considers every life as his own" (3; Mariyajōcap n.d., 2). It is therefore important to point out altruistic traits and morally appropriate behavior as preconditions for vital spot students.

In order to select acceptable students by detecting such desirable characteristics, some manuscripts advise practitioners to subject aspiring candidates to testing (*cōtaṉai*) their state of mind systematically (Irājēntiraṉ 2006, 16). Only after testing a student, should an *ācāṉ* consider "hand[ing] over the treatise [of the vital spots]," notes the *Varmakkaṇṇāṭi* (3; Mariyajōcap n.d., 2). Manuscripts may even contain sets of questions to be asked of prospective apprentices, in order to assess their suitability. According to one informant, Samuel *ācāṉ*, who practices on the outskirts of Nagercoil town, such testing should enquire into a student's aggression potential. For instance, confronted with threats, a "good student" should never fight back, but choose to abstain from violence.[14] This is also

14. Citing a North Indian ayurvedic practitioner, who eclectically incorporates *marmma cikitsā* into his regimen, Langford (2002, 213) provides a similar statement.

reflected in the *Varmakkaṇṇāṭi*: "On earth, whoever may oppose you, be cool-headed and recede just like an honorable person [would]. Talk in a friendly way with him and withdraw, without revealing the acclaimed loci" (4; Mariyajōcap n.d., 2).

Many contemporary practitioners furthermore suggest that they had to undergo frequent and repeated testing even during much of their apprenticeship period, while many aspects, such as how to attack a vital spot, were withheld from them. The tendency of some *gurus* to refuse to teach particular aspects even to their own apprentices is a particularly familiar experience of former students. Many *ācāṉs* thus recollected their instruction with mixed feelings, evocative of testing and hardships (*kaṣṭam*). The following occurrence was narrated to me by Palani *ācāṉ*, who had learned *varmakkalai* while simultaneously enrolled in a homeopathy course in a government college. Primarily practicing siddha medicine and administering a thriving *varmam* hospital situated a one-hour bus ride north of Thackalai in West Kanyakumari today, Palani reflected on his apprenticeship as follows:

> Once, my *guru* had called me to come to his hut one morning. I was about to take an exam in Homeopathy on this very day. Although he knew that I had to go to my college, he advised me to collect some medicinal plants, which he said he had run out of. As he was my *guru*, I could not refuse. But to find the right herb, I had to walk a considerable distance. It took me long, and when I returned, it had become very late. My *guru* told me to put the plants where he stored all his medicines. What did I see there? The very same plant was already there in abundance! When I reached my college that day it was too late to take my exam and I had to retake it on another day. That was one way of him testing me.

Accounts of how *ācāṉs* allegedly deceive their students to prevent them from observing a certain technique or knack are frequently encountered. Chidambarathanu Pillai (1995, 27) states that many practitioners did not teach important therapeutic spots to their own students directly: "The student who follows in his foot-steps may come to know these techniques. Those who do not have the blessings of the Guru may not come to know these." One of Zarrilli's (1998, 156) informants was adamant that he would only pass on to his most trusted student the secrets of a particular technique for reviving unconscious patients when he himself was on his deathbed! Now as before, *varmakkalai* masters are reported to be reluctant to transmit their knowledge for fear of misuse by many young people (Jeyrāj 2000, 3). Learning *varmam* is therefore described by apprentices as long and strenuous. Students whom I interviewed often complained that they were allowed to do only "unimportant work," and several full-fledged *ācāṉ*s reminisced about their apprenticeship as hard times, during which they had been expected to serve their *guru*s as servants, especially during the initial stages of learning.

It appears that practitioners link teaching of specific aspects of their knowledge to the moral development and trustworthiness of their students, which may frequently be verified through tests. Most *ācāṉ*s emphasize loyalty and obedience as crucial aspects of studentship, and also as the first principles of a *guru*-disciple relationship in general. But a *guru* also bears a certain kind of responsibility toward an apprentice and, as we shall see, informed by the particular moral notions involved, develops a distinct economy of knowledge transmission.

A Moral Economy of Knowledge Transmission

Students have to fulfill demanding criteria and are carefully selected; they are required to have a virtuous character, and to be devoted to god and to their teachers. If the character as prescribed is assessed favorably in an apprentice, a *guru* can accept the student's vow, *kurutīṭcai* (Skt. *dīkṣā*), and accept a stipulated gift or fees, *taṭciṇam* (*dakṣiṇa*), so the manuscripts note (*Varma cūttiram*, 3; Subramaniam 1994, 14). While I will address the initiatory process of *tīṭcai* shortly, it is important to enquire into reasons for the testing and the concealing. Velayudhan explained that a period of twelve years and tests were important, as only then will a student have "felt hardships," an experience important for forming a practitioner's personality. An *ācāṉ* should of course possess in-depth knowledge of martial and therapeutic applications, and, most importantly, a practitioner's character should be defined by sympathy with all beings, pure thoughts, calmness, self-control, absence of bad thoughts and of bad habits (Irājēntiraṉ 2006, 21; Maṇiyaṉ 2012, 47), such as quarreling, telling lies, boasting, murder, or theft, but rather should feed ascetics, and revere elders, *gurus*, and gods (*Varmakkaṇṇāṭi*, 99–101; Mariyajōcap n.d., 46–48). The same ethical regulations do not concern only apprentices, but also form an important part of the code of conduct for any full-fledged *ācāṉ* as well.

Let me quote and explain here two proverbs, commonly cited by *ācāṉ*s, which describe the relationship between teacher and student in a nutshell. One goes: "The *guru*'s curse is the student's ruin" (*kuru cāpam ciṣyiaṉukku kēṭu*). The disciple, according to one practitioner, was highly dependent on his or her teacher. *Guru* are for their part responsible for what to instruct and how. Many vital spot techniques are designed as therapeutic measures, with the objective of curing people. Yet vital spot combat methods are always prone to be (mis)used against others, and are potentially lethal. A *guru* is hence responsible for what and how something is taught, as the reputation and possibly even the life of a student may be at stake. Furthermore, if the *guru* curses a student, it may be for a terrible transgression on the latter's part, and the saying therefore contains a warning to the disciple against any kind of misconduct or disobedience. Another phrase is often encountered exactly when *ācāṉ*s refer to the possibility of misuse of martial techniques or of (medical) malpractice. This saying expresses that if, for instance, a student misuses the knowledge and kills a person by applying pressure to a vital spot, then not the student, but the respective *guru*, would be blamed: "the blame is the *guru*'s, not the student's" (*kuruvukku paḻi ciṣiyaṉukku paḻi illai*). As Velayudhan explained:

> [i]f one passes [this knowledge] on and something happens, who will be blamed? The *guru* will be blamed, not the student. So if I taught you some vital spots now and you went out on the streets and attacked someone using these spots, he might die. Whose fault would this be then? It would be my fault; people would blame me!

A *guru* is thus ultimately responsible for the doings of a student, a student's actions, deeds, and misdeeds ultimately rebound on the teacher. For this very reason, a student has responsibility toward the *guru* as well, and this is largely due to the dangerous nature of the practices involved. One unidentified manuscript notes, in cautioning the practitioner to carefully select apprentices: "[the vital spot knowledge] is to be handed on to none other than a *Śivayogin*. Should you [divulge this information] to the mischievous of this world, then you will live in a most terrible hell [in a state] like dying. I am telling you: do not hand over [this knowledge] to the sinners of this world" (Mariyajōcap n.d., xii; compare also Maṇiyaṉ 2012, 13).

Instruction of vital spots was and is often a system of filial apprenticeship and in many cases *guru* and disciple are cognates. Velayudhan's own son, about ten years old, spends every Saturday and Sunday and virtually all school holidays in his father's dispensary, playfully engaged in the proceedings inside the dispensary, a playful learning through mimicry, a modality of education which has been considered of utmost importance by numerous scholars (Benjamin [1933] 2007; Taussig 1993; Wulf 2002; Downey 2010). The *ācāṉ*'s two students at the time I was visiting the dispensary—Murugan, aged thirty, and Manikandhan, twenty-four—were both close relatives of Velayudhan as well, Murugan being the *ācāṉ*'s elder sister's son, and Manikandhan the son of Velayudhan's wife's brother. *Guru* and student may thus share a close, intimate relationship on many grounds: they live together, often are from one family, and they are importantly bound by a relationship of mutual responsibility. Student always have to keep in mind their *guru* and remind themselves constantly that the wrongs and mistakes they commit are not only theirs; this ultimately includes the responsibility not to spoil the reputation of the *guru* or lineage, *paramparā*. To revere and respect one's *guru* is hence a concept of utmost importance, constantly related by manuscripts and by practitioners as well. This is called "respect for the *guru*," *kuru mariyātai*, a concept that the manuscripts and the present-day *ācāṉ*s frequently stress.

"Treat without Arrogance, Thinking of Your Guru"

In *varmakkalai*, as in most traditional learning relationships in India, from forms of music and dance to artisanship, reverence is paid to the person who is responsible for transmitting the knowledge: the *guru*. Some of Velayudhan's former teachers would frequently come for a visit, and invariably the *ācāṉ* would give them some money upon their departure. Although these "old *ācāṉ*s" did not practice any more, they could still depend on their former students. It is stated that for students, the *guru* should come only next to god in devotion and gratefulness (Subramaniam 1994, 93; Pillai 1986, 65). In *varmakkalai*, this is reflected in manuscripts that advise practitioners to contemplate the preceptor before starting any therapeutic technique or martial training. Such homage includes repeating the *guru*'s name inwardly while bearing his or her image in mind, as in a prayer. Some *ācāṉ*s would approach a picture of their *guru*, close their eyes and pray for a short moment, before even turning their attention to me to talk about the vital spots. Likewise, practitioners may start their consultation only after having prayed to their respective *guru*(s) and god(s), unconcerned at the crowd of patients gathered outside. Irājēntiraṉ (2006,

309) notes that in order to efficiently cure, an *ācāṉ* must "treat without arrogance [*āṇavam*], thinking of one's *guru*."

Indeed, a practitioner's devotion toward the *guru*, I was told, was even of therapeutic value. The skill of their teacher is expected to positively affect their own healing (and fighting), and to this end, *ācāṉ*s may seek the blessing of their lineage and their preceptor. The *Varmakkaṇṇāṭi* (156; Mariyajōcap n.d., 75–76) notes that those practitioners who applaud themselves foolishly claiming to be capable of vital spot mastery would merely amass vast amounts of *karma*. If, on the other hand, a student had learned from an experienced *ācāṉ*, then it was a good practice; and the *Varmapīraṅkicūttiram* (5; Nicivilcaṉ 2003, 36) adds that, in order to prevent such skill from "falling prey to the fire [of hell]," a practitioner should always revere his or her *guru*. Meditating on a preceptor's name and image, by literally "keeping the *guru* in mind" (*kuruvai maṉacukkuḷḷē vaiccakka*), for Agasthiyar *ācāṉ* also meant remembering his period of apprenticeship. In doing so, he even appeared to refresh his memory to some extent. Explaining that his *guru*, long passed away, was constantly teaching him, and intervening if he was ever about to commit a mistake in treating a patient, the remembrance of his late *ācāṉ* for Agasthiyar *ācāṉ* has become almost a mnemonic device.[15]

For the Knowledge to Stand

The special relationship between student and teacher is exemplified in a rite of initiation, in the course of which an apprentice is accepted by an *ācāṉ* and instruction is commenced thereafter. This is called *guru tīṭcai*. After two months of having been an observer in Velayudhan's dispensary, I was astonished when the *ācāṉ* one day announced that I had to perform a *guru tīṭcai*, a "vow to the teacher." A little while earlier, the *ācāṉ* had started me on hands-on instruction on the reading of *nāṭi* pulse, the only way he said to learn the different aspects of pulse examination. Three days later, he declared: "I cannot teach you about all this any further. If you want to learn, then we have to conduct *guru tīṭcai* first." This initiation, Velayudhan declared, was the right way to demonstrate "respect for the *guru*," *kuru mariyātai*. If I wished to further understand vital spot practice,

15. Similarly, Sujatha, Aruna, and Balasubramanian (1991, 75) report that South Indian healers often draw on supernatural guidance, like receiving advice from a deity or a deceased forefather.

conducting *tīṭcai* was inevitable. Of course, I was not only willing to learn more, but was also thrilled to experience an initiation.

Thursday is the most auspicious day of the week for conducting *tīṭcai*, as this is the day of the *guru*, Velayudhan elucidated. Thursday, *viyāḻakkiḻamai* in Tamil, is connected closely to any initiation, as it is the weekday named for the planet Jupiter, *viyāḻam*, the preceptor of the gods (Skt. *bṛhaspati*). Velayudhan indeed often referred to Thursday simply as "*guru*" in everyday speech, thereby reflecting the Sanskrit term for Thursday: *guru vāsara*, "day of the teacher." On a Thursday morning chosen by Velayudhan, I was to go to the Nagercoil market to purchase the following items: a bundle of bananas, one coconut, betel leaves, areca nuts, a ripe mango, flowers, frankincense, and a clay lamp. Upon arrival at the *ācāṉ*'s house, his two students helped me place all the items on a plate, plus a copper vessel filled with water. I was further instructed to add the amount of 101 rupees.[16] We presented the plate to a small idol of Śiva, installed inside the dispensary, and lit the clay lamp from another lamp already burning at the idol's feet. I was directed to take the tray, and to present it to Velayudhan, who took the lamp from it, to circulate it in front of the idol. The *ācāṉ* held his hand shortly over the flame and then brought the same hand close to my eyes, so I could feel the fire's warmth. He then received the whole tray from my hands, and I was told to prostrate myself on the ground, lying flat in front of the *ācāṉ*, while touching his feet with my hands. This posture is called *aṣṭāṅganamaskāra*, a form of obeisance made by prostrating oneself in such a way as to touch the ground with eight (*aṣṭa*) parts (*aṅgam*) of the body (feet, hands, shoulders, breast, and forehead). Handing over the tray to one of his students, Velayudhan bowed down toward me, grasped my hands, and raised me up to a standing position. Now he placed his hands on my head and moved thumb and ring finger of his right hand as if inscribing on my scalp, after which he applied sandal-paste, *vipūti* or cow dung ash, and red *kuṅkumam* powder on my forehead. Leaning toward me, the *ācāṉ* whispered into my right ear. What he whispered was a *mantra*, the "words of the *guru*" (*kuru vārttai*) which, as he cautioned me later, I was never to reveal to anyone under any circumstances. Velayudhan now took the coconut and split it open by smashing it on the hard floor. The water from inside the coconut was offered to the deity, and we shared the

16. See also Aleksāṇṭar Ācāṉ (1998, 4) for mentioning similar items used in *tīṭcai*. At the time of this event, 101 rupees equated to about €1.50.

flesh of the coconut later. The *ācāṉ* handed the tumbler containing water to me to drink, and explained that henceforth, concluding the ritual, I was accepted by him as student, and I had accepted him as my *guru* (compare Aleksāṇṭar Ācāṉ 1998, 4). In fact, I did feel accepted and welcome. Accepted by an *ācāṉ* well versed in his practice, who had demonstrated his willingness to have me around to observe and even to learn from him. But I also felt responsible now: responsible not to misuse this relationship, but also responsible not to disappoint him. I was eager to fulfill expectations Velayudhan potentially had in me.

The *ācāṉ* later elucidated that when accepting a student, a *guru* starts to change the fate, *viti*, of the apprentice. Tamils assume that fate is inscribed on a person's forehead (*talaiyeḻuttu*) at the time of birth by the god Brahmā. The gesture of inscribing a new fate on the student's head may be said to be performed during *tīṭcai*, and Velayudhan had done so, by writing with his fingers on my head. He also explained that, having received the words of the *guru*, which I was never to disclose, the knowledge of the vital spot would henceforth "stand in my mind": *maṉacule nikkum*. Similar pledges of secrecy by the initiate are found in many South Asian rites of initiation, especially regarding esoteric knowledge (Levy 1990, 314). Proceeding otherwise, teaching without performing *tīṭcai*, "knowledge would not stand, but fall," said Velayudhan. That is, knowledge transmitted without due rites might be disrespected or fall into the wrong hands. This, the *ācāṉ* explained, was the reason to perform an initiation. It may be necessary to analyze some of the steps of this initiation individually with regard to this aim of ensuring that "knowledge will stand."

The student prostrates on the ground, and touches the *guru*'s feet, a performance called "to greet by touching the feet," *kāl toṭṭu vaṇaṅku-tal*, by which devotion or highest respect is accorded (Alex 2008, 537) to the *guru*. The *guru* thus revered acknowledges and reciprocates this gesture, by touching the head of the apprentice. This is called "touching the head," *talai toṭu-tal*, which expresses acknowledgment both of the reverence paid, and thus of a superior status, and of one's courtesy, or blessing. *Kāl toṭṭu vaṇaṅku-tal* and *talai toṭu-tal* can be described as successional parts of a contiguous performative social gesture. In the context of initiation, this gesture entails the request of a student to be accepted and taught by a *guru*, and the *guru*'s acceptance of the student. It is important to note the hierarchy embodied in this performance, which is emblematic of the relationship between teacher and student. In the Hindu, Indian context, where different body parts are inscribed with different values and (im) purities, the feet are accorded the highest degree of impurity. Persons are understood to be constantly influenced by myriad substances by which they are permeated (Marriott 1990), and the feet absorb the greatest degree of impurity of the human body. Therefore, touching someone else's feet includes being permeated by the impurities and sharing in this person's attributes (Alex 2008, 537). In contrast to the feet, the head, which is touched by a *guru*, is regarded as the purest body part, and the touching symbolizes a blessing and acceptance.

The act of touching the feet of an elder or a teacher and the act of prostrating oneself before deities symbolize humility and faith. The latter posture forms an important part of *pūjā*, prayer conducted by Hindus. *Pūjā* includes *darśan* or "perceiving" of a deity, by bringing the warmth of a flame, which has been presented before a god's idol, toward one's eyes with the hands. As Diana Eck (1998) has pointed out in her study of *darśan*, this visual experience includes not only "seeing a deity," but also "being seen by the deity" (see also Babb 1981). Through "seeing a deity," devotees establish contact with their god, whom they admire, while at the same time they are "being seen" by the deity, who thus gives his or her blessing. In this way, through the vision and the flame, a contact between god and devotee is established, a contact which is experienced as intimate and as almost tactile in nature (Eck 1998). In temples, the flame is normally presented first before the god and then before devotees by an official priest (*pūjāri*). While the *darśan* in my case was that of god Śiva, the conveyor was Velayudhan in a *pūjāri*'s stead. It is important to note in this context that the items used in *tīṭcai* correspond to the items used in Hindu *pūjā* (Jeanes 1982, 2). What are offered as gifts to deities in the sphere of temple ritual are offered by students in a parallel way to *gurus* in initiation. While prospective apprentices thus devote themselves to a preceptor, *gurus* acknowledge this and accept them as students in return. But also, the students take the part of the devotees who offer oblations and who receive the leftovers (*piracātam*) of the deity from the hands of a *guru*. The *guru* might therefore be seen as taking over the mediatory position of *pūjāri*. Moreover, and more intriguingly, the *guru* also becomes homologous to the deity in being revered by the student, after which the *ācāṉ* offers blessing and acceptance.

I had expected Velayudhan to use this opportunity to demand money from me, a kind of course fee. Handing over the items mentioned as an initial present given by students to teachers when commencing instruction is also known as *guru dakṣiṇa*, "*guru*'s gift, fee" (Jeanes 1982, 30), or as *ācā<u>n</u> kāṇikkai* (Raj 1977, 95) with regard to *varmakkalai*, the "offering to the *ācā<u>n</u>*." Many informants reported that they had spent large amounts of money on their education in *varmakkalai*. Some practitioners indeed seem to understand the term *tīṭcai* as tantamount to "study fees." Velayudhan however maintained that such practitioners, for whom *varmam* was a "business," did not deserve being called *ācā<u>n</u>*, since they completely misunderstood the meaning of an initiation. This was not about money, or about receiving a gift, or about paying a teacher to receive education, and hence he never asked me for any money, either during my initiation or on any other occasion. Rather, as I experienced it, *tīṭcai* enacts a substantial and moral relationship, in which the *guru* is simultaneously like a god and like a father. It is an act of bonding a student to a teacher and is, in fact, similar to brahmanical-hinduistic initiations, which enact a kind of birth (Glaser 1912, 13; Michaels 1998, 102). The initiator is described by the *Atharvaveda* as accommodating the adept in his or her uterus, and as ritually giving birth to the student afterwards. The *guru* of such a ritual can be said to become a new figure of attachment and reverence replacing the adept's parents. Indologists therefore have argued that the relationship between *guru* and disciple is best compared to that between mother or father and child (Steinmann 1986, 36). In other words, a strong, personal, and intimate bond between student and teacher is being established. The initiation in my case clearly was conducted out of concerns by Velayudhan of ethical justifications of passing on certain details of his knowledge to me. By performing this initiatory rite, he was establishing a substantial and moral relationship with me. The words, *vārttai*, which the *guru* had uttered, marked this acceptance by the *ācā<u>n</u>*. At the same time, the term *vārttai*, apart from "word," also means "undertaking" or "promise," a most appropriate connotation of the word—the *ācā<u>n</u>* solemnly promised to accept me into his care, and to teach me, while I promised to obey the *guru* and carry out his instructions faithfully. As has been remarked before, the relation between *guru* and disciple thus becomes an intensely personal one (Mandelbaum 1970, 529), built on mutual responsibilities.

Tacit Knowledge and Moral Economies of Learning

As described earlier, vital spot knowledge is somatic; it is acquired through a student's body and senses, and may be termed "tacit." Tacit knowledge, according to Michael Polanyi (1974; 1985), is knowledge that cannot be verbalized or has not yet been verbalized, a nonlinguistic form of knowledge which is embedded in individual experiences, and which, in Polanyi's words, "indwells" the body. Tacit knowledge is opposed to explicit knowledge, information that can be written down or explained, but similar to implicit knowledge, which "takes place largely independently of conscious attempts to learn and largely in the absence of explicit knowledge about what was acquired" (Reber 1993, 5). But implicit knowledge and tacit knowledge are not synonymous, according to Stephen Gourlay (2004, 86), as "[i]mplicit knowledge is something we might know, but do not wish to express, while tacit knowledge is something that we know but cannot express; it is personal, difficult to convey, and which does not easily express itself in the formality of language and is thus non-communicable." For this reason, tacit knowledge "is always ahead of the capability of its possessor to explicate it" (Reber 1993, 64). It may be said to pertain to a "practical consciousness," but not to a "discursive consciousness," which includes "those forms of recall which the actor is able to express verbally," in the words of Anthony Giddens (1984, 49). Apprenticeship learning in particular has been often described as the acquisition of bodily skills, and as being in contrast to the didactic schooling models, which are more concerned with verbal and abstract knowledge. The former involves "the *ability to do* rather than the *ability to talk about* something, and indeed, it may be impossible to verbally elicit from people operating in this mode what they know (how to do)," according to Jordan (1993, 192).

Ways of acquiring tacit knowledge include observation, mimesis, and extensive and repetitious physical practice, such as in learning how to ride a bike or speak a language (Polanyi 1967, 50; Downey 2010), and importantly, a sensory, bodily engagement. Mayan bonesetters, with whom Hinojosa has worked, emphasize that their knowledge of the body and of diagnosing broken bones cannot be taught, but can only be detected by "the hands [that] make contact with the suffering bodies" (Hinojosa 2002, 27). They accordingly may be said to know in "a bodily, multisensorial way, lacking the language and categories of human experience" (27). *Varmakkalai* being itself a body-based, sense-based practice, its knowledge and techniques are therefore not transmitted primarily through texts. Rather, vital spot knowledge transmission must be recognized as a process of "carnal and sensual learning," parallel to "carnal and sensual knowing," as described by Shilling and Mellor (1995). Treatment and martial applications are directed by a practitioner's body and repeated by a student's body, and the knowhow is internalized in these bodies and is not, and cannot be, externalized. Within this, senses are of great importance, the first of which are a student's tactility and kinesthesia, but not so much the sense of sight, which has received a lot of scholarly attention in recent decades in the West (Foucault 1977), but to which many *ācāṉ*s would rather deny educative effectiveness with regard to the vital spots. For *varmakkalai* practitioners, therapeutic and martial practices become, with experience, a "bodily being-in-the-world." Csordas (1999, 143) has argued for such a concept of embodiment as "an existential condition in which the body is the subjective source or intersubjective ground of experience." As Polanyi, the first to have used the term "tacit knowledge" has stated, "it is one thing to learn a list of bones, arteries, nerves and viscera and quite another to know how precisely they are intertwined inside the body" (1967, 89).

On this ground I argue that, in the case of *varmakkalai* and for siddha medicine in general, textual sources such as the palm-leaf manuscripts have to be complemented with practical observation and experience. Manuscripts generally only give short descriptions of treatment procedures, if at all, and leave a vast space for interpretations. With regard to vital spots, textual sources often remain conspicuously vague or ambiguous, and may even contradict other vital spot manuscripts. The same is true for practitioners, who exhibit vastly differing perceptions of, discourses on, and methods of vital spots. This can in part be explained by the closed, lineage-based learning and teaching, which create differing corpuses of knowledge, but which also answer to the requirements of teaching a highly embodied, tacit knowledge. A considerable gap exists between the texts in the possession of many *ācāṉ*s and their practice. I would argue that the key to this gap is to be found in the "traditional" educational system, or *guru-śiṣya-paramparā*. This way of teaching, learning, and ultimately practicing outweighs textual education. It is informative in this context to note that the Sanskrit word for education, *śikṣā*, which is the root for the Sanskrit and Tamil words for "student," *śiṣya*, means *practice* (Crook 1996b, 9). As should have become clear above, *varmam* learning and practice are highly touch-based.

Furthermore, and important for our understanding of secrecy, in accepting *varmakkalai* as pertaining to a large degree to tacit knowledge, we must acknowledge that *ācāṉ*s may indeed *know more than they can tell* (Polanyi 1967, 4). The difficulty in objectifying and thus talking or writing about tactile experience has already been acknowledged by Merleau-Ponty ([1962] 1996, 316), who noted that: "tactile experience . . . adheres to the surface of our body; we cannot unfold it before us and it never quite becomes an object." As tactile perception and experience are twofold, a two-tier process, consisting of both touching and being touched, the distinction between touching subject and touched object blurs; touching, as Glen Mazis (1998, 147) has pointed out, drawing on Merlau-Ponty, is not unidirectional: that is, "one cannot neatly bisect the experience of touch into the act of touching and the passively touched object." And according to Hsu (2000a, 252), it is "precisely this involvement between subject and object [that] makes it difficult to account for touch in a detached and descriptive way." While such sensory, somatic factors handicap attempts at scholarly description, the same is true for *ācāṉ*s' (re)presentations of their practices. Following Polanyi's (1967, 4) argument, *ācāṉ*s *know more than they can tell*, and this is, I argue, an important aspect of the particular type of secrecy which surrounds the vital spots. But such a connection between knowledge that cannot be articulated and concealed knowledge has largely been overlooked by scholars. Simmel (1907), for instance, claimed that remaining silent on something supposed to be kept concealed was unnatural, and therefore had to be learned under difficulties. On the other hand, acknowledging that some secrets pertain to tacit dimensions allows for recognizing that secrecy may *by definition* be silent.

Moreover, there is a strong connection between tacit knowledge, sensory learning, and moral constraints; analyzing the apprenticeship mode of instruction, Polanyi has hinted at such a correlation:

> To learn by example is to submit to authority. You follow your master because you trust his manner of doing things even when you cannot analyse and account in detail for its effectiveness. By watching the master and emulating his efforts in the presence of his example, the apprentice unconsciously picks up the rules of the art. ... These hidden rules can be assimilated only by a person who surrenders himself to that extent uncritically to the imitation of another.
>
> (Polanyi 1967, 53)

Sure enough, in the case of hereditary instruction of vital spots, *ācāṉ*s demand from their students submission to their authority regarding all aspects of practice and secrecy. Furthermore, experience of concealment, it has been pointed out (Luhrmann 1989, 161), may be educational itself. Sissela Bok (1984, 37) has noted that learning to keep a secret may be central to children's development with regard to childhood individualization and in conveying control over one's own life. People who have secrets decide what to tell and to whom. *Ācāṉ*s are required, and demand of their students, to keep vital spots secret, since the knowledge they embody can be used to heal and harm. It is thus with regard to potential misuse that the vital spots are taught in the intimate, close, and life-long relationship of *guru-śiṣya-paramparā*, which is characterized by testing and hardships. It is for this reason that *ācāṉ*s not only guide students in manual techniques and applications of vital spots, but also convey moral implications and make sure that knowledge "will stand" and does not fall into wrong hands.

But why do I term this relationship a "moral economy" of knowledge transmission? Admittedly, learning or teaching is not normally described as an economic process, at least not according to conservative notions of "economy." On the other hand, recent studies in economic anthropology and sociology have argued for including the "general economy of being" (Das and Das 2010, 21). Knowledge transmission in the case of *varmakkalai* is a process of exchange, rather than a lopsided, unidirectional "passing down." The intricacies of hereditary knowledge transmission of vital spots in Kanyakumari are probably nowhere better observed than in the rite of initiation, the request of a student to be affiliated and his or her acceptance by a *guru*. It marks the beginning of a close and often arduous relationship. Such intimate proximity is necessary as *ācāṉ*s assess their apprentices' adequacy for vital spot practices. This includes a student's character, as aggressive natures are more prone to misuse a potentially lethal technique. Therefore, the readiness of a student is constantly tested by preceptors, with regard to their moral development. What a student is not deemed to be ready to know will be kept concealed. Once a *guru* evaluates an apprentice as morally ready to be allowed access to a certain technique, it may be revealed to him or to her. Teachers share their expertise with their students, but students also contribute to this exchange by subscribing to specific values and by obeying their *guru*, thus proving themselves worthy to be taught. It is in this sense that I am using the term "moral economy."

However, secrecy has been identified not with morality, but with crime and immoral conduct, and as representing the "dark side of man" (Spitznagel 1998, 28), which dreads the light of day and publicity. Secrecy is commonly viewed as morally reprehensible (Kippenberg and Stroumsa 1995, xii; Nedelmann 1995, 1), and it has been stated that "the border between secrecy and lying is tenuous" (Fainzang 2005, 44).[17] Simmel (1906, 463) has defined immorality as one of the intrinsic values pivotal in bringing secrecy into play, and has added that "the immoral hides itself" and that "secrecy is not in immediate interdependence with evil, but evil with secrecy." Alternatively it has been argued, that secrets serve purposes of assuring the power of the powerful, the *arcana imperii* (Spitznagel 1998, 31), and that concealment of practices and knowledge, especially with regard to transmission of knowledge in lineages or families, must be regarded as maintaining economic prowess. Keeping special processes of manufacture or a medical recipe secret is thus understood to fulfill primarily economic objectives (23). But in the case of *ācāṉs*, concealment of knowledge is not necessarily connected with immoral conduct, nor can secrecy here be depicted as unethical behavior. On the contrary, secrecy is partly necessitated by practitioners' moral responsibility to protect what they know in order to protect others. Safeguarding their knowledge from being misused means protecting patients from being ill-treated, securing fellow beings from receiving ill-effects of a potentially dangerous knowledge, and also shielding their own students from any harm they could cause. Hence, for *ācāṉs*, I would argue, secrecy is not only about property, but also about proper deeds, and hence ultimately about righteous, morally approvable conduct. Simmel's (1906, 463) statement that "[s]ecrecy is . . . also the sociological expression of moral badness" appears misplaced in the case of *varmakkalai*. Furthermore, his opinion that "[s]ecrecy is a universal sociological form, which, as such, has nothing to do with the moral valuations of its contents" cannot be supported.

Conclusion

Instruction of the vital spots, a highly kinesthetic, tactile practice, is conducted nonverbally, but deploys and stimulates a student's senses. Massaging of patients, stimulation of vital spots, important to both martial and therapeutic techniques, is done almost exclusively manually, and instructions on how to do it draw heavily on physical experience and sensations. This is a carnal mode of learning, and especially the knack of stimulating vital spots and the resultant effects are impossible to practice

17. However, with the Hippocratic Oath, biomedical doctors pledge to keep confidentiality—albeit with the aim of respecting the privacy of patients.

on the basis of words alone and difficult to express verbally. Secrecy, in this regard, attains a deeper meaning, as the vital spots pertain to a nonverbalized and nonverbalizable sphere. *Varmam* knowledge is both tacit and implicit: knowledge which practitioners cannot express and which they do not wish to express. The fact that their knowledge eludes a verbalizable sphere may account for much of the secrecy to which vital spots are subjected. Secrecy in hereditary *varmakkalai* is thus characterized in at least two respects. "You see," one practitioner told me, "our secret has two meanings: On the one hand, it is a secret because it is kept hidden [*maṟaiñcu veccatu*] to prevent its misuse. On the other hand, it is a secret, because it is that which cannot be comprehended [*aṟiya muṭiyātu*]." Secrecy in this sense relates to the Greek terms *apporheton*, "forbidden to say," and *arrheton*, "unsayable" (Burkert 1995, 83).

The connection between morality, that is, a particular altruistic worldview, and behavior, a particular judgment of what is wrong and what is right, is central to *varmakkalai* and pivotal with regard to a number of questions, most notably the attainment and possibility of efficacy of vital spot practices. Secrecy in *varmakkalai*, and by extension in siddha medicine and possibly in other esoteric practices to some extent, can be an expression of a particular notion of morality. Moreover, and surprisingly enough, secrecy can be shown as intrinsic not just to the effect of keeping a corpus of knowledge restricted—in fact, this study shows that the knowledge under consideration is a particularly fluid, nonstandardized one. Secrecy, alongside moral behavior and ethics, must be recognized as intrinsic to the therapeutic and to the martial practice of the vital spots. Charles Leslie (1976, 3) had interpreted ethical codes and instructions for practitioners to dress in white, to be hygienic, and so on—advice which is regularly found in textual sources on medicine—as rationalization or sign of aspiration for a high social status by practitioners, but I am not entirely convinced by this on the basis of my research. The case of the vital spots shows rather that such guidance and ethical codes may be precondition for and epiphenomenon of successful therapeutic (and martial) practice.

But to concede to and realize both the moral and tacit features of this particular account of secrecy as found in the practices of vital spot practitioners in Kanyakumari, it is indispensable to consider not only the *form* of secrecy but also its *content*. As I would argue, isolating forms of secrecy from its content, and allocating to the latter a subordinate or negligible role, has fostered limited, reductionist analyses, which have led to secret traditions and esotericism being insufficiently understood. As several scholars have lucidly pointed out, there are a number of methodological snarls involved in trying to understand secret traditions. These include epistemological and ethical problems and questions (Urban 1998). First, is it possible to unravel the content of a secret, and, second, should such a challenging task be attempted? These are important considerations. The methodological entanglement involved can possibly never be disentangled. Nevertheless, would not a neglect of the contents of secrecy, and of the nature of that which is concealed, reduce any account to only superficial, shallow attempts at representation? Are not other methodological, ethical, and epistemological questions raised by compartmentalizing secret traditions into their form and their content on the one hand, and by then assuming that such secrets are or may be actually empty? The former approach forestalls any bid toward a holistic representation or understanding of a secret tradition, and the latter is a form of almost colonial paternalism. Therefore, I argue that without incorporating at least the particular nature of that which is concealed—that is, the specific character of a secret tradition or of what is being concealed and how—any analysis is doomed to be superficial and limited at best, and distorting at worst.

Varmakkalai in many regards exhibits features of an esoteric, tantric tradition. A similar view has been advanced for siddha medicine in general (Sujatha 2009, 80), amongst others, due to the heavy use of metallic and poisonous substances for its pharmacopoeia and the surrounding secrecy. Siddha texts are known for an esoteric, difficult language that makes extensive use of codes and jargon. It has been remarked that this aspect might be a deliberate attempt at circumventing the knowledge contained from becoming known publicly (Trawick 1983, 939; Zvelebil 1973, 229). On the other hand, it has been speculated that such codes are empty, their content devoid of any meaning, ephemeral (Weiss 2009, 161). But such a notion is highly debatable, and the case of the vital spots sheds a different light on secrecy. It shows that, apart from the texts, an initiation is needed, as vital spots require an experiential understanding, which happens via the physicality of life, of the body, but not via the physicality of texts. As we have seen here, a reductionist approach to secrecy is inadequate to explain how secrecy is being utilized and to what outcome. Besides, while secrecy may indeed be ephemeral or even void of content in a purely semantic sense, there may be considerable embodied meaning. In the case of *varmakkalai*, this meaning is embodied because it consists of tacit rather than of verbally explicit and semantic content, and because it relates to moral responsibilities rather than to public knowledge.

The analysis of secrecy in this chapter therefore shows it to be structured and preconditioned by moral considerations and constraints and by the corporeal, tacit nature of knowledge and skills involved in the vital spots and their medical and martial applications. Interestingly, therefore, this instance of secrecy also demonstrates how far the social aspects of moral concerns and biological, neurological issues at stake in the physicality of *ācāṉs*' skills are inseparably linked. As Luhrmann (2010, 213) argues, this is the strength of the concept and methodology of embodiment, as "it resists the binary distinction between culture and the body and the insistence that culture alone is the proper focus of the anthropologist."

Epilogue

FROM TACTILITY TO TEXTUALITY, FROM KANYAKUMARI TO THE WORLD

ON THE OCCASION of the Fourth National Siddha Doctor's conference 2006 in Chennai, N. Shanmugom, a Tamil lecturer from Coimbatore, delivered a paper titled "Tamil Vital Spot Medicine for the Medicines of the World." Shanmugom explained that in a world where people are in need of affordable, safe remedies, it was the duty of Tamils to share their healthcare modalities. He appealed to the siddha practitioners who were present in the following words: "The medical world expectantly looks to you siddha doctors. Vital spot medicine will elevate you and *varmam* itself will be elevated; it will be a marvelous gift to the world."[1]

More than 650 participants attended another event: the First International Conference on Medical Varmalogy, held in Coimbatore in May 2012, and organized by the Arts Research Institute (ARI). According to its organizers, the aim of this conference was "to bring to the world stage this hitherto hidden knowledge [of vital spots], to showcase the results obtained by modern-day registered medical practitioners using this science and to give . . . a first-hand taste of some of its techniques, through demonstrations by highly skilled experts."[2] Speakers described how *varmam*-trained doctors successfully treat about twenty-seven diseases, including arthritis, spondylosis, diabetes, and asthma. On this basis,

1. "Ulaka maruttuvattiṟkut tamiḻariṉ varma maruttuvam"; http://www.varmam.org/articles/Tamils-Varma-Therapy-for-World-Medical-Field.pdf.

2. http://www.vethasatthi.in.

some demanded official recognition for vital spot medicine. Meer Mustafa Hussain, former vice-chancellor of the Tamil Nadu Dr. MGR Medical University, even urged the Indian government to recognize varmalogy as an independent system of medicine, and went so far as to demand to rename the department of AYUSH as VAYUSH, where the first letter would represent "varmalogy," the scientific use of vital spot therapies (*The Hindu*, May 15, 2012).[3]

In order to understand such reasoning, it is necessary to discern how in recent decades indigenous Indian medical practices have received increasing awareness and patronage, from Indian as well as international individuals, networks, and policies. The successive five-year plans published by the planning commission of the government of India testify to a steady increase of expenditure on Indian systems of medicine (H. Madhavan 2010, 88). While this does not even come close to the amount spent on biomedicine, it still points to a heightened support for indigenous healthcare. Despite biomedicine occupying a much favored position in India, where it is widely preferred, especially for acute health issues, traditional medicines are important and patients extensively patronize the plurality of healing practices and the associated healthcare choices. At the same time, traditional Asian medical practices in particular enjoy popularity even beyond Asia, as their use in clinics, health resorts, and spas in regions such as North America and Europe shows.

In this context, *varmam* and *marma(m)* vital spots, related exercises, and therapies are gaining a rapidly growing popularity as well, as international workshops, recent publications, and their presence on the Internet indicate. For instance, a quick appraisal of "ayurveda marma" in September 2010 yielded 50,900 results on Google and 29,100 results for "marma massage." Only about seven months later, in April 2011, the search engine provided 332,000 results for "ayurveda marma" and 160,000 results for "marma massage"—an increase of about 500 percent. In December 2012, the same terms yielded as many as 1,660,000 and 439,000 results, respectively. Spas, hotels, and private massage practitioners, both in India and abroad, advertise relaxing "ayurveda marma massages." This includes the Hale Clinic in London, a facility for alternative medical practices and

3. AYUSH is part of the Ministry of Health and Family Welfare, government of India. It was created in 1995 as the Department of Indian Systems of Medicine and Homoeopathy (ISM&H), and renamed AYUSH in 2003. The acronym means Department of Ayurveda, Yoga & Naturopathy, Unani, Siddha and Homeopathy.

massage, where, among others, "marma-puncture" is offered at £70 for a half-hour treatment.[4] Vital spots are moreover becoming interesting for medical research, as clinical trials regarding the effects and applicability of such manual treatment modalities show.[5] Complementary health circles reinterpret ayurvedic *marman* spots as points of therapeutic attention, despite authoritative ayurvedic compendia clearly ruling this out (Wujastyk 2009, 242). Nonetheless, *marman* have been compared to Chinese acupuncture points, and several writers have hypothesized that all therapeutic needling may have been invented in India (Ros 1994; Frawley, Ranade, and Lele 2005; Lad and Durve 2008). The fact that same shops that sell energy pyramids, books on pranic healing, reiki, or urine therapy in larger South Indian cities offer such recent publications on vital spot treatments in Tamil, Malayalam, and English (Nātarācaṉ in Kaṇṇaṉ Rājārām 2007a, 2–3) shows that vital spots are increasingly being marketed for urban, and middle- and upper-class clients or patients.

Concurrently, the World Health Organization (WHO) has since the late 1970s urged its member states to utilize and integrate traditional medicines (TRM) into their national healthcare systems (WHO 1978; 1981; 2008; Akerele 1987, 177). It has recommended that governments supplement biomedical facilities, which are often expensive, technocentric, and confined to urban areas in developing countries, with traditional healthcare practitioners, who cover rural areas with generally cost-effective treatments (Choi 2008). This includes local, informally trained physicians, such as midwives, called "traditional birth attendants," and manual health practitioners, termed "traditional bonesetters" (Shankar and Unnikrishnan 2004). Possibly influenced by this, vital spot medical practices are increasingly perceived as siddha medicine and diverse actors demand its incorporation into the siddha medical curriculum as well as its global spread.

These complex developments have ensured that vital spot therapies, alongside other so-called traditional forms of healthcare, are the focal point of recent attention and of remarkable reinterpretations. This epilogue

4. http://www.haleclinic.com/treatment/marmapuncture.

5. Fox and colleagues (2006) is a report on a pilot trial study assessing the rehabilitative value of *marman* spot stimulations in post-stroke patients. While this study was found inconclusive, its investigators nevertheless found therapies to be "safe…, tolerable and acceptable to the majority of patients" (Fox et al. 2006, 271), and therefore to provide ground for further trials.

describes some endeavors at forging novel ways of *varmam* transmission and practice. At the core of these are processes of translation, and interrelated movements from tactility to textuality and from secrecy to an apparent openness. A requisite for this is a transformation or reinterpretation of secrecy and its portrayal as individualistic, egoistic possession in the hands of a few, to the treatment of vital spots as common good, or at least as Tamil property.

Into the Siddha Curriculum?

One reason for the promotion of vital spot therapy may be its potential as emergency treatment, a field that is allegedly less developed in indigenous medicine (Mariyajōcap n.d., v). Vital spot medicine has therefore been variously described as emergency or first-aid medicine (Irājēntiraṉ 2006, 27; Kaṇṇaṉ Rājārām 2007a). This is remarkable insofar as alternative healing practices are stereotypically denied an effective emergency medical value (Naraindas 2006); their uses are generally seen to lie in long-term treatments rather than in quick responses to urgent health issues (Nichter 1992). This may explain why siddha physicians and colleges are increasingly attentive to *varmam*, since it potentially allows for competing with biomedicine in this regard, while trumping other traditional medicines which allegedly lack similar emergency therapies. Official syllabi indicate that "Special Medicine including Yoga & Varmam" is an essential part of instruction in all siddha medical colleges, covered during the final trimester of the four-and-a-half-years Bachelor of Siddha Medicine and Surgery (BSMS) course.[6] However, formally trained siddha practitioners recurrently denounce the lack of concise teaching of vital spots in siddha medical colleges (Narayanaswami 1975, 46; Vasanthakumar 2004, 35). Considering the fact that the siddha curriculum has remained unchanged for forty years (*Deccan Chronicle*, July 8, 2013), this may not surprise. Both students and faculty of siddha colleges confided in me during interviews that *varmam* instruction in their facilities was not conducted in a comprehensive way.[7] Rather, vital spots appear to be restricted to a theoretical study in siddha colleges. This is exemplified by the BSMS syllabus, which

6. http://web.tnmgrmu.ac.in/syllabus/bsmssyllabus2007-2008.pdf.

7. Interviews with siddha students and faculty conducted in Kanyakumari on March 3, 2009, and in Thirunelveli on May 14, 2009.

illustrates that examinations exclusively consist of theoretical tests, but not of practical tuitions.

Noteworthy is therefore a special type of instruction adopted by the Government Siddha College in Palayamkottai, where *varmam* can be studied as a postgraduate degree course. For this, an off-campus program utilizes hereditary practitioners, who live and practice around Tirunelveli town. Postgraduates who select *varmam* as their main subject visit one or several *ācāṉ*s on a regular basis in order to receive instruction from these hereditary practitioners. However, students conveyed to me a largely negative picture of this type of instruction; several postgraduates lamented that *ācāṉ*s withheld information from them. One student complained that he had been treated as a servant or assistant, rather than as a student. The students are used to concise textual learning, which *ācāṉ*s, whose methods of knowledge transmission rely on hands-on practice and observation, are unlikely to provide. *Ācāṉ*s require apprentices to assist them on a long-term basis and to prove their worthiness to learn. This situation is exacerbated by the circumstance that the college students are siddha postgraduates, who have already attained a BSMS degree, and therefore feel in no way subordinate to hereditary practitioners. Such a state of affairs is prone to provide for conflict and to complicate teaching.

It is this situation which has led Irācāmaṇi (1996, 41), author of an AYUSH-sponsored publication on vital spots, to lament that *varmam* was like "a gem that lies in a heap of waste, its greatness not known even to the Tamils themselves." He portrays hereditary practitioners, who selfishly conceal their knowledge and treat it as private or family property, as an obstacle to a thorough utilization of techniques and as putting the vital spots at risk of becoming lost. Siddha practitioners and Tamil scholars alike argue that *varmam* should rightly be the property of all Tamils, not least since they claim that the art originated in Tamil Nadu and has been documented entirely in the Tamil language (Caṇmukam 2010, 3; 2006; Rajamony 1983, 482; Aleksāṇṭar Ācāṉ 1998, 2; Vasanthakumar 2004, ix). Private possession of knowledge has been decried as "unscientific" and as hampering the progression of Indian medicines since independence (Brass 1972, 344). Proponents of a scientific development of siddha have suggested that the ancient Siddhars in fact used their knowledge for altruistic healing with egalitarian, rationalist objectives, and thus were ideal scientists (Jeyrāj 2000, 3; Weiss 2009, 51), and they juxtapose this with the alleged egoistic, selfish conduct of hereditary practitioners, who conceal their practices.

Transmitting, Translating, and Transnationalizing Varmam

In this absence of a comprehensive vital spot instruction in government siddha medical colleges, a number of private education facilities have begun offering certificate courses in siddha-related topics. Increasingly, this includes courses on vital spots, which are established or assisted by hereditary *ācāṉ*s. In marked contrast to the hereditary mode of *varmam* knowledge transmission stands a course offered by the International Thanu Foundation in Chennai.[8] This institution was founded by Chidambarathanu Pillai, who is an author of more than twenty books on vital spot therapies, for which he has coined the term "Thanuology." His institute offers a Diploma in Siddha Medicine (DSM), a Doctorate in Siddha Medical Sciences (DSMS), and a Doctorate in Varma Medical Sciences (DVMS). All these function as correspondence courses (Chidambarathanu Pillai 1995b, 4), an instructional modality which is rapidly growing in popularity in India. Moreover, the DVMS courses appear to be tailor-made to satisfy the needs of students outside of Tamil Nadu and especially abroad, as study materials are in English and textbooks and even exam questions are provided by mail or, more recently, by e-mail.

Chidambarathanu Pillai was born in Kanyakumari district in 1934 and claims to hail from a family of *ācāṉ*s which can look back to forty-six generations of practice (Citamparatāṇuppiḷḷai 1991, 76).[9] He insists that *varmam*, or rather, Thanuology, needs to be recognized, especially since he perceives vital spot injuries to relate to about 19 percent of all diseases. The same percentage of ailments according to him can be treated through Thanuology (Chidambarathanu Pillai 1996, 3). However, as Chidambarathanu Pillai regrets, the vital spots have remained concealed by egoistic practitioners. To counter an alleged fading away of *varmam*, he has been collecting, translating, and publishing manuscripts dealing with the vital spots during the last three decades and has set up his own treatment, research, and education institute in Chennai, the International Thanu Foundation.

8. For a detailed analysis of this case of transnational transmission of vital spots, see Sieler (2013).

9. From: http://varmam.com. Estimating twenty-five years for a generation, Chidambarathanu Pillai claims to be standing in a line of practitioners more than a thousand years old.

To be eligible for the Doctorate in Varma Medical Sciences course, an applicant is required to be "a Graduate from a recognised College or University or Diploma holder in Medical science with 2 years experience," according to an application brochure. On the other hand, I was assured in personal interviews that, even without medical experience or degree, enrolment for the courses was possible at any time, and it seems therefore that virtually everybody has access to the courses offered.[10] Overall costs for foreign students amount to $1,500 US and to 26,500 rupees for Indian Nationals (International Thanu Foundation 2009). Whereas the duration of the course is specified as four years on the foundation's homepage and the application form for the DVMS course explains that "an average student devoting 12 hours a week" would complete the course in four and a half years, a much faster completion is possible, Chidambarathanu Pillai told me. For instance, he lauded the efforts exerted by some outstanding students of his, such as one Japanese student, who had completed the DVMS course in less than nine months. Chidambarathanu Pillai claims to have instructed as many as 500 students in siddha and *varma* diploma courses and 200 in *varma* doctorate courses at his institute. Half of these are from India, the other half, about 100 diploma holders and 250 *varmam* doctorates, come from various parts of the world: the United States, the United Kingdom, France, Belgium, Japan, and Malaysia. Chidambarathanu Pillai has not yet achieved state accreditation of his institution or the degrees he offers, which he keeps on striving for despite his advanced age. However, he is convinced that he will achieve recognition for his program within the next few years.

Publicizing and Globalizing the Vital Spots

In attempts to publicize it, the concept of the vital spots as figuring in Chidambarathanu Pillai's courses has undergone several shifts during the last decades. Interestingly, this was partly conducted in a merger of notions of "tradition" and "modernity," Hindu religious belief and "science." The front cover of the DVMS application form displays an image of a dancing god Śiva under which reads: *Medicina origini*[*s*], Latin for "medicine of the beginning." The term "Thanuology" to denote *varmam* is also interesting. The degree awarded to successful candidates was

10. Personal interview with Chidambarathanu Pillai in Chennai on March 27, 2009.

earlier called ThD, Diploma in Thanuology, probably emulating the PhD degree of doctor of philosophy.[11] Thanu is a name of lord Śiva, albeit rarely used beyond Kanyakumari. Śiva is often perceived as having created the vital spots (*Varma Oṭimuṟivu Cara Cūttiram*, 5; cited in Jēms 2010, 75), and Chidambarathanu Pillai therefore holds that the related therapies should be identified by his name, Thanu.[12] The term Thanuo-*logy*, moreover, makes *varmam* look akin to physio-*logy* or neuro-*logy*, and uses a terminology familiar to recognized academic subjects. At the same time he coined the term, Chidambarathanu Pillai approached the ministers of health for both the Central and Tamil Nadu governments to achieve recognition of Thanuology as a separate medical entity. As early as 1982 he demanded the establishment of a National Institute of Varmam (Thanuology) for this purpose, albeit in vain (Citamparatāṇuppiḷḷai 1991, 48). During the eighties and nineties the Thanu Foundation tried to urge the Universities of Madras, Mysore, and Pune directly to consider the introduction of Thanuology as a new discipline into the academic curriculum. After having been presented with a syllabus designed by Chidambarathanu Pillai, the universities expressed their appreciation, but declined for financial reasons (58).

Chidambarathanu Pillai thereupon changed the framework of Thanuology; he approached the International Olympic Committee (IOC) as early as the mid-eighties and tried to get Thanuology accepted as a recognized sports therapy. He suggested developing Thanuology or "Indian Sports Medicine," as he now called it, with financial aid of the IOC, for utilization during Olympic sports events. An interested IOC asked him to submit a report for evaluation by the Olympic Committee (Citamparatāṇuppiḷḷai 1991, 55). After having assessed a report of the Thanu Foundation titled *Thanuology as Sports Medicine*, the IOC wrote in a letter to Chidambarathanu Pillai that it was very impressed by the practice of Thanuology. However, the letter made clear that "as a general rule the IOC Medical Commissioner or indeed the IOC is unwilling to promote any one particular type of sports medicine for use during the Olympic Games."[13] Nevertheless, the IOC bibliography of sports

---

11. http://varmam.com/.

12. Notably, Chidambarathanu Pillai's name contains *Thanu* as well. In earlier publications, he uses the term "varmology" (Chidambarathanu Pillai 1970). Others have coined similar terms for denoting *varmam*, including "varmalogy," a term used by the Thirumoolar Varmalogy Institute in Coimbatore; see http://www.varmam.org/aboutus.

13. Letter by the chairman, Medical Commission, International Olympic Committee, October 31, 1987; cited in Citamparatāṇuppiḷḷai (1991, 56).

medicine, a publication series called *IOC Medical Commission: Collection of Sports Medicine and Sports Sciences*, mentions Chidambarathanu Pillai's report, which is kept in the library of the Olympic Museum in Lausanne, noted as "Indian Sports Medical Science" (IOC 2006, 69; Citamparatāṇuppiḷḷai 1991, 56).

Recently, the Thanu Foundation has promoted *varmam* as emergency medicine and as a therapeutic specialization worthy of being incorporated into different medical systems (Chidambarathanu Pillai 2009, 20). Furthermore, Chidambarathanu Pillai (2008, 53) has urged the inclusion of vital spots in forensic analyses; in cases of doubt pertaining to the cause of death, for instance, a skilled Thanuologist could be of help.

Translating the Vital Spots

The correspondence course materials illustrate an underlying rendition of the vital spots, which involves linguistic translations, such as the coinage of the term Thanuology. The *varmam* loci are generally called "life centers" or "nerve centers" throughout the instruction material (Chidambarathanu Pillai 1995b; 1995a; 1996). While most hereditary practitioners would agree on a *varmam* being a location of life, the case is more complicated with regard to "nerve centers," the term primarily used in DVMS textbooks. As the material is in English, it is unclear whether the "nerves" of these "nerve centers" correspond to *narampu* (nerves) in Tamil. This is of importance insofar as *narampu* are indeed recognized by *ācāṉ*s as important to their practice. Some vital spots are nerve-related, as these coincide with *narampu* nerves. But other spots are related to bones, *elumpu*. Translating *varmam* as "nerve centers" gives to a particular physical category the appearance of being dominant over others, whether or not this is intended, while other anatomical categories, such as bones or joints are, at least taxonomically, misrepresented. The same holds true for the concept of *pirāṇam*, which in DVMS textbooks is translated as "oxygen" (Chidambarathanu Pillai 1994, 12). Possibly to be intelligible globally, Chidambarathanu Pillai has translated many concepts which figure in the practices and the textual sources of *varmam*, and some of these appear to have been replaced with biomedical equivalents from anatomy and pathology.

However, the biggest leap in translation can be recognized in the respective modality of transmission of *varmam* knowledge. Whereas hereditary transmission of knowledge presupposes the student living with a *guru*, in the teacher's house, the *tutors* of the DVMS correspondence course are "as near as [a student's] corner Post Box" (International Thanu Foundation 2009). Students are required to pass exam papers, not partake in hands-on instruction. In this mode of knowledge transmission, *gurus* have become *tutors*, and learning happens through reading and writing rather than through touching. Hence one of the most crucial translations is found in the transition of the senses utilized in learning: from tactility and kinesthesia to the sense of vision and to the faculty of reading.

Linda Harasim (1990, 7) has described online education as a "new environment," which "requires new approaches to understand, design and implement [instruction]." This environment is the "virtual classroom," a space—cyberspace, to be precise—which requires adaptations and new approaches to teaching a subject matter. Studies of online education have pointed out various transformations happening in the processes of instruction: the different forms of teaching available through the Internet for instance, or the new possibilities of virtual textbooks (Rossman 1992). Cyberspace thus offers new forms of learning and practice by providing a virtual classroom and has become a thriving and increasingly active place for evolving forms of practice and knowledge transmission for siddha medicine.[14] The DVMS correspondence course uses comparatively short-term courses, material in text form, and the Internet to bridge long, sometimes transnational distances between instructor and learner. But this virtual classroom is similar to the academic world: it is highly "ocularcentrist" and "logocentrist" (Foucault 1965; 1977), which means it prioritizes the vision and the logic of the word or text. Regina Bendix (2005, 7) seems to be correct in noting that "logocentrism, generated in conjunction with ocularcentrism, has contributed to a certain amount of neglect of culturally shaped sensory knowledge." It understandably favors theoretical knowledge and training over hands-on instruction and tacit knowledge.

---

14. For instance, *Deva Vidya* is an Internet platform, which offers franchise opportunities for providing siddha and ayurveda services worldwide, and "Tele Medicine," which includes medical consultations via phone and video chat. This company offers training in Traditional Siddha Science (TSS) through its *Deva Vidya* Siddha Gurukulam. Its homepage depicts a collage of a stethoscope next to Indian palm-leaf manuscripts and a drawing of a Siddhar besides a white, female student with a laptop (http://www.devavidya.org/). Students can study "Traditional Siddha Science" in a four-year online course. An Applied Siddha Marmam (ASM) degree can be obtained through a six-month online course, for an overall course fee of $600 US. This course utilizes tools, such as an online library of electronic textbooks and online video chat, through which students can interact with faculty by "exchanging written messages in real-time," e-mail, and presence on social networks such as "LinkedIn, Facebook, MySpace, Twitter, YouTube, and Ning" (http://www.siddhagurukulam.org/).

Secrecy exhibited by *ācāṉs* can be explained partially by their wish to conceal potentially lethal spots from misuse. These ethical considerations appear not to have influenced the design and the promotion of the DVMS course. Virtually anybody may enroll, a process in which interest and solvency of a student are decisive factors, rather than trust and moral considerations. This is an instance of a learning relationship being transplanted from a moral economy into a market economy. Secrecy is here ignored or contested, deemed as ignorance and egoism, while the necessary spread of valuable knowledge is postulated instead. Moreover, as I have argued previously, secrecy in vital spot practice also results from the nonverbalizable, somatic nature of practices and loci, which for this reason are largely transmitted through hands-on methods by most practitioners in Kanyakumari. It is interesting to acknowledge that in shifting the focus of attention in instructing *varmam* from the tactile, sensory capacity of students to discursive, mental, and visual faculties, secrecy is being considerably deemphasized. At the same time, it is precisely this shift from secrecy to openness that enables the translation from an instruction based on the physicality of life or the body to a physicality of texts and pictures in the first place.

Lastly, it seems plausible to say that it is not only the practice of medicine and medicinal substances that are being viewed as marketable commodities, but also the knowledge required to produce them. This may seem obvious, but the commodification of Asian medicines and of their knowledge has not attracted adequate attention. Thanuology can, in this regard, be compared to other innovations of traditional knowledge, especially in transnational contexts, such as "transnational commercial yoga," a phenomenon which has been described by several scholars (Alter 2004; De Michelis 2004) as a particular type of yoga to have arisen out of international commercial exchange (Fish 2006, 190). The example of commercial forms of yoga, a multibillion-dollar industry, in this regard may be of vital importance for giving rise to entrepreneurial transnational efforts in traditional medicine. Entrepreneurial forces, though, have largely not been acknowledged with regard to traditional knowledge; not with regard to siddha medicine, at least, the promotion and spread of which have been described as largely defined by Tamil nationalist agendas and development strategies. But the modes of the transnational transmissions described here can result in major modifications in the way siddha medicine is perceived, and presumably in the way it is practiced. It becomes apparent that it is the interests of the person(s), groups, or institutions of instruction, based on the *assumed* perceptions and interests of the potential foreign recipients of the courses, that shape the subject of instruction. Such perceptions therefore influence the way siddha is transmitted and communicated.

Transnationalism in healthcare terms has been understood largely as the promotion and spread of medicines and medical practices beyond the borders of a conceived area from which a particular medicine is thought to have originated.[15] This is a notion which in itself is awkward, as it regards nation-states and particular medicines as congruent (Alter 2005b). The case presented here, however, shows that knowledge itself becomes transmuted. This happens not only in the course of such transfer, but it may also become a *necessity for the transfer of knowledge*. In the case of the vital spots, a long-term instruction by apprenticeship as well as the retaining of esoteric, secret lineages seem hardly practicable in a transnational scenario, and therefore the instruction offered by the Thanu Foundation appears as one alternative, feasible option. In this respect, Marshall McLuhan's well-known dictum, "the medium is the message" (1973), holds true. The case of *varmam* distance education exemplifies how an instruction medium may influence how the content is perceived, and how, for instance, the Internet shapes the kind of knowledge that can be transmitted. This happens, for example, by selecting from the corpus and thereby transforming it, but also by translating a particular concept so that it may be transmittable, receivable, and understood through a medium such as the Internet.

---

15. Such transnational movements are no recent phenomenon. Movements of medical knowledge, as historians of Asian medicines show, have been a decisive mode of shaping its forms, and "[c]ontemporary trends are best viewed as a continuation of a long ongoing historical process" (Høg and Hsu 2002, 209–210). Interestingly, *ācāṉs* frequently narrate a global history of vital spots, holding that both martial art aspects and therapies of the vital spots, after originating in South India, were transported to China, Japan, and other, mostly East Asian, countries (Balakrishnan 1995, 34; Sarma 2007, 120; Varghese 2003). The art is said to have strived in these foreign countries, while at the same time it was forgotten and perished in India. Bodhidharma, widely accepted to have been a fifth-century Buddhist monk and prince of the South Indian Paḷḷava dynasty of Kanchipuram (Faure 1986), is often credited with having transported *varmakkalai* to the Chinese regions (Varghese 2003). And in China, Bodhidharma is said not only to have founded *chian* Buddhism (in Japanese known as *Zen*, both terms being derived from Sanskrit *dhyāna*, meditation), but also to have lived at the famous Shaolin temple, where it is believed he taught the monks martial exercises, which today are known and popular as Shaolin *ch'uan-fa*, or *gung-fu*.

Networks of Vital Spot Promotion and Regulation

At least two positions with respect to vital spots frame their promotion and regulation. Critical notions are mostly expressed by biomedical, orthopedic practitioners, and associations, while supportive views are exhibited by NGOs, which are actively involved in a revival of "tradition." Despite their apparently opposing attitudes regarding nonformal healthcare practices, the initiatives of these two camps are strikingly similar. Both work to assess and document "good practices," and to educate traditional practitioners. Both recommend scientific evaluation of nonformal healthcare due to an alleged "lack of sound scientific evidence concerning the efficacy of many of its therapies" (Choi 2008, 153). Such evaluation is expected to eventually lead to "standardization with evidence-based approaches" (154). This has prompted the development of educational initiatives for traditional practitioners, including training of midwives in aseptic delivery techniques and antenatal care, and instructing manual practitioners in basic orthopedics and anatomy, especially in the use of graphic methods for diagnosis (Raju and Hariramamurthy 2004). Many have suggested special designations such as "Traditional Orthopaedic Attendant (TOA)," or "Trained Bone Setters (TBS)" for practitioners who have undergone additional training, with a view to eventually legalizing the medical practice of only thus designated physicians (Agarwal and Agarwal 2010). This is an important aspect, not least since there is a considerable ambiguity regarding the recognition of physicians of "traditional" medicines in India. For noninstitutionally trained practitioners in Tamil Nadu, the requirements for obtaining a medical license are highly ambiguous and keep on changing (Sébastia 2010). Since most *ācāṉ*s have enjoyed a hereditary, noninstitutionalized training and hence are not in possession of a medical certificate, they often actively seek and participate in conferences and education programs, hoping to achieve some form of official recognition.

NARDEP is one example of an NGO that gathers data on traditional medicine, conducts training, and provides a network for traditional healthcare providers. NARDEP, the acronym stands for Natural Resources Development Project, is a division of Vivekanada Kendra in Kanyakumari.[16] It aims to generate rural development, promote organic farming methods,

16. According to Pralay Kanungo (2013), Vivekananda Kendra is a Hindutva-sponsored organization. Hindutva, meaning Hinduness, is the umbrella term for various Hindu nationalist movements.

and revitalize traditional medicine.[17] As part of this, NARDEP regularly offers free *varmam* medical treatment, with the help of local *ācāṉ*s. In the words of Dr. Ganapathi, a college-trained siddha doctor who is in charge of projects on medicine, NARDEP strives for "a rejuvenation of vital spot medicine" through documentation, standardization, and promotion of vital spots, and through connecting hereditary physicians with siddha students, doctors, and the general public.[18]

In the beginning of 2008, NARDEP started a series of four "*varmam* conferences." I was able to visit one of these, held at Kanyakumari and attended by about 200 participants: *ācāṉ*s, siddha physicians and students of both institutional and hereditary backgrounds, and laypersons. In his reception speech, Ganapathi drew attention to the efficiency and cost-effectiveness of vital spots as both "first aid remedial measure" and "all-purpose therapy." To counter the drawback that vital spots were generally kept concealed and not comprehensively taught, NARDEP had been surveying *ācāṉ*s of Kanyakumari and Tirunelveli, recording their practices. Parts of the outcome of this, a collection of film material, were presented to the audience at the conference. The clips showed about ten practitioners, each exhibiting different treatment procedures for similar cases of shoulder joint dislocation. After the last sequence had ended, Ganapathi addressed the present practitioners, requesting them to present and share with the audience their own methods. Several *ācāṉ*s entered the small stage set up in front of the venue to explain individual techniques, exhibiting an astonishing variety in deploying pulling, pushing, turning, and twisting manipulations. Together with the movie clips shown before, they impressively attested to the diversity of techniques utilized by *varmam* practitioners. Participants were next asked to demonstrate vital spots for the treatment of asthmatic conditions. One *ācāṉ* took the microphone to explain that for curing asthma, it was important to assure proper circulation of both blood and *pirāṇam* in a patient. Hence, *meykālavarmam*, which activated both, was an important spot to be stimulated. More contributions by practitioners followed, who all agreed that asthma could not just be managed, but easily cured by *varmam*—especially as it was an ailment connected to *pirāṇam* life force circulation, which could be

17. http://vknardep.org/services/holistic-health/89-cost-effective-bone-setting-techniques.html.

18. Interview with V. Ganapathi in Kanyakumari on November 16, 2008.

activated by respective stimulations. Several spots, which different *ācāṉs* held to be beneficial for treating asthmatic conditions, came to be listed on a blackboard. Using such data gathered from documenting and recording of techniques, NARDEP produces manuals which it provides to *ācāṉs* and interested siddha students. Ganapathi concluded the *varmam* conference by handing out such a manual, which lists important spots, together with symptoms and treatment methods, alongside a list of techniques for massage and manual stimulation (Kaṇapati n.d.), and a poster depicting names and locations of 108 vital spots. This chart is intended to be posted in practitioners' dispensaries, as a visual form of orientation.

The conductors of the conference stressed the need to form an association for vital spot practitioners. The main objectives of such an association would be to achieve attention and financial support for practitioners, to record treatment methods and medicines, and to provide education to members on this basis. Hence, before concluding the conference, contact details of participants were collected and all attendants who would participate in all four conferences were promised to be awarded a "*varmam* passport" along with a certificate, which would label its bearer "knowledgeable in vital spot treatments." NARDEP hence has been actively researching, compiling, standardizing, and instructing manual vital spot therapies, as well as connecting and promoting, but also regulating its practitioners.[19]

Notably, such efforts may provide practitioners with something long years of studying with hereditary *gurus* cannot: recognition in the form of a certificate. Licensing of physicians is conducted statewide, and the Tamil Nadu Board of Indian Medicine is in charge of registration and monitoring of practitioners of Indian medicines in Tamil Nadu. Only being registered and licensed with this board characterizes practitioners as "qualified." It also prevents conviction or punishment for illegal, unlicensed practice. In the case of siddha medicine, only the graduates of the recognized siddha medical colleges, with a BSMS degree, receive unquestioned state recognition as physicians. "Traditional," hereditary practitioners, who have not visited any of the accredited educational institutions, and who are therefore not in possession of accepted certificates, are exempted from registering. Different Tamil Nadu governments have instead set up enlistment provisions for such physicians. The central authority in this regard, the

19. The Arts Research Institute (ARI), located in Coimbatore, is engaged in a similar endeavor, see http://www.ari.org.in/.

Central Council of Indian Medicine, Delhi, however, considers this procedure as illegal (Sébastia 2010, 7–8), and does not recognize traditional practitioners as legitimate medical specialists by its account. A certificate is an institutionalized form of cultural capital; it constitutes or, in the words of Bourdieu (1986, 51), institutes an individual's cultural capital. That is, it attests to the capability of its holder. Such recognition by means of a degree is required by vital spot practitioners, like all other medical practitioners in India, to openly and legally practice and to maintain a dispensary. The ambiguous and constantly shifting situation with regard to medical registration in Tamil Nadu is one reason why many hereditary siddha practitioners appear to collect certificates such as that offered by NARDEP and may utilize opportunities to participate in diploma courses, distance education courses, and so on.

All these are important aspects of the process of governing traditional medicine in general and vital spot practices in particular. These often conflict, but converge in one important aspect; secret possession of *varmam* is wrong. Governing the vital spots and its practitioners is also influenced by notions of traditional healthcare. Both critics and advocates demand documentation, utilization but also standardization and monitoring. Also, there are both governmental and nongovernmental organizations that are actively involved in reviving supposedly endangered indigenous medical practices. Such groups organize conferences and workshops for hereditary practitioners in order to both collect and record their knowledge and to help them abide by medical regulations. Collection of data, translations of manuscripts, compilation of manuals, conducting of workshops, and facilitation of practitioner associations, all constitute one form of governance.

Bruno Latour's notion of "inscription devices" (Latour and Woolgar 1986, 51) is noteworthy in this regard. By means of inscription, Latour holds, reality is made stable, comparable, debatable, and criticizable. Such inscription devices include surveys, statistical data, reports, drawings, pictures, numbers, charts, graphs, and so on. But information provided by inscriptions is not the outcome of a neutral recording function, "it is itself a way of acting upon the real, a way of devising techniques for inscribing it in such a way as to make the domain in question susceptible to evaluation, calculation and intervention" (Rose and Miller 2008, 65–66). Inscription devices include even the labels and appellations such as TBS, "Trained Bone Setter," which are being awarded to bonesetters and *ācāṉs* trained in using imaging devices and basic orthopedic techniques, and which are supposed to designate "good" practitioners, and thus simultaneously allegedly "bad" practitioners—categories of persons who henceforth are perceived to embody bad and good practices, respectively. Such inscription devices also include lists of vital spots and charts which show their locations, and which thus establish their number and sites in a comparable, scrutinizable, concrete, and definite way.

This regulation of vital spots and practitioners is not entirely of a top-down type, but rather develops through the dynamic interplay and discourses of multitudinous actors. For instance, endeavors for promotion of *varmam* may contribute to standardization and control of related knowledge and practices through the compilation of charts of vital locations. Nongovernmental organizations, private research institutes, practitioner associations, and individual practitioners complement the efforts of government agencies in defining "traditional" healthcare and in regulating vital spot therapies. Governance of the vital spots is a continuum, extending from political government to forms of self-regulation, rather than top-down control (Lemke 2001, 201; see also Foucault 1991). This, alongside *ācāṉs*' active involvement in institutionalizations and standardizations of *varmam*, challenges the alleged binary polarities of state and subject, power and subjectivity, and of modernity and tradition.

Lost in Translation? Vital Spot Martial Arts

In all these discourses and attempts to promote and transmit *varmam*, martial aspects which draw on vital spots seem irrelevant. In its description as medical science, martial implications of the vital spots are eliminated. In a publication of the Arts Research Institute, Coimbatore, which is devoted to research and revitalization of the vital spots, Shanmugom writes that the Siddhars had created vital spot techniques with curing people in mind. In contemporary Tamil Nadu, however, *varmakkalai* was largely misunderstood as martial arts (Caṇmukam 2010, 17). Increasingly, *cilampam* staff fencing, *varma aṭi* techniques, and so on, are taught in separate institutions and courses, where medical applications are absent (Caṇmukam 2006).

T. Jeyrāj, nicknamed "Dragon," descends from a family of hereditary practitioners of *varmakkalai* from Kanyakumari and is the founder of "Jey varmakkaḷari," or Jay Varmakkalai Training Centre, in Coimbatore (Jeyrāj 1999, 3). Witnessing the boom of East Asian martial arts in South India beginning in the eighties, with *gung-fu* movies being popular and *karate* schools setting up, Jeyrāj felt the urge to present and teach vital spot combat methods to a wider population. However, as he elucidates (Jeyrāj 2007, 42), this was entirely against the will of his family, to whom he had sworn never to reveal secrets of the vital spots to anyone else. He writes that, "[f]eeling that everyone in this land should learn [*varmam*], I disregarded my family's opposition and founded the 'Jay Varmakkalai Training Centre' on April 18th 1991" (Jeyrāj 2000, 3). He modeled his training center on the style of *karate* schools, which were mushrooming in South India. Students learn in a way that resembles instruction in *judo* and *karate*, and are entitled to wear a skill-specific colored belt on an obligatory white *karate*-style dress. Jeyrāj himself, grand master in his institution, is the bearer of a gold belt.

Vital spot martial arts therefore appear to be promoted as competitors of other martial arts, notably better-known East Asian martial practices, as is also evidenced in several publications (Caravaṇakaṇēṣ 2009, 3; Vasanthakumar 2004, 36–37). What is more, and what seems to make such a shift possible, is the fact that medical practices of *varmam* are disconnected from martial practices related to vital spots, even though these are part and parcel of a combined practice for hereditary *ācāṉ*s.

Some Concluding Reflections

As this book shows, the vital spots are a lived practice. This is seen in the corporeality of the practice; being a body-based, rather than a textual, logocentric practice, knowledge of the vital spot is an ongoing, fluent activity, inseparable from its practice. Concealment, the social implications of secrecy, and the discursive and performative articulations of dissimulation and disclosure are important parts of these practices: discourse on therapies, diagnosis, and treatment procedures of vital spot medicine are secretive procedures, just as information on vital spot combat applications is kept concealed. They are conducted and passed on "behind drawn curtains" averting visual participation of patients and witnesses. Practitioners do not verbally communicate their diagnostic insights to patients, even if this is importantly not the result of a deliberate move on the side of practitioners to disempower their patients, but rather a prerequisite of the manual, body-based therapies which deploy vital spots. These are entities "hidden" inside the body.

Similar notions or practices of "vital spots" can be traced in various parts and regions of India and in different aspects of society spread over most periods and extending to the present times. Some of these vital spots have not only medical but also martial applications, and are of theoretical and philosophical importance as well. This aspect appears to highlight connections between ayurveda and siddha, something which is often overlooked today, since these traditions are generally described and practiced as clearly demarcated and bounded medical systems. Vital spots moreover attest to the fact that the borders between these and so-called folk medical practices were drawn comparatively recently. To speak of "medical systems" in this regard may be misleading, insofar as this suggests neatly defined and bounded medical subjects. In the case of the South Indian vital spot theory and practice, at least, manuscripts and practitioners render multiple, often conflicting accounts. Moreover, the amalgamation of medical and martial concepts in hereditary practice is so complete that it is difficult to imagine one without the other. The analytical framework of a "medical system" is clearly inadequate for *varmakkalai*. This may be also true of other healing practices; as Alter (2005b, 3) cautions, the term "medicine" itself might be a distorting analytical concept in South Asian therapeutic contexts. The vital spots and their diverse theories, which incorporate not only aspects of healing, but facets that might at first glance appear to conservative Western minds as nontherapeutic, such as yoga or astrology, or even as diametrically opposed, such as combat exercises, underscore this. It also accentuates the fact that healing includes more than what is perceived as medicine or as therapeutically relevant according to a Western taxonomy—a basic assumption of medical anthropology. Laurent Pordié (2007, 9) seems right in demanding that with regard to anthropological theory in South Asia, a "culture of healing must be distinguished from medicine, not only from biomedicine but from medicine as a category." This may hold true for other regions as well. In the West, medicine is constantly redrawn and reconfigured. Currently, various therapeutic modes are being explored for their efficacies, including dance, exercise, or music therapy, kinesiatrics, and other treatment forms. It is high time we reconsider medicine as a category and social practice.

Multiplicity must be considered a crucial aspect if one wants to describe and analyze *varmakkalai*: there is no codified, unitary, or consistent system—at least, not as yet. This is an important point to consider in the light of *varmam* therapies being appraised as a subbranch and part of siddha medicine today. In efforts to integrate vital spots into the syllabus of the siddha colleges in Tamil Nadu and into an institutionalized curriculum, the heterogeneous practices of *varmakkalai* have to be adjusted to a new kind of knowledge transmission. These heterogeneous practices are becoming codified, by documenting spots and isolating those practices that are considered more valuable and therapeutically relevant than other, partly opposing practices, such as martial arts or yogic exercises. This becomes apparent when we look at recent attempts to institutionalize *varmam* within a codified siddha medical system, or at efforts to systematize the vital spots to fit a modern curriculum, which represent the recent development of siddha medicine and ayurveda into "medical systems" according to academic frames. Vital spot martial activities do not easily fit into the latter, and hence are taught separately, in distinct schools, usually run as private for-profit businesses. The incorporation of *varmam* into institutionalized, curricula-oriented and thus standardized instruction frameworks requires and presupposes a translation of both the mode of knowledge transmission and its practice. This translation is not (merely) a linguistic one. It is one which requires a more dramatic form of adaptation of information. The translation in modern educational institutions is a movement away from tactility toward textuality; this is expressed in attempts to forge the vital spot practices and knowledge into texts, charts, and figures. In other words, the medium here dictates what the message is, and how it is communicated. The case of *varmakkalai* highlights that such a step involves a crucially transformative process. A requirement for this is a devaluation of secrecy.

The discussion here may briefly reconsider the notions of "tradition" and "modernity." Volker Scheid (2006), in a thoughtful discussion of Chinese medicine, depicts how "tradition" is often considered synonymous with "culture." Tradition further tends to be perceived as static, while change is generally understood as cognate with "modernity," and hence tradition and modernity are thought to be diametrically opposed. Another, related controversial distinction has been created in recent scholarship, between genuine and invented traditions—some more authentic and old, others radically new and unauthentic. This may go back to Hobsbawm and Ranger's edited volume *The Invention of Tradition* (1983), which argues that tradition can be a tool to forge communities or to legitimize status. But the categories of modernity and tradition have been overtaxed and are artificial when taken to demarcate binary opposites. And "traditional" here does not merely mean "a thing from the past"; it also helps to distinguish "traditional medicine" from "modern medicine." And more often than not, "modern medicine" refers to nothing other than biomedicine. The tradition-modernity divide thus camouflages power relations, which have emanated from a colonial world and which are continued in contemporary fiscal and economic environments.

To counter the dividing approaches that use the tradition-modernity binary, Scheid argues for a dynamic interpretation of traditions as living traditions. In doing so, he draws on Alasdair MacIntyre (1984), who saw living traditions as continually, and as a prerequisite, open to change. Practices and differing strands of vital spots therefore may be acknowledged as signs of just such a living tradition, and, perceived as such, there is no tradition-modernity divide involved. All practices reflect the "complex interplay between continuity and change, identity and agency" (Scheid 2006, 67). There is, furthermore, no fissure between modernizers and traditionalists; indeed, they are likely to be the same persons. As we have seen, hereditary *ācāṉ*s actively contribute to the institutionalization of *varmam* in colleges in Tamil Nadu; they edit and publish manuscripts, organize and partake in conferences, or conceptualize their own diploma courses for transnational distance education. The modernity-tradition divide is blurred, as actors are never either traditional or modern, modernizers or traditionalists. Moreover, an interpretation of "traditional" as old, static, and unchanging leads one to overlook the manifold dynamic developments these medical practices are undergoing today. Besides, and given the synergetic nature of *varmakkalai*, comprising as much therapy as martial practice—something which might be argued to be very "modern," in light of recent trends to incorporate movement or dance therapies into standard biomedical procedures—do we not have to fundamentally reconsider the concept of "traditional medicine," if not of "medicine" altogether? I would argue that the analysis of the vital spots provides an impetus for doing so.

Bibliography

Adams, Vincanne. 2001. "The Sacred in the Scientific: Ambiguous Practices of Science in Tibetan Medicine." *Cultural Anthropology* 16 (4): 542–575.

———. 2002. "Establishing Proof: Translating "Science" and the State in Tibetan Medicine." In *New Horizons in Medical Anthropology: Essays in Honour of Charles Leslie*, edited by Charles M. Leslie, Mark Nichter, and Margaret M. Lock, 200–220. London: Routledge.

Agarwal, A., and R. Agarwal. 2010. "The Practice and Tradition of Bonesetting." *Education for Health* 23 (1): 1–8.

Akerele, Olayiwola. 1987. "The Best of Both Worlds: Bringing Traditional Medicine up to Date." *Social Science & Medicine* 24 (2): 177–181.

Aleksāṇṭar Ācāṉ, Es. Em. 1998. *V(m)armakkalai Kaḷañciyam* [*The Treasury of the Art of the Vital Spots*]. Karuṅkal: Ē. Jē Patippakam.

Alex, Gabriele. 2008. "A Sense of Belonging and Exclusion: 'Touchability' and 'Untouchability' in Tamil Nadu." *Ethnos* 73 (4): 523–543.

Alter, Joseph S. 1989. "Pehlwani: Identity, Ideology and the Body of the Indian Wrestler." PhD diss., University of California, Berkeley.

———. 1992a. "The Sannyasi and the Indian Wrestler: The Anatomy of a Relationship." *American Ethnologist* 19 (2): 317–336.

———. 1992b. *The Wrestler's Body: Identity and Ideology in North India*. Berkeley: University of California Press.

———. 2004. *Yoga in Modern India: The Body between Science and Philosophy*. Princeton, NJ: Princeton University Press.

———. 2005a. "Introduction: The Politics of Culture and Medicine." In *Asian Medicine and Globalization*, edited by Joseph S. Alter, 1–20. Philadelphia: University of Pennsylvania Press.

———. 2005b. "Āyurvedic Acupuncture—Transnational Nationalism: Ambivalence about the Origin and Authenticity of Medical Knowledge." In *Asian Medicine and Globalization*, edited by Joseph S. Alter, 21–44. Philadelphia: University of Pennsylvania Press.

Anderson, Robert. 2004. "Indigenous Bonesetters in Contemporary Denmark." In *Healing by Hand: Manual Medicine and Bonesetting in Global Perspective*, edited by Katherine S. Oths and Servando Z. Hinojosa, 5–22. Walnut Creek, CA:Altamira.

Anderson, Robert, and Norman Klein. 2004. "Two Ethnographers and One Bonesetter in Bali." In *Healing by Hand: Manual Medicine and Bonesetting in Global Perspective*, edited by Katherine S. Oths and Servando Z. Hinojosa, 157–170. Walnut Creek, CA: Altamira.

Anonymous. n.d. *Varma Cūṭcā Cūṭcam* [*The Supreme Subtlety of the Vital Spots*]. Manuscript on palm-leaves.

Aptullā Cāyapu, Hakkīm Mukammatu. 1888. *Yūnāni Tāruṭya Virutti Pōtiṉi*. Cennai: Mataras Rippan Piras.

Aruḷmiku paḻaṉi taṇṭāyutapāṇi cuvāmi tirukkōyil [Holy Palani Dandayudhapani Swami Temple]. 1976. *Varma Viti* [*Vital Spot Conduct*]. Ceṉṉai: Aruḷmiku paḻaṉi taṇṭāyutapāṇi cuvāmi tirukkōyil.

Aybin Raj, P. 2008. "Fundamentals and Role of Varmam in Forensic Medicine," unpublished manuscript.

Ayurveda Art of Being. 2007. Film documentary directed by Pan Nalin, Germany; India: Pandora Film production.

Babb, Lawrence A. 1981. "Glancing: Visual Interaction in Hinduism." *Journal of Anthropological Research* 37 (4): 387–401.

Baer, Hans A., Merrill Singer, and Ida Susser. 2003. *Medical Anthropology and the World System*. Westport, CT: Praeger.

Balakrishnan, P. 1995. *Kalarippayattu: The Ancient Martial Art of Kerala*. Trivandrum: C. V. N. Kalari.

Balasubramaniam, A. V., ed. 1991. *Marma Chikitsa in Traditional Medicine*. Madras: Lok Swasthya Parampara Samvardhan Samithi.

Balasubramaniam, A. V., ed. 2004. "Building a Bridge between Local Health Cultures and Codified Traditions." In *Challenging the Indian Medical Heritage*, edited by Darshan Shankar and P. M. Unnikrishnan, 63–75. Ahmedabad: Centre for Environment Education.

Balasubramaniam, A. V., and V. Dharmalingam. 1991. "'Varma kalai': An Interview with Vaidya Dharmalingam." In *Marma Chikitsa in Traditional Medicine*, edited by A. V. Balasubramaniam, 20–50. Madras: Lok Swasthya Parampara Samvardhan Samithi.

Barrett, B., with L. Marchand, J. Scheder, M. B. Plane, R. Maberry, D. Appelbaum, D. Rakel, and D. Rabago. 2003. "Themes of Holism, Empowerment, Access, and Legitimacy Define Complementary, Alternative, and Integrative Medicine in Relation to Conventional Biomedicine." *Journal of Alternative and Complementary Medicine* 9 (6): 937–47.

Barth, Fredrik. 1975. *Ritual and Knowledge among the Baktaman of New Guinea*. Oslo: Universitetsforlaget.

Bataille, Georges. 1986. *Erotism: Death and Sensuality*. San Francisco: City Lights.

Beattie, Angela Gwen. 2004. "How do Your Babies Grow? Infant Massage, Media, Markets and Medicine in North India." PhD diss., University of California, San Francisco.

Bellman, Beryl L. 1981. "The Paradox of Secrecy." *Human Studies* 4 (1): 1–24.

———. 1984. *The Language of Secrecy: Symbols and Metaphors in Poro Ritual*. New Brunswick, NJ: Rutgers University Press.

Bendix, Regina. 2005. "Introduction: Ear to Ear, Nose to Nose, Skin to Skin—The Senses in Comparative Ethnographic Perspective." *Etnofoor* 18 (1): 3–14.

Benjamin, Walter. (1933) 2007. "On the Mimetic Faculty." In *Beyond the Body Proper: Reading the Anthropology of Material Life*, edited by Margaret Lock and Judith Farquhar, 130–132. Durham, NC: Duke University Press.

Blackburn, Stuart H. 1988. *Singing of Birth and Death: Texts in Performance*. Philadelphia: University of Pennsylvania Press.

Blake, Rosemary. 2011. "Ethnographies of Touch and Touching Ethnographies: Some Prospects for Touch in Anthropological Enquiries." *Anthropology Matters* 13 (1). Available at: http://www.anthropologymatters.com/index.php/anth_matters/article/view/224/409.

Bok, Sissela. 1984. *Secrets: On the Ethics of Concealment and Revelation*. New York: Vintage America.

Bourdieu, Pierre. 1977. *Outline of a Theory of Practice*. Translated by Richard Nice. Cambridge: Cambridge University Press.

———. 1984. *Distinction: A Social Critique of the Judgement of Taste*. Translated by Richard Nice. Cambridge, MA: Harvard University Press.

———. 1986. "The Forms of Capital." In *Handbook of Theory and Research for the Sociology of Education*, edited by John G. Richardson, 241–258. New York: Greenwood.

———. 1990. *The Logic of Practice*. Translated by Richard Nice. Cambridge: Polity.

———. 2003. "Participant Objectivation." *Journal of the Royal Anthropological Institute* 9 (2): 281–294.

Brass, Paul, R. 1972. "The Politics of Ayurvedic Education: A Case Study of Revivalism and Modernization in India." In *Education and Politics in India: Studies in Organization, Society, and Policy*, edited by Susan H. Rudolph and Lloyd I. Rudolph, 342–371. Delhi: Oxford University Press.

Broom, A., A. Doron, and P. Tovey. 2009. "The Inequalities of Medical Pluralism: Hierarchies of Health, the Politics of Tradition and the Economies of Care in Indian Oncology." *Social Science & Medicine* 69 (5): 698–706.

Burkert, Walter. 1995. "Der Geheime Reiz des Verborgenen." In *Secrecy and Concealment: Studies in the History of Mediterranean and Near Eastern Religions*, edited by Hans G. Kippenberg and Guy G. Stroumsa, 79–100. Leiden: Brill.

Burrow, Thomas, and Murray B. Emeneau. 1984. *A Dravidian Etymological Dictionary*. Oxford: Clarendon Press.

Caldwell, Robert. 1849. *The Tinnevelly Shanars: A Sketch of their Religion, and Their Moral Condition and Characteristics, as a Caste*. Madras: Christian Knowledge Society.

Canetti, Elias. 1963. *Crowds and Power*. Translated by Carol Stewart. New York: Viking.

Caṇmukam, Na. 2006. "Ulaka maruttuvattiṟkkut tamilariṉ varma maruttuvam: Tamil Varma Medicine for the World." Paper presented at the 4th National Siddha Doctor's conference, Chennai, November 25.

———. 2010. *Vētacatti Eṉṉum Varmakkalai* [*The Art of the Vital Spots, or the Hidden Power*]. Kōvai: Kalaikaḷiṉ āyvu niṟuvaṉam (Arts Research Institute).

Caravaṇakaṇēṣ. 2009. *Varmakkalai Rakaciyam* [*Secrets of the Art of the Vital Spots*]. Ceṉṉai: Kavitā papḷikēśaṉ.

Cārōjā, V. 1995. *Nāṭṭuppuṟa Varaital Kalai: Pacai Kuttalum Kōlamum* [*Rural Graphic Arts: Tattoos and Floor Designs*]. Peṅkalūr: Kāvyā.

Chidambarathanu Pillai, S. 1970. *Varma Kaimuṟai Ēṭu* [*Handbook of Varmology*]. Madras: International Institute of Thanuology.

———. 1994a. *The Origin of Thanuology*. Madras: International Institute of Thanuology.

———. 1994b. *Philosophy of Thanuology* [*Varma Kuravanji*]. Madras: International Institute of Thanuology.

———. 1994c. *Vital Life-Centres in Thanuology* [*Paduvarma Thirattu*]. Madras: International Institute of Thanuology.

———. 1995a. *Intellection in Thanuology*. Madras: International Institute of Thanuology.

———. 1995b. *Retrieval Techniques in Thanuology*. Madras: International Institute of Thanuology.

———. 1995c. *Wisdom on Dislocations, Breakages and Damages in Thanuology*. Madras: International Institute of Thanuology.

———. 1996. *Pulse Reading in Thanuology* [*Varma Naadi*]. Madras: International Institute of Thanuology.

———, ed. 2008. *Siddha System of Life* 32 (4). Chennai: Siddha Medical Literature Research Centre.

———, ed. 2009. *Siddha System of Life* 33 (1). Chennai: Siddha Medical Literature Research Centre.

Choi, Seung-Hoon. 2008. "WHO Traditional Medicine Strategy and Activities 'Standardization with Evidence-Based Approaches.'" *Journal of Acupuncture and Meridian Studies* 1 (2): 153–154.

Citamparatāṇuppiḷḷai, S. 1991. *Taṭṭuvarmat Tiraṭṭu: Striking Nerve Centres in Varmam*. Ceṉṉai: International Institute of Thanuology.

Classen, Constance. 2005. *The Book of Touch*. New York: Berg.

Coy, Michael W., ed. 1989. *Apprenticeship: From Theory to Method and Back Again* (SUNY Series in the Anthropology of Work). Albany: State University of New York Press.

Crego, Robert. 2003. *Sports and Games of the 18th and 19th Centuries*. Westport, CT: Greenwood.

Crook, Nigel. 1996a. *The Transmission of Knowledge in South Asia: Essays on Education, Religion, History, and Politics*. Delhi: Oxford University Press.

———. 1996b. "The Control and Expansion of Knowledge: An Introduction." In *The Transmission of Knowledge in South Asia: Essays on Education, Religion, History, and Politics* edited by Nigel Crook, 1–27. Delhi: Oxford University Press.

Csordas, Thomas J. 1990. "Embodiment as a Paradigm for Anthropology." *Ethos* 18 (1): 5–47.

———. 1993. "Somatic Modes of Attention." *Cultural Anthropology* 8 (2): 135–156.

———. 1994. *Embodiment and Experience: The Existential Ground of Culture and Self.* Cambridge: Cambridge University Press.

———. 1999. "Embodiment and Cultural Phenomenology." In *Perspectives on Embodiment: The Intersections of Nature and Culture*, edited by Gail Weiss and Honi Fern Haber, 143–162. New York: Routledge.

Cukumāraṉ, P. 2006. *Citta Rakaciyam* [*Secrets of Siddha*]. Ceṉṉai: Nalam.

Daniel, E. Valentine. 1984a. *Fluid Signs: Being a Person the Tamil Way*. Berkeley: University of California Press.

———. 1984b. "The Pulse as an Icon in Siddha Medicine." *Contributions to Asian Studies* 18: 115–126.

Daniel, Sheryl B. 1983. "The Tool Box Approach of the Tamil to the Issues of Moral Responsibility and Human Destiny." In *Karma: An Anthropological Inquiry*, edited by Charles Fenton Keyes, 27–62. Berkeley: University of California Press.

Das, Veena, and Ranendra K. Das. 2010. "The Moral Embedding of Economic Action: An Introduction." In *The Moral Embedding of Economic Action*, edited by Veena Das and Ranendra K. Das, 1–30. New Delhi: Oxford University Press.

Davies, James. 2010. "Introduction: Emotions in the Field." In *Emotions in the Field: The Psychology and Anthropology of Fieldwork Experience*, edited by James Davis and Dimitrina Spencer, 1–31. Stanford, CA: Stanford University Press.

Deccan Chronicle. 2013. "Physiotherapists under Scanner." March 30.

———. 2013. "Malaysia Seeks to Start Siddha Course." July 8.

De Michelis, Elizabeth. 2004. *A History of Modern Yoga: Patañjali and Western Esotericism*. London: Continuum.

Department of Ayurveda, Yoga & Naturopathy, Unani, Siddha and Homeopathy (AYUSH). 2010. "Summary of Infrastructure Facilities under AYUSH [Ayurveda, Yoga and Naturopathy, Unani, Siddha and Homeopathy]," January 1, 2010. http://indianmedicine.nic.in/showfile.asp?lid=44.

Derrida, Jacques. 1986. *Glas*. Translated by John P. Leavey Jr. and Richard Rand. Lincoln: University of Nebraska.

Devereux, George. 1967. *From Anxiety to Method in the Behavioural Sciences*. The Hague: Mouton.

Dharmalingam, V., Mani Radhika, and Angarai Venkataraman Balasubramaniam, eds. 1991. *Marma Chikitsa in Traditional Medicine*. Madras: Lok Swasthya Parampara Samvardhan Samithi.

Doniger, Wendy. 1973. *Asceticism and Eroticism in the Mythology of Siva*. London: Oxford University Press.

Downey, Greg. 2010. " 'Practice without Theory': A Neuroanthropological Perspective on Embodied Learning." *Journal of the Royal Anthropological Institute* 16 (1): 22–40.

Dunn, Frederick L. 1976. "Traditional Asian Medicine and Cosmopolitan Medicine as Adaptive Systems." In *Asian Medical Systems: A Comparative Study*, edited by Charles Leslie, 133–158. Berkeley: University of California Press.

Dutta, Sristidhar. 2006. "Thang-Ta: The Traditional Martial Art of Manipur." In *Martial Traditions of North East India*, edited by B. Tripathy and S. Dutta, 251–262. New Delhi: Concept.

Eck, Diana L. 1998. *Darśan: Seeing the Divine Image in India*. New York: Columbia University Press.

Ekbote, Gopal Rao. 2007. "The Indian National Movement in Retrospect: Role of National Language: Hindi." In *Indian National Movement in Retrospect*, edited by N. G. Rajurkar, 15–24. Secunderabad: R. K. Printing Press and Publication Centre.

Eliade, Mircea. 1970. *Yoga: Immortality and Freedom*. Princeton, NJ: Princeton University Press.

Fabrega, Horacio, and Daniel B. Silver. 1973. *Illness and Shamanistic Curing in Zinacantan: An Ethnomedical Analysis*. Stanford, CA: Stanford University Press.

Fainzang, Sylvie. 2005. "When Doctors and Patients Lie to Each Other. Lying and Power within the Doctor-Patient Relationship." In *Lying and Illness: Power and Performance*, edited by Els Van Dongen and Silvie Fainzang, 36–55. Amsterdam: Hel Spinuis.

Faure, Bernard. 1986. "Bodhidharma as Textual and Religious Paradigm." *History of Religions* 25 (3): 187–198.

Fedorova, Mariana. 1990. "Die Marmantheorie in der Klassischen Indischen Medizin." PhD diss.,Ludwig-Maximilians-Universität München.

Feuerstein, Georg. 1990. *Encyclopedic Dictionary of Yoga*. New York: Paragon House.

———. 2008 *The Yoga Tradition: Its History, Literature, Philosophy and Practice*. Prescott, AZ: Hohm.

Fine, Gary Alan, and Lori Holyfield. 1996. "Secrecy, Trust, and Dangerous Leisure: Generating Group Cohesion in Voluntary Organizations." *Social Psychology Quarterly* 59 (1): 22–38.

Fish, Allison. 2006. "The Commodification and Exchange of Knowledge in the Case of Transnational Commercial Yoga." *International Journal of Cultural Property* 13 (2): 189–206.

Flood, Gavin D. 2006. *The Tantric Body: The Secret Tradition of Hindu Religion*. London: I. B. Tauris.

Foucault, Michel. 1965. *Madness and Civilization: A History of Insanity in the Age of Reason*. New York: Pantheon.
———. 1973. *The Birth of the Clinic: An Archeology of Medical Perception*. New York: Random House Vintage.
———. 1977. *Discipline and Punish: The Birth of the Prison*. New York: Pantheon.
———. 1988. "Technologies of the Self." In *Technologies of the Self: A Seminar with Michel Foucault*, edited by Luther H. Martin, 16–49. Amherst: University of Massachusetts Press.
———. 1990. *The History of Sexuality*. Vol. 2, *The Use of Pleasure*. London: Penguin.
———. 1991. "Governmentality." In *The Foucault Effect: Studies in Governmentality*, edited by G. Burchell, C. Gordon, and P. Miller, 87–104. London: Harvester/Wheatsheaf.
Fox, Mary, Andy Dickens, Colin Greaves, Michael Dixon, and Martin James. 2006. "Marma Therapy for Stroke Rehabilitation: A Pilot Study." *Journal of Rehabilitation Medicine* 38: 268–271.
Frawley, David, with Subhash Ranade and Avinash Lele. 2005. *Ayurveda & Marma Therapy: Energy Points in Yogic Healing*. Delhi: Chaukhamba Sanskrit Pratishthan.
Freidson, Eliot. 1970. *Profession of Medicine: A Study of the Sociology of Applied Knowledge*. Michigan: Dodd, Mead.
Fuller, C. J. 1980. "The Calendrical System in Tamilnadu (South India)." *Journal of the Royal Asiatic Society of Great Britain and Ireland* 112 (1): 52–63.
Gafni, Amiram, with Cathy Charles and Tim Whelan. 1998. "The Physician-Patient Encounter: The Physician as a Perfect Agent for the Patient Versus the Informed Treatment Decision-Making Model." *Social Science & Medicine* 47 (3): 347–354.
Ganapathy, T. N. 1993. *The Philosophy of the Tamil Siddhas*. New Delhi: Indian Council of Philosophical Research.
———. 2008. *The Contribution of Tamil Siddhas to Dravidian Thought*. Kuppam: Prasaranga, Dravidian University.
Geertz, Clifford. 1973. *The Interpretation of Cultures: Selected Essays*. New York: Basic Books.
———. 1986. "Making Experience, Authoring Selves." In *The Anthropology of Experience*, edited by Victor Turner and Edward Bruner, 373–380. Urbana: University of Illinois Press.
Geetha, G. 1983. "Kaya Kalpa Mooligai in Siddha Medicine." In *Heritage of the Tamils: Siddha Medicine*, edited by S. V. Subramaniam and V. R. Madhavan, 132–145. Madras: International Institute of Tamil Studies.
Gibson, James J. 1966. *The Senses Considered as Perceptual Systems*. Boston: Houghton Mifflin.
Giddens, Anthony. 1984. *The Constitution of Society: Outline of the Theory of Structuration*. Cambridge: Polity.
Giri, Rajneesh V. 2007. *Synopsis of Suśruta Saṃhitā*. Varanasi: Chaukhambha Orientalia.

Glaser, Karl. 1912. "Der Indische Student." *Zeitschrift der Deutschen Morgenländischen Gesellschaft* 66: 1–37.

Good, Byron J. 1996. *Medicine, Rationality, and Experience: An Anthropological Perspective.* Cambridge: Cambridge University Press.

Goody, Esther N. 1989. "Learning: Apprenticeship and the Division of Labor." In *Apprenticeship: From Theory to Method and Back Again,* edited by Michael W. Coy, 233–256. Albany: State University of New York Press.

Gourlay, Stephen. 2004. "Knowing as Semiosis: Steps Towards a Reconceptualization of 'Tacit Knowledge.'" In *Organizations as Knowledge Systems: Knowledge, Learning and Dynamic Capabilities,* edited by Hardimos Tsoukas and Nikolaos Mylonopoulos, 86–108. New York: Palgrave Macmillan.

Govindan, S. V. 2005. *Massage Therapy for Diseases of Vital Areas: Marma Treatment.* New Delhi: Abhinav.

Gray, David B. 2005. "Disclosing the Empty Secret: Textuality and Embodiment in the Cakrasamvara Tantra." *Numen* 52 (4): 417–444.

Gurumurthy, S. 1979. *Education in South India: Ancient and Medieval Periods.* Madras: New Era.

Hahn, Robert A., and Arthur Kleinman. 1983. "Biomedical Practice and Anthropological Theory: Frameworks and Directions." *Annual Review of Anthropology* 12: 305–333.

Halliburton, Murphy. 2002. "Rethinking Anthropological Studies of the Body: Manas and Bodham in Kerala." *American Anthropologist* 104 (4): 1123–1134.

Harasim, Linda M. 1990. *Online Education: Perspectives on a New Environment.* New York: Praeger.

Haraway, Donna. 1988. "Situated Knowledges: The Science Question in Feminism and the Privilege of Partial Perspective." *Feminist Studies* 14 (3): 575–599.

Hardgrave, Robert L. 1968. "The Breast-Cloth Controversy: Caste Consciousness and Social Change in Southern Travancore." *Indian Economic and Social History Review* 5 (2): 171–187.

———. 1969. *The Nadars of Tamilnad: The Political Culture of a Community in Change.* Berkeley: University of California Press.

Hart, George L. 1973. "Woman and the Sacred in Ancient Tamilnad." *Journal of Asian Studies* 32 (2): 233–250.

Hausman, Gary J. 1996. "Siddhars, Alchemy, and the Abyss of Tradition: 'Traditional' Tamil Medical Knowledge in 'Modern Practice.'" PhD diss., University of Michigan, Ann Arbor.

Herzfeld, Michael. 2001. *Anthropology: Theoretical Practice in Culture and Society.* Malden: Blackwell.

———. 2009. "The Performance of Secrecy: Domesticity and Privacy in Public Spaces." *Semiotica* 175 (4): 135–162.

Hiltebeitel, Alf. 1999. *Rethinking India's Oral and Classical Epics: Draupadī among Rajputs, Muslims, and Dalits.* Chicago: University of Chicago Press.

Hinojosa, Servando Z. 2002. "'The Hands Know': Bodily Engagement and Medical Impasse in Highland Maya Bonesetting." *Medical Anthropology Quarterly* 16 (1): 22–40.

———. 2004a. "The Hands, the Sacred, and the Context of Change in Maya Bonesetting." In *Healing by Hand: Manual Medicine and Bonesetting in Global Perspective*, edited by Kathryn S. Oths and Servando Z. Hinojosa, 107–130. Walnut Creek, CA: Altamira.

———. 2004b. "Bonesetting and Radiography in the Southern Maya Highlands." *Medical Anthropology* 23 (4): 263–293.

Hobsbawm, Eric J., and Terence Ranger, eds. 1983. *The Invention of Tradition*. Cambridge: Cambridge University Press.

Høg, Erling, and Elisabeth Hsu. 2002. "Introduction. Theme Issue, 'Countervailing Creativity: Patient Agency in the Globalisation of Asian Medicines.'" *Anthropology & Medicine* 9 (3): 205–221.

Holdrege, Barbara A. 1998. "Body Connections: Hindu Discourses of the Body and the Study of Religion." *International Journal of Hindu Studies* 2 (3): 341–386.

Hsu, Elisabeth. 1999. *The Transmission of Chinese Medicine*. Cambridge: Cambridge University Press.

———. 2000a. "Towards a Science of Touch, Part I: Chinese Pulse Diagnostics in Early Modern Europe." *Anthropology & Medicine* 7 (2): 251–268.

———. 2000b. "Towards a Science of Touch, Part II: Representations of the Tactile Experience of the Seven Chinese Pulses Indicating Danger of Death in Early Modern Europe." *Anthropology & Medicine* 7 (3): 319–333.

———. 2005. "Acute Pain Infliction as Therapy." *Etnofoor* 18 (1): 78–96.

———. 2006. "Participant Experience: Learning to Be an Acupuncturist, and Not Becoming One." In *Critical Journeys: The Making of Anthropologists*, edited by Geert De Neve and Maya Unnithan-Kumar, 149–163. Aldershot: Ashgate.

———, ed. 2008a. "The Senses and the Social." Special issue, *Ethnos* 73 (4).

———. 2008b. "The Senses and the Social: An Introduction." *Ethnos* 73 (4): 433–443.

Huber, Brad R., and Robert Anderson. 1996. "Bonesetters and Curers in a Mexican Community: Conceptual Models, Status, and Gender." *Medical Anthropology* 17 (1): 23–38.

Illich, Ivan. 1975. *Medical Nemesis: The Expropriation of Health*. London: Calder and Boyars.

Immanuel, M. 2002. *The Dravidian Lineages: The Nadars through the Ages*. Nagercoil: Historical Research and Publications Trust.

———. 2007. *Kanniyakumari: Aspects and Architects*. Nagercoil: Historical Research and Publications Trust.

International Olympic Committee (IOC). 2006. *IOC Medical Commission: Collection of Sports Medicine and Sports Sciences*. Lausanne: International Olympic Committee.

International Thanu Foundation. 2009. *Doctorate in Varma Medical Sciences: Brochure cum Application Form*. Madras: Thanu Foundation.

Intiyaṉ [*Indian*]. 1996. Movie directed by S. Shankar, India.

Irācāmaṇi, S. 1996. *Citta Maruttuvattil Varma Parikāramum Cikiccai Muṟaikaḷum* [*Vital Spot Remedies and Curing Methods in Siddha Medicine*]. Ceṉṉai: Intiya maruttuvam maṟṟum ōmiyōpati iyakkam.

Irājēntiraṉ, T. 2006. *Varmamum Taṭavumuṟai Aṟiviyalum* [*The Vital Spots and Massage Science*]. Mūlaccal: Teṉṟal Patippakam.

———. n.d. *Caracūkṣattiṟavukōl—36* [*36 Verses of the Key to the Garland of Subtlety*]. Maṇali: Kastūri piras.

Jackson, Michael. 1983. "Knowledge of the Body." *MAN* 18 (2): 327–345.

———. 2010. "From Anxiety to Method in Anthropological Fieldwork." In *Emotions in the Field: The Psychology and Anthropology of Fieldwork Experience*, edited by James Davis and Dimitrina Spencer, 35–53. Stanford, CA: Stanford University Press.

Jaggi, Om Prakash. 1979. *Yogic and Tantric Medicine*. Delhi: Atma Ram.

Jeanes, Rosemary A. 1982. "Tradition and Learning in Odissi Dance of India: Guru-Sisya-Parampara." MA thesis, York University.

Jekatā. 2005. *Cittarkaḷ Kaṇṭa Varmakkalai Marmaṅkaḷ* [*The Secrets of the Art of the Vital Spots as Discovered by the Siddhars*]. Ceṉṉai: Rāmpiracānt Papḷikēṣaṉs.

Jēms, Tē. Ka. 2010. *Varma Oṭimuṟivu Cara Cūttiram—1500: Maruttuvac Cuvaṭip Patippu Nūl* [*The 1500 Verses of the Treatise on Vital Spot Fractures and Breakages: A Medical Palm-Leaf Manuscript*]. Ceṉṉai: Cēkar Patippakam.

Jeyrāj, Ṭirākaṉ T. 1999. *Varmacāstiram* [*Vital Spot Treatise*]. Ceṉṉai: Kumaraṉ patippakam.

———. 2000. *Varmayuttam* [*Vital Spot Combat*]. Ceṉṉai: Kumaraṉ patippakam.

———. 2007. *Aṭaṅkal Varmam* [*Varmam Therapeutic Spots*]. Ceṉṉai: Kumaraṉ patippakam.

Johari, Harish. 1984. *Ancient Indian Massage: Traditional Massage Techniques based on the Ayurveda*. New Delhi: Munshiram Manoharlal.

Johnson, Paul Christopher. 2002. *Secrets, Gossip, and Gods: The Transformation of Brazilian Candomblé*. New York: Oxford University Press.

Jonas, Hans. 1981. *Macht oder Ohnmacht der Subjektivität? Das Leib-Seele-Problem im Vorfeld des Prinzips Verantwortung*. Frankfurt am Main: Insel-Verlag.

Jones, David E. 2002. *Combat, Ritual, and Performance: Anthropology of the Martial Arts*. Westport, CT: Praeger.

Jordan, Brigitte. 1993. *Birth in Four Cultures: A Crosscultural Investigation of Childbirth in Yucatan, Holland, Sweden, and the United States*. Prospect Heights, Ill: Waveland Press.

Kaṇapati, Vē. n.d. *Varmap Payiṟci Kaiyēṭu*. I: *Naṭaimuṟai Viḷakkam* [*Handbook of Vital Spot Practice. Vol. 1: Illustration of Conduct*]. Kaṉṉiyākumari: Vivēkāṉanta kēntiram, Nārṭep.

Kaṇṇaṉ Rājārām, T. 2005. *Varma Aḷavai Nūl Maṟṟum Varma Muṟaikaḷ* [*Book on Measurements and Methods of the Vital Spots*]. Ceṉṉai: Tamiḻ maruttuvak kaḻakam.

———. 2007a. *Varma Maruttuvam (Ciṟappu)* [*Varma Medicine (Special)*]. Muṉciṟai: ATSVS Citta Maruttuvakkallūri.

———. 2007b. *Varma Maruttuvattiṉ Aṭippaṭaikaḷ* [*Fundamentals of Varma Medicine*]. Muṉciṟai: ATSVS Citta Maruttuvakkallūri.

———. 2007c. *Varma puḷḷikaḷiṉ iruppiṭam* [*Location of Varma Points*]. Muṉciṟai: ATSVS Citta Maruttuvakkallūri.

Kanungo, Pralay. 2013. "Another Avatar of Hindu Nationalism: Vivekanada Kendra, Kanyakumari." Paper presented at the International Institute for Asian Studies, Amsterdam, November 7.

Katre, S. M. 1969. "The Official Language and the National Languages of India." In *Language and Society in India*, edited by A. Poddar, 165–187. Simla: Indian Institute of Advanced Study.

Kēcavappiḷḷai, Pi. 1983. "Varma Maruttuvam" [Vital spot medicine]. In *Heritage of the Tamils: Siddha Medicine*, edited by S. V. Subramaniam and V. R. Madhavan, 29–57. Madras: International Institute of Tamil Studies.

Kember, Sarah. 1991. "Medical Diagnostic Imaging: The Geometry of Chaos." *New Formations* 15: 55–66.

Khan, Ruqayya Yasmine. 2008. *Self and Secrecy in Early Islam*. Columbia: University of South Carolina Press.

Kingston, C., B. S. Nisha, S. Kiruba, and S. Jeeva. 2007. "Ethnomedicinal Plants used by Indigenous Community in a Traditional Healthcare System." *Ethnobotanical Leaflets* 11: 32–37.

Kippenberg, Hans G. 1995. "Introduction: Secrecy and Its Benefits." In *Secrecy and Concealment: Studies in the History of Mediterranean and Near Eastern Religions*, edited by Hans G. Kippenberg and Guy G. Stroumsa, xiii–xxiv. Leiden: Brill.

Kippenberg, Hans G., and Guy G. Stroumsa, eds. 1995. *Secrecy and Concealment: Studies in the History of Mediterranean and Near Eastern Religions*. Leiden: Brill.

Kleinman, Arthur. 1980. *Patients and Healers in the Context of Culture: An Exploration of the Borderland between Anthropology, Medicine, and Psychiatry*. Berkeley: University of California Press.

Kleinman, Arthur, and Erin Fitz-Henry. 2007. "The Experiential Basis of Subjectivity: How Individuals Change in the Context of Societal Transformation." In *Subjectivity: Ethnographic Investigations*, edited by João Biehl, Byron Good, and Arthur Kleinman, 52–65. Berkeley: University of California Press.

Kleinman, Arthur, and Joan Kleinman. 1991. "Suffering and Its Professional Transformation: Toward an Ethnography of Experience." *Culture, Medicine and Psychiatry* 15 (3): 275–301.

Krishnamurthy, K. H., and G. Chandra Mouli. 1984. "Siddha System of Medicine: A Historical Appraisal." *Indian Journal of History of Science* 19 (1): 43–53.

Krishna Rao, P. V. (1937) 2007. *Comparative Study of the Marmas*. New Delhi: Rashtriya Sanskrit Sansthan.

Kutumbiah, P. 1969. *Ancient Indian Medicine*. Bombay: Orient Longman.

Lad, Vasant D., and Anisha Durve. 2008. *Marma Points of Ayurveda: The Energy Pathways for Healing Body, Mind and Consciousness.* Albuquerque: Ayurvedic Press.

Lambert, Helen. 1995. "Of Bonesetters and Barber-Surgeons: Traditions of Therapeutic Practice and the Spread of Allopathic Medicine in Rajasthan." In *Folk, Faith and Feudalism: Rajasthan Studies,* edited by N. K. Singhi and R. Joshi, 92–111. Jaipur: Rawat.

———. 2012. "Medical Pluralism and Medical Marginality: Bone Doctors and the Selective Legitimation of Therapeutic Expertise in India." *Social Science & Medicine* 74 (7): 1029–1036.

Langford, Jean M. 2002. *Fluent Bodies: Ayurvedic Remedies for Postcolonial Imbalance.* Durham, NC: Duke University Press.

Latour, Bruno, and Steve Woolgar. 1986. *Laboratory Life: The Construction of Scientific Facts.* Princeton, NJ: Princeton University Press.

Lemke, Thomas. 2001. "The Birth of Bio-Politics: Michel Foucault's Lecture at the Collège de France on Neo-Liberal Governmentality." *Economy and Society* 30 (2): 190–207.

Leslie, Charles M. 1976. *Asian Medical Systems: A Comparative Study.* Berkeley: University of California Press.

Leder, Drew. 1992. "A Tale of two Bodies: The Cartesian Corpse and the Lived Body." In *The Body in Medical Thought and Practice,* edited by Drew Leder, 17–36. Dordrecht: Kluwer Academic.

Levy, Robert I. 1990. *Mesocosm: Hinduism and the Organization of a Traditional Newar City in Nepal.* Berkeley: University of California Press.

Lincoln, Bruce. 1994. *Authority: Construction and Corrosion.* Chicago: University of Chicago Press.

Little, Layne Ross. 2006. "Bowl Full of Sky: Story-Making and the Many Lives of the Siddha Bhogar." PhD diss., University of California, Berkeley.

Lock, Margaret, and Vinh-Kim Nguyen. 2011. *An Anthropology of Biomedicine.* Malden, Mass.: Wiley-Blackwell.

Luhrmann, Tanya M. 1989. "The Magic of Secrecy." *Ethos* 17 (2): 31–165.

———. 2010. "What counts as Data?" In *Emotions in the Field: The Psychology and Anthropology of Fieldwork Experience,* edited by James Davis and Dimitrina Spencer, 212–238. Stanford, CA: Stanford University Press.

Luijendijk, D. H. 2007. "Kalarippayat: The Structure and Essence of an Indian Martial Art." PhD diss., Department for Study of Religions, University of Nijmegen.

MacIntyre, Alasdair C. 1984. *After Virtue : A Study in Moral Theory.* 2nd ed. Notre Dame, IN: University of Notre Dame Press.

Madhavan, Harilal. 2010. "Growth, Transition and Globalisation of a Traditional Medicine: Ayurvedic Manufacturing with Special Focus on Kerala." PhD diss., Jawaharlal Nehru University, New Delhi.

Madhavan, V. R. 1984. *Siddha Medical Manuscripts in Tamil.* Madras: International Institute of Tamil Studies.

———. 1986. "Medical Education of the Tamils." In *Heritage of the Tamils: Education and Vocation*, edited by S. V. Subramaniam, 222–232. Madras: International Institute of Tamil Studies.

Majno, Guido. 1975. *The Healing Hand: Man and Wound in the Ancient World.* Cambridge: Harvard University Press.

Makovicky, Nicolette. 2010. "'Something to Talk About': Notation and Knowledge Making amongst Lace Makers in Central Slovakia." *Journal of the Royal Anthropological Institute* 16 (1): 80–99.

Mandelbaum, David Goodman. 1970. *Society in India.* Berkeley: University of California Press.

Maṇiyaṉ, Pa. Cu. 2012. *Akastiyariṉ Varmacūttira Viḷakkam* [*Explanation of Agasthiyar's Vital Spot Treatise*]. Kōyamputtūr: Vijayā patippakam.

Manu Vaidyar, S. 2007. "Siddha Vaidyam." In *Healing Traditions of India*, edited by Todd Pesek, 61–72. Thiruvananthapuram: Olive.

Marchand, Trevor Hugh James, ed. 2010. *Making Knowledge: Explorations of the Indissoluble Relation between Mind, Body and Environment.* Malden, MA: Wiley-Blackwell.

Mariyajōcap, A. n.d. *Varmak Kaṇṇāṭi—500: Mūlamum Uraiyum* [*The 500 Verses of the Mirror of the Vital Spots: Source Text and Commentary*]. Maṇalikkarai: Muttu nūlakam.

Marriott, McKim. 1955. "Little Communities in an Indigenous Civilization." In *Village India: Studies in the Little Community*, edited by McKim Marriott, 171–222. Chicago: University of Chicago Press.

———. 1990. *India through Hindu Categories.* New Delhi: Sage.

Marx, Gary T., and Glenn W. Muschert. 2009. "Simmel on Secrecy: A Legacy and Inheritance for the Sociology of Information." In *Soziologie als Möglichkeit: 100 Jahre Georg Simmels Untersuchungen über die Formen der Vergesellschaftung*, edited by Cécile Rol and Christian Papilloud, 217–236. Wiesbaden: VS Verlag für Sozialwissenschaften.

Mauss, Marcel. 1934. "Les Techniques du Corps." *Journal de Psychologie* 32 (3–4): 271–293.

May, Shannon. 2010. "Rethinking Anonymity in Anthropology: A Question of Ethics." *Anthropology News* 51 (4): 10–13.

Mazis, Glen A. 1998. "Touch and Vision: Rethinking with Merleau-Ponty Sartre on the Caress." In *The Debate between Sartre and Merleau-Ponty*, edited by Jon Stewart, 144–153. Evanston, IL: Northwestern University Press.

McLuhan, Marshall. 1973. *Understanding Media: The Extensions of Man.* London: Abacus.

Meenakshi, K. 2001. "The Siddhas of Tamil Nadu: A Voice of Dissent." In *Tradition, Dissent and Ideology: Essays in Honour of Romila Thapar*, edited by Radha Champakalakshmi, 111–134. New Delhi: Oxford University Press.

Mehra, Raakhee. 2008. *Significance of Ayurvediya Marma: Vital Body Points: Based on Suśruta śārīra.* New Delhi: Readworthy.

Merleau-Ponty, Maurice. (1962) 1996. *Phenomenology of Perception*. Delhi: Motilal Banarsidass.

Meulenbeld, Gerrit Jan. 1974. *The Mādhavanidāna and its Chief Commentary*. Leiden: Brill.

———. 2000. *A History of Indian Medical Literature*. Groningen: Forsten.

Michaels, Axel. 1998. *Der Hinduismus: Geschichte und Gegenwart*. Munich: Beck.

Miller, Robert J. 1966. "Button, Button. . . Great Tradition, Little Tradition, Whose Tradition?" *Anthropological Quarterly* 39 (1): 26–42.

Mishra, J. N. 2005. *Marma and Its Management*. Varanasi: Chaukhambha Orientalia.

Mojumdar, Atindra. 1973. *The Caryapadas: A Treatise on the Earliest Bengali Songs*. Calcutta: Naya Prokash.

Mol, Annemarie. 2002. *The Body Multiple: Ontology in Medical Practice*. Durham, NC: Duke University Press.

———. 2008. *The Logic of Care: Health and the Problem of Patient Choice*. London: Routledge.

Mol, Annemarie, with Ingunn Moser and Jeannette Pols. 2010. *Care in Practice: On Tinkering in Clinics, Homes and Farms*. Bielefeld: Transcript.

Monier-Williams, Monier. 1899. *A Sanskrit-English Dictionary: Etymologically and Philologically Arranged with Special Reference to Cognate Indo-European Languages*. New edition, greatly enlarged and improved with the collaboration of E. Leumann, C. Cappeller, and other scholars. Oxford: Clarendon Press.

Mukharji, Projit Bihari. 2007. "Structuring Plurality: Locality, Caste, Class and Ethnicity in Nineteenth-Century Bengali Dispensaries." *Health and History* 9 (1): 80–105.

Muraleedharan, V. R. 1992. "Professionalising Medical Practice in Colonial South-India." *Economic and Political Weekly* 25: 27–37.

Nagarajan, Vijaya Rettakudi. 1998. *Hosting the Divine: The Kōlam as Ritual, Art and Ecology in Tamil Nadu, India*. Berkeley: University of California.

Nair, Chirakkal T. Sreedharan. 1957. *Marmmadarppanam*. Calicut: P. K. Brothers.

———. 2007 *Kalarippayattu: The Complete Guide to Kerala's Ancient Martial Art*. Chennai: Westland.

Nair, K. N., with P. Sivanandan, and V. C. V. Retnam. 1984. "Education, Employment, and Landholding Pattern in a Tamil Village." *Economic & Political Weekly* 19 (24–25): 948–955.

Naraindas, Harish. 2006. "Of Spineless Babies and Folic Acid: Evidence and Efficacy in Biomedicine and Ayurvedic Medicine." *Social Science & Medicine* 62 (11): 2658–2669.

Narayanaswami, V. 1975. *Introduction to the Siddha System of Medicine*. Madras: Pandit S. S. Anandam Research Institute of Siddha Medicine.

Natarajan, K. 1984. "Purification Processes in Siddha System." In *Heritage of the Tamils: Siddha Medicine*, edited by S. V. Subramaniam and V. R. Madhavan, 117–131. Madras: International Institute of Tamil Studies.

Nedelmann, Brigitta. 1995. "Geheimhaltung, Verheimlichung, Geheimnis: Einige Soziologische Vorüberlegungen." In *Secrecy and Concealment: Studies in the History of Mediterranean and Near Eastern Religions*, edited by Hans G. Kippenberg, 1–16. Leiden: Brill.

Neuber, Erika. 2006. "Die Guru-Sisya-Beziehung." In *Ethnohistorie: Empirie und Praxis*, edited by Hermann Mückler, Werner Zips, and Manfred Kremser, 145–155. Wien: WUV Universitätsverlag.

Nichter, Mark. 1980. "The Layperson's Perception of Medicine as Perspective into the Utilization of Multiple Therapy Systems in the Indian Context." *Social Science & Medicine* 14 (4): 225–233.

———. 1992. "Of Ticks, Kings, Spirits, and the Promise of Vaccines." In *Paths to Asian Medical Knowledge*, edited by Charles Leslie and Allan Young, 224–253. Berkeley: University of California Press.

———. 2002. "Social Relations of Therapy Management." In *New Horizons in Medical Anthropology: Essays in Honour of Charles Leslie*, edited by Charles M. Leslie, Mark Nichter, and Margaret M. Lock, 81–110. London: Routledge.

———. 2008. "Coming to Our Senses: Appreciating the Sensorial in Medical Anthropology." *Transcultural Psychiatry* 45 (2): 163–197.

Nicivilcan̲, W. 2003. *Varmapīraṅki—100; Varmapīraṅki Cūttiram; Varmapīraṅki Tir̲avukōl* [*100 Verses of the Vital Spot Canon; The Vital Spot Canon Treatise; The Key to the Vital Spot Canon*]. Karuṅkal: Ammā patippakam.

———. 2004. *Varma Cūṭāmaṇi Pañcīkaraṇa Pin̲n̲al—1500* [*1500 Verses of the Garland of Songs on the Creation of the Precious Vital Spots*]. Karuṅkal: Ammā patippakam.

Nyamongo, Isaac K. 2004. "Borana Bonesetters: Integrating Modernity and Tradition in a Northern Kenyan Pastoral Community." In *Healing by Hand: Manual Medicine and Bonesetting in Global Perspective*, edited by Kathryn S. Oths and Servando Z. Hinojosa, 221–236. Walnut Creek, CA: Altamira.

Okely, Judith. 2007. "Fieldwork Embodied." In *Embodying Sociology: Retrospect, Progress and Prospects*, edited by Chris Shilling, 65–79. Malden: Blackwell.

Onuminya, J. E. 2004. "The Role of the Traditional Bonesetter in Primary Fracture Care in Nigeria." *South African Medical Journal* 94 (8): 652–658.

Oths, Kathryn S., and Servando Z. Hinojosa, eds. 2004. *Healing by Hand: Manual Medicine and Bonesetting in Global Perspective*. Walnut Creek, CA: Altamira.

Pandian, Jacob. 1983. "Political Emblems of Caste Identity: An Interpretation of Tamil Caste Titles." *Anthropological Quarterly* 56 (4): 190–197.

Pappas, Gregory. 1990. "Some Implications for the Study of the Doctor-Patient Interaction: Power, Structure, and Agency in the Works of Howard Waitzkin and Arthur Kleinman." *Social Science & Medicine* 30 (2): 199–204.

Parsons, Talcott. 1951. "Illness and the Role of the Physician: A Sociological Perspective." *American Journal of Orthopsychiatry* 21 (3): 452–460.

Pati, George. 2009. "Body as Sacred Space in Kaḷari cikitsā of Kerala, South India." *Religions of South Asia* 3 (2): 235–250.

Pati, George. 2010. "Kalari and Kalarippayattu of Kerala, South India: Nexus of the Celestial, the Corporeal, and the Terrestrial." *Contemporary South Asia* 18 (2): 175–189.

Payne, Peter. 1981. *Martial Arts: The Spiritual Dimension*. London: Thames and Hudson.

Pechilis, Karen. 2006. "The Story of the Classical Tamil Woman Saint, Kāraikkāl Ammaiyār: A Translation of Her Story from Cēkkiḻār's 'Periya Purāṇam.'" *International Journal of Hindu Studies* 10 (2): 171–184.

Pigg, Stacy Leigh. 1996. "The Credible and the Credulous: The Question of 'Villagers' Beliefs' in Nepal." *Cultural Anthropology* 11 (2): 160–201.

Pillai, J. K. 1986. "Teacher, Students and Teaching-Learning Process in ancient Tamil Educational System." In *Heritage of the Tamils: Education and Vocation*, edited by S. V. Subramaniam, 56–68. Madras: International Institute of Tamil Studies.

Pitchai, A. 1986. "Curriculum of Ancient Tamil's Educational System and Its Uses." In *Heritage of the Tamils: Education and Vocation*, edited by S. V. Subramaniam, 135–150. Madras: International Institute of Tamil Studies.

Polanyi, Michael. 1967. *The Tacit Dimension*. New York: Anchor.

———. 1974. *Knowing and Being: Essays*. Chicago: University of Chicago Press.

———. 1985. *Implizites Wissen*. Frankfurt am Main: Suhrkamp.

Pordié, Laurent. 2007. "Presentation: Ethnographies of 'folk healing.'" *Indian Anthropologist* 37 (1): 1–12.

Prasad, Amit. 2005. "Making Images/Making Bodies: Visibilizing and Disciplining through Magnetic Resonance Imaging (MRI)." *Science, Technology, & Human Values* 30 (2): 291–316.

Purecha, Sandhya. 2003. *Theory and Practice of Āṅgikābhinaya in Bharatanāṭyam*. Mumbai: Bharatiya Vidya Bhavan.

Rācā. (1997) 2002. *Nīṅkaḷum Varmakkalai Kaṟkalām* [*You Too Can Learn the Art of the Vital Spots*]. Ceṉṉai: Śrī caṅkītavāṇi.

Raj, J. David Manuel. 1975. *Silambam Fencing from India*. Eugene, OR: J. David Manuel Raj.

———. 1977. "The Origin and the Historical Development of Silambam Fencing: An Ancient Self-Defense Sport of India." PhD diss., University of Oregon.

Rajam, V. S. 1986. "Aṇaṅku: A Notion Semantically Reduced to Signify Female Sacred Power." *Journal of the American Oriental Society* 106 (2): 257–272.

Rajamony, S. 1983. "Varma & Neurology in Siddha." In *Heritage of the Tamils: Siddha Medicine*, edited by S. V. Subramaniam and V. R. Madhavan, 473–483. Madras: International Institute of Tamil Studies.

Rājēntiraṉ, Ār. 1998. *Maraṇaviti Varmam* [*The Deadly Varmam Spots*]. Maturai: Ār. Rājēntiraṉ.

———. 2008. *Varmakkalai: Putumaiyāṉa Taṟkāppu Muṟaikaḷ* [*The Art of the Vital Spots: A Wondrous Self-Defense Method*]. Ceṉṉai: Caparīś pārati.

———. 2009. *Piṭivarmam* [*Grappling Vital Spot*]. Maturai: Śrīlekṣmi piras.

Raju, G., and G. Hariramamurthy. 2004. "Health at Our Doorstep: Reviving Home Remedies." In *Challenging the Indian Medical Heritage*, edited by Darshan Shankar and P. M. Unnikrishnan, 128–170. New Delhi: Foundation.

Ram, Kalpana. 2001a. "Modernity and the Midwife: Contestations over a Subaltern Figure, South India." In *Healing Powers and Modernity: Traditional Medicine, Shamanism, and Science in Asian Societies*, edited by Linda Connor and Geoffrey Samuel, 64–84. Westport: Begin & Garvey.

———. 2001b. "The Female Body of Possession: A Feminist Perspective on Rural Tamil Women's Experiences." In *Mental Health from a Gender Perspective*, edited by Bhargavi V. Davar, 181–216. London and New Delhi: Sage.

———. 2008. "The Mukkuvars of Kanyakumari: On the Margins of Caste Society." In *Caste in History*, edited by Ishita Banerjee-Dube, 136–152. New Delhi: Oxford University Press.

———. 2010. "Class and the Clinic: The Subject of Medical Pluralism and the Transmission of Inequality." *South Asian History and Culture* 1 (2): 199–212.

Ramalingam, A., and G. Veluchamy. 1983. "Elements of Medical Science in Sangam Literature." In *Heritage of the Tamils: Siddha Medicine*, edited by S. V. Subramaniam and V. R. Madhavan, 44–53. Madras: International Institute of Tamil Studies.

Ramaswamy, Sumathi. 1997. *Passions of the Tongue: Language Devotion in Tamil India 1891–1970*. Berkeley: University of California Press.

Rao, S. K. Ramachandra. 1987. *Encyclopedia of Indian Medicine*. Vol. 2, *Basic concepts*. Bangalore: Parameshvara Charitable Trust.

Rao Siripuram, Dattatraya. 2009. "Marmas (The Vital Parts in the Body) and Their Relevance in Yogic Practices." In *Yoga: The Ancient Tradition in the New Millennium*, edited by Kolla Chenchulakshmi, 54–66. Ambala Cantt.: Associated.

Rāya, Rāma Kumāra. 1982. *Encyclopedia of Yoga*. Varanasi: Prachya Prakashan.

Reber, Arthur S. 1993. *Implicit Learning and Tacit Knowledge: An Essay on the Cognitive Unconscious*. New York: Oxford University Press.

Redfield, Robert. 1956. *The Little Community and Peasant Society and Culture*. Chicago: University of Chicago Press.

Rhodes, Lorna A., with Carol A. McPhillips-Tangum, Christine Markham, and Rebecca Klenk. 1999. "The Power of the Visible: The Meaning of Diagnostic Tests in Chronic Back Pain." *Social Science & Medicine* 48 (9): 1189–1203.

Ros, Frank. 1994. *The Lost Secrets of Ayurvedic Acupuncture: An Ayurvedic Guide to Acupuncture*. Twin Lakes, WI: Lotus.

Rose, Nikolas, and Peter Miller. 2008. *Governing the Present: Administering Economic, Social and Personal Life*. Cambridge: Polity.

Rossman, Parker. 1992. *The Emerging Worldwide Electronic University: Information Age Global Higher Education*. Westport, CT, and London: Greenwood.

Roşu, Arion. 1978. *Les Conceptions Psychologiques dans les Textes Médicaux Indiens*. Paris: Institute de Civilisation Indienne.

Roşu, Arion. 1981. "Les Marman et les Arts Martiaux Indiens." *Journal Asiatique* 269: 417–451.

Rudolph, Lloyd I., and Susanne Rudolph. 1984. *The Modernity of Tradition: Political Development in India.* Chicago: University of Chicago Press.

Salati, Sajad Ahmad, and Ajaz Rather. 2009. "Bonesetter's Gangrene of Hand: A Preventable Disaster." *Journal of Surgery Pakistan* 14 (3): 143–144.

Sambasivam Pillai, T. V. 1993. *Introduction to Siddha Medicine: Portions selected from the Introduction of Thiru T. V. Sambasivam Pillai's Tamil-English Dictionary.* Madras: Directorate of Indian Medicine and Homeopathy.

———. 1991–1998. *Tamil-English Dictionary of Medicine, Chemistry, Botany, and Allied Sciences.* 5 vols. Madras: Research Institute of Siddhar's Science.

Sampath, C. K. 1983. "Evolution and Development of Siddha Medicine." In *Heritage of the Tamils: Siddha Medicine,* edited by S. V. Subramaniam and V. R. Madhavan, 155–166. Madras: International Institute of Tamil Studies.

Samudra, Jaida Kim. 2008. "Memory in our Body: Thick Participation and the Translation of Kinesthetic Experience." *American Ethnologist* 35 (4): 665–681.

Sarma, Shudhananda. 2007. *Tamil Siddhas: A Study from Historical, Socio-cultural, and Religio-philosophical Perspectives.* New Delhi: Munshiram Manoharlal Publications.

Sax, William S. 2009. *God of Justice: Ritual Healing and Social Justice in the Central Himalayas.* New York: Oxford University Press.

———. 2010. "Introduction: Ritual and the Problem of Efficacy." In *The Problem of Ritual Efficacy,* edited by William S. Sax, Johannes Quack, and Jan Weinhold, 3–16. New York: Oxford University Press.

Sax, William S., and Johannes Quack. 2010. "Introduction: The Efficacy of Rituals." *Journal of Ritual Studies* 24 (1): 5–12.

Sayer, Andrew. 2004. Moral Economy. Published by the Department of Sociology, Lancaster University, Lancaster at http://www.lancaster.ac.uk/fass/sociology/research/publications/papers/sayer-moral-economy.pdf, accessed November 24, 2014, pp. 1–15.

Scarry, Elaine. 1985. *The Body in Pain: The Making and Unmaking of the World.* New York: Oxford University Press.

Scharfe, Hartmut. 1999. "The Doctrine of the Three Humours in Traditional Indian Medicine and the Alleged Antiquity of Tamil Siddha Medicine." *Journal of the American Oriental Society* 119 (4): 609–629.

———, ed. 2002. *Education in Ancient India.* Leiden: Brill.

Scheid, Volker. 2006. "Chinese Medicine and the Problem of Tradition." Asian Medicine 2 (1): 59–71.

Scheper-Hughes, Nancy, and Margaret Lock. 1987. "The Mindful Body: A Prolegomenon to Future Work in Medical Anthropology." *Medical Anthropology Quarterly* 1 (1): 6–41.

Scott, James C. 1976. *The Moral Economy of the Peasant: Rebellion and Subsistence in Southeast Asia*. New Haven, CT: Yale University Press.

Sébastia, Brigitte. 2010. "Governmental Institutions vs. Associations: The Multifaceted Expression of Siddha Medicine in Tamil Nadu." *Sciences de l'Homme et de la Société*. https://halshs.archives-ouvertes.fr/halshs-00408677/document.

Shah, R. K., with V. K. Thapa, D. H. Jones, and R. Jones. 2003. "Improving Primary Orthopaedic and Trauma Care in Nepal." *Education for Health* 16 (3): 348–356.

Shankar, Darshan. n.d. "Traditional Bone Setting: Planning Commission Report on Health Systems." http://planningcommission.nic.in/reports/sereport/ser/seeds/seed_helth.pdf, accessed July 16, 2007, 403–410.

Shankar, Darshan, and P. M. Unnikrishnan, eds. 2004. *Challenging the Indian Medical Heritage*. Ahmedabad: Centre for Environment Education.

Shanmuga Velan, A. 1992. *Siddhar's Science of Longevity and Kalpa Medicine of India*. Madras: Directorate of Indian Medicine and Homoeopathy.

Sharma, Ajay Kumar. 2002. *The Pancakarma Treatment of Ayurveda including Keraliya Pancakarma*. Delhi: Sri Satguru.

Shilling, Chris, and Philip Mellor. 1995. *Re-forming the Body: Religion, Community and Modernity*. London: Sage.

Sieler, Roman. 2013. "From Lineage Transmission to Transnational Distance Education: The Case of Siddha Varmam Medicine." *European Journal of Transnational Studies* 5 (1): 112–143.

Simmel, Georg. 1906. "The Sociology of Secrecy and of Secret Societies." *American Journal of Sociology* 11 (4): 441–498.

———. 1907. "Das Geheimnis: Eine sozialpsychologische Skizze." *Illustrierte Zeitung* [Leipzig], December 12.

———. 1950. *The Sociology of Georg Simmel*. Translated, edited, and with an introduction by Kurt H. Wolff. Glencoe, IL: Free Press.

Singer, Milton. 1968. *Krishna: Myths, Rites, and Attitudes*. Chicago & London: University of Chicago Press.

Singer, Milton B. 1972. *When a Great Tradition Modernizes: An Anthropological Approach to Indian Civilization*. London: Praeger.

Singleton, John, ed. 1998. *Learning in Likely Places: Varieties of Apprenticeship in Japan*. Cambridge and New York: Cambridge University Press.

Spitznagel, Albert. 1998. "Einleitung." In *Geheimnis und Geheimhaltung: Erscheinungsformen—Funktionen—Konsequenzen*, edited by Albert Spitznagel, 19–51. Göttingen and Bern: Hogrefe.

Srinivas, M. N. 1966. *Social Change in Modern India*. Berkeley: University of California Press.

Staal, Frits. 1979. "The Meaninglessness of Ritual." *Numen* 26 (1): 2–22.

———. 1996. *Ritual and Mantras: Rules without Meaning*. New Delhi: Motilal Banarsidass.

Stafford, Barbara Maria. 1991. *Body Criticism: Imaging the Unseen in Enlightenment Art and Medicine*. Cambridge, MA: MIT Press.

Steever, Stanford B. 1994. "Civavākkiyar's Abecedarium Naturae." *Journal of the American Oriental Society* 114 (3): 363–382.

Steinmann, Ralph Marc. 1986. *Guru-śiṣya-sambandha: Das Meister-Schüler-Verhältnis im traditionellen und modernen Hinduismus*. Stuttgart: Steiner.

Stoller, Paul. 1989. *The Taste of Ethnographic Things: The Senses in Anthropology*. Philadelphia: University of Pennsylvania Press.

Stuckrad, Kocku von. 2010. *Locations of Knowledge in Medieval and Early Modern Europe: Esoteric Discourse and Western Identities*. Leiden: Brill.

Subrahmanyam, Padma. 2003. *Karaṇas: Common Dance Codes of India and Indonesia*. Chennai: Nrithyodaya.

Subramaniam, P. 1994. *Varma Cūttiram [A Tamil Text on Martial Art from Palm-Leaf Manuscript]*. Madras: Institute of Asian Studies.

Subramanian, S. V. 1986. *Heritage of the Tamils: Education and Vocation*. Madras: International Institute of Tamil Studies.

Sujatha, V. 2003. *Health by the People: Sociology of Medical Lore*. Jaipur: Rawat.

———. 2007. "Pluralism in Indian Medicine: Medical Lore as a Genre of Medical Knowledge." *Contributions to Indian Sociology* 41 (2): 169–202.

———. 2009. "The Patient as a Knower: Principle and Practice in Siddha Medicine." *Economic & Political Weekly* 44 (16): 76–83.

Sujatha, V., with R. Aruna, and A. V. Balasubramanian. 1991. *Nidaana: Diagnosis in Traditional Medicine*. Madras: Lok Swasthya Parampara Samvardhan Samithi.

Suresh, A., and G. Veluchamy. 1983. "Surgery in Siddha System." In *Heritage of the Tamils: Siddha Medicine*, edited by S. V. Subramaniam and V. R. Madhavan, 461–471. Madras: International Institute of Tamil Studies.

Svātmārāma, Yogīndra. 2005. *The Hatha Yoga Pradipika*. New Delhi: New Age.

Tambiah, Stanley J. 1974. "From Varna to Caste through Mixed Unions." In *The Character of Kinship*, edited by Jack Goody, 191–230. Cambridge: Cambridge University Press.

Tamil Lexicon. (1924–1936) 1982. Madras: University of Madras.

Taussig, Michael T. 1980. "Reification and the Consciousness of the Patient." *Social Science & Medicine* 14 (2): 3–13.

———. 1984. "History as Sorcery." *Representations* 7: 87–109.

———. 1986. *Shamanism, Colonialism, and the Wild Man: A Study in Terror and Healing*. Chicago: University of Chicago Press.

———. 1993. *Mimesis and Alterity: A Particular History of the Senses*. New York: Routledge.

———. 1998. "Transgression." In *Critical Terms for Religious Studies*, edited by Mark C. Taylor, 349–364. Chicago: University of Chicago Press.

———. 1999a. "Viscerality, Faith and Scepticism: Another Theory of Magic." In *In Near Ruins: Cultural Theory at the End of the Century*, edited by Nicholas Dirks, 221–265. Minneapolis: University of Minnesota Press.

———. 1999b. *Defacement: Public Secrecy and the Labor of the Negative*. Stanford, CA: Stanford University Press.

Templeman, Dennis. 1996. *The Northern Nadars of Tamil Nadu: An Indian Caste in the Process of Change*. Delhi and New York: Oxford University Press.

Thakkur, Chandrashekhar G. 1965. *Introduction to Ayurveda (Basic Indian Medicine)*. Bombay: Ancient Wisdom.

Thatte, D. G. 1983. "Anatomical and Physiological Significance of Marmas." In *Ayurvedaprabhandhavali*, vol. 9, 47–59. Kottakkal: Kottakkal Ayuvredashala.

———. 1988. *Acupuncture, Marma and Other Asian Therapeutic Techniques*. Varanasi: Chaukhamba Orientalia.

Thirugnanasambandhan, P. 1986. "The Ancient Indian Education of North India and Tamilnadu: A Comparative Study." In *Heritage of the Tamils: Education and Vocation*, edited by S. V. Subramaniam, 120–134. Madras: International Institute of Tamil Studies.

Thompson, Edward P. 1991. *Customs in Common: Studies in Traditional Popular Culture*. New York: New Press.

Throop, Jason C. 2003. "Articulating Experience." *Anthropological Theory* 3 (2): 219–241.

———. 2010. *Suffering and Sentiment: Exploring the Vicissitudes of Experience and Pain in Yap*. Berkeley: University of California Press.

Thurston, Edgar. (1909) 1965. *Castes and Tribes of Southern India*, vol. 6. New York: Johnson Reprint.

Tilak, Srinivas. 2007. "Prana: Healing Powers of Prana in Yoga and Ayurveda." In *Healing Traditions of India*, edited by Todd Pesek, 17–60. Thiruvanthapuram: Olive.

Times of India. 2010. "Govt. Whets Its Scalpel to End Quackery," July 29.

Tirumūlar. 1991. *Tirumantiram: A Tamil Scriptural Classic*. Translated by B. Natarajan. Madras: Sri Ramakrishna Math.

Trawick, Margaret. 1983. "Death and Nurturance in Indian Systems of Healing." *Social Science & Medicine* 17 (14): 935–945.

———. 1992. "An Ayurvedic Theory of Cancer." In *Anthropological Approaches to the Study of Ethnomedicine*, edited by Mark Nichter, 207–222. Philadelphia, PA: Gordon & Breach.

Turner, Victor, and Edward Bruner. 1986. *The Anthropology of Experience*. Urbana: University of Illinois Press.

Urban, Hugh B. 1998. "The Torment of Secrecy: Ethical and Epistemological Problems in the Study of Esoteric Traditions." *History of Religions* 37 (3): 209–248.

———. 2001a. "The Adornment of Silence: Secrecy and Symbolic Power in American Freemasonry." *Journal of Religion & Society* 3: 1–29.

———. 2001b. *The Economics of Ecstasy: Tantra, Secrecy, and Power in Colonial Bengal*. Oxford: Oxford University Press.

Vāgbhaṭa. 1999. *Aṣṭāṅga Saṃgraha: The Compendium of Eight Branches of Āyuveda*. Delhi: Sri Satguru.

Valiathan, M. S. 2007. *The Legacy of Suśruta*. Chennai: Orient Longman.

Vālmīki. 1927. *Kishkindhya & Sundara Kandam*. Calcutta: Oriental.

Van Dongen, Els, and Riekje Elema. 2001. "The Art of Touching: The Culture of 'Body Work.'" *Nursing. Anthropology & Medicine* 8 (2–3): 149–162.

Varghese, Mathew. 2003. "Cross-Cultural Relations between Dravidian India and Central China: New Evidences from the Tradition of Martial Art." *Indian Folklore Research Journal* 1 (3): 15–34.

Varier, M. R. Raghava. 2002. *The Rediscovery of Ayurveda: The Story of Arya Vaidya Sala, Kottakkal.* New Delhi: Viking Penguin.

Vasanthakumar, T. 2004. *Siddha V(m)armology: A Study.* Adaikkakuzhi: T. Vasanthakumar.

Vedavathy, S. 2003. "Folk Medicinal Wisdom of Chittoor District, Andhra Pradesh." *Indian Folklife* 13: 19–20.

Vēlappaṉ, Tē. 2000. *Nāñcil Nāṭu: Varalāṟu, Marapukaḷ, Poruḷnilai* [*Kanyakumari: History, Customs, State of Affairs*]. Nākarkōvil: Rōkiṇi ējeṉcīs.

Venkatachalapathy, V. R. 2012. *The Province of the Book: Scholars, Scribes, and Scribblers in Colonial Tamil Nadu.* Ranikhet: Permanent Black.

Venkatraman, Ramaswamy. 1990. *A History of the Tamil Siddha Cult.* Madurai: ENNES.

Wacquant, Loïc J. D. 2004. *Body and Soul: Notebooks of an Apprentice Boxer.* Oxford: Oxford University Press.

Walkley, Susan. 2004. "When the Body Leads the Mind: Perspectives on Massage Therapy in the United States." In *Healing by Hand: Manual Medicine and Bonesetting in Global Perspective*, edited by Kathryn S. Oths and Servando Z. Hinojosa, 23–42. Walnut Creek, CA: Altamira.

Warren, Carol, and Laslett, Barbara. 1980. "Privacy and Secrecy: A Conceptual Comparison." In *Secrecy: A Cross-Cultural Perspective*, edited by Stanton K. Tefft, 25–34. New York: Human Sciences.

Weiss, Richard S. 2003. "The Reformulation of a Holy Science: Siddha Medicine and Tradition in South India." PhD diss., University of Michigan, Ann Arbor.

———. 2008. "Divorcing Ayurveda." In *Modern and Global Ayurveda: Pluralism and Paradigms*, edited by Dagmar Wujastyk and Frederick M. Smith, 77–99. Albany: State University of New York Press.

———. 2009. *Recipes for Immortality: Medicine, Religion, and Community in South India.* New York: Oxford University Press.

White, David Gordon. 1996. *The Alchemical Body: Siddha Traditions in Medieval India.* Chicago: University of Chicago Press.

Wikan, Unni. 1991. "Toward an Experience-Near Anthropology." *Cultural Anthropology* 6 (3): 285–305.

Wilke, Annette, and Oliver Moebus. 2011. *Sound and Communication: An Aesthetic Cultural History of Sanskrit Hinduism.* Berlin: Walter de Gruyter.

Wittgenstein, Ludwig. (1922) 2003. *Tractatus Logico-Philosophicus.* New York: Barnes and Noble.

Wolfson, Elliot R. 2002. "Assaulting the Border: Kabbalistic Traces in the Margins of Derrida." *Journal of the American Academy of Religion* 70 (3): 475–514.

———. 2005. *Language, Eros, Being: Kabbalistic Hermeneutics and Poetic Imagination.* New York: Fordham University Press.

Wood, Ananda E. 1985. *Knowledge before Printing and After: The Indian Tradition in Changing Kerala.* Delhi: Oxford University Press.

Woodburne, A. Stewart. 1992. "The Evil Eye in South Indian Folklore." In *The Evil Eye*, edited by Alan Dundes, 55–65. Madison: University of Wisconsin Press.

World Health Organization (WHO). 1978. *Primary Health Care: A Joint Report by the Director-General of the World Health Organization and the Executive Director of UNICEF.* Geneva: World Health Organization.

———. 1981. *Global Strategy for Health for All by the Year 2000.* Geneva: World Health Organization.

———. 2008. *The World Health Report 2008: Primary Health Care: Now More Than Ever.* Geneva: World Health Organization.

Wujastyk, Dagmar, and Frederick M. Smith. 2008. *Modern and Global Ayurveda: Pluralism and Paradigms.* Albany: State University of New York Press.

Wujastyk, Dominik. 1998. *The Roots of Āyurveda: Selections from Sanskrit Medical Writings.* London: Penguin.

———. 2009. "Interpreting the Image of the Human Body in Premodern India." *International Journal of Hindu Studies* 13 (2): 189–228.

Wulf, Christoph. 2002. *Anthropology of Education.* Münster: Lit-Verlag.

———. 2003. *Educational Science: Hermeneutics, Empirical Research, Critical Theory.* Münster, Munich, and Berlin: Waxmann.

Zarrilli, Phillip B. 1989. "Three Bodies of Practice in a Traditional South Indian Martial Art." *Social Science &Medicine* 28 (12): 1289–1309.

———. 1992a. "To Heal and/or to Harm: The Vital Spots (Marmmam/Varmam) in Two South Indian Martial Traditions. Part I: Focus on Kerala's Kalarippayattu." *Journal of Asian Martial Arts* 1 (1): 36–67.

———. 1992b. "To Heal and/or to Harm: The Vital Spots (Marmmam/Varmam) in Two South Indian Martial Traditions. Part II: Focus on the Tamil Art, Varma Ati." *Journal of Asian Martial Arts* 1 (2): 1–15.

———. 1994. "Actualizing 'Power(s)' and 'Crafting a Self' in Martial Practice: Kalarippayattu, a South Indian Martial Art and the Yoga and Ayurvedic Paradigms." *Journal of Asian Martial Arts* 3 (3): 10–51.

———. 1995. "Traditional Kerala Massage Therapies." *Journal of Asian Martial Arts* 4 (1): 67–78.

———. 1998. *When the Body Becomes All Eyes: Paradigms, Discourses and Practices of Power in Kalarippayattu, a South Indian Martial Art.* New Delhi: Oxford University Press.

———. 2005. "'Kalarippayattu is Eighty Percent Mental and Only the Remainder is Physical': Power, Agency and Self in a South Asian Martial Art." In *Subaltern Sports: Politics and Sport in South Asia*, edited by James H. Mills, 19–46. London: Anthem.

Zempléni, Andras. 1976. "La Chaîne du secret." *Nouvelle revue de psychanalyse* 14: 313–324.

Zimmermann, Francis. 1978. "From Classical Texts to Learned Practice: Methodological Remarks on the Study of Indian Medicine." *Social Science & Medicine* 12B: 97–103.

———. 1980. "Ṛtu-Sātmya: The Seasonal Cycle and the Principle of Appropriateness." *Social Science & Medicine* 14B (2): 87–105.

Zvelebil, Kamil V. 1973. *The Poets of the Powers: Magic, Freedom, and Renewal.* London: Rider.

Zysk, Kenneth G. 1991. *Asceticism and Healing in Ancient India: Medicine in the Buddhist Monastery.* New York: Oxford University Press.

———. 1993. "The Science of Respiration and the Doctrine of the Bodily Winds in Ancient India." *Journal of the American Oriental Society* 113 (2): 198–213.

———. 2008. *Siddha Medicine in Tamil Nadu.* Tranquebar Initiativets Skriftserie, no. 4. Copenhagen: Nationalmuseet.

Index